X-Ray Department
Royal United Hospital
Bath

ARTHROGRAPHY

ARTHROGRAPHY

Robert H. Freiberger, M.D.

Professor of Radiology
Cornell University Medical College
Director of Radiology
Hospital for Special Surgery
New York, New York

Jeremy J. Kaye, M.D.

Professor of Radiology
Director, Division of Diagnostic Radiology
Vanderbilt University Medical School
Nashville, Tennessee

Jill Spiller

Editorial Consultant

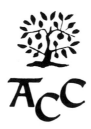

APPLETON-CENTURY-CROFTS / New York

79 80 81 82 83 / 10 9 8 7 6 5 4 3 2 1

Prentice-Hall International, Inc., London
Prentice-Hall of Australia, Pty. Ltd., Sydney
Prentice-Hall of India Private Limited, New Delhi
Prentice-Hall of Japan, Inc., Tokyo
Prentice-Hall of Southeast Asia (Pte.) Ltd., Singapore
Whitehall Books Ltd., Wellington, New Zealand

Library of Congress Cataloging in Publication Data
Freiberger, Robert H.
    Arthrography

    Includes index.
    1. Joints—Diseases—Diagnosis.   2.   Joints—
Radiography.   3.   Contrast media.   I.   Kaye,
Jeremy J., 1939-   joint author.   II.   Spiller, Jill,
1941-   joint author.   III.   Title.
[DNLM: 1.   Joint—Radiography.   WE 300.3F862a]
RC 933.F74   616.7′2-16952   79-16952
ISBN   0-8385-0423-X

Design: Robert Bull
PRINTED IN THE UNITED STATES OF AMERICA

Contributors

Bernard Ghelman, M.D.
Attending Radiologist, Hospital for Special Surgery;
Assistant Professor of Radiology, Cornell University Medical College;
Assistant Attending Radiologist, New York Hospital
New York, New York

Amy Beth Goldman, M.D.
Associate Attending Radiologist, Hospital for Special Surgery;
Associate Professor of Radiology, Cornell University Medical College;
Associate Attending Radiologist, New York Hospital
New York, New York

Terry M. Hudson, M.D.
Assistant Professor of Radiology and Orthopaedics
College of Medicine, University of Florida
Gainesville, Florida

Helene Pavlov, M.D.
Assistant Attending Radiologist, Hospital for Special Surgery;
Assistant Professor of Radiology, Cornell University Medical College;
Assistant Attending Radiologist, New York Hospital
New York, New York

Robert Schneider, M.D.
Attending Radiologist, St. Vincent's Hospital
New York, New York

Contents

Preface

Arthrographic examination of the joints, most commonly the knee, but also the shoulder, hip, elbow, ankle, and wrist, has in the past 15 years grown from an occasional to a common radiologic procedure. Arthrography can yield much accurate information, heretofore unavailable, about joints and joint spaces. Our experience with knee arthrography at the Hospital for Special Surgery began in 1963 in enthusiastic response to the demonstrations of the visiting Swedish radiologist, Dr. Lars Andrén. Later that same year, a study trip to his hospital in Malmö, Sweden, indoctrinated me in the technique. I was able to observe how knee arthrograms were routinely performed. Back in New York, with the help of the hospital carpentry shop, we constructed the simple devices we needed for knee arthrograms with the horizontal beam technique—a small table and a film holder—and began working with the knee. The menisci and the other cartilaginous structures became visible in a totally new and different perspective.

Initially, the very complex attachments of the lateral meniscus and the normal variants of those attachments were confusing to interpret on the roentgenograms, so we began to dissect fresh cadaver knees in an attempt to better understand the anatomy. By also examining frozen knee specimens that had been cut into vertical radial sections to resemble the arthrographic appearance of the knee, we became familiar with the normal anatomy, and the arthrogram held less terror.

The first contrast media used routinely for these examinations were sodium salt contrast agents. When they leaked from the joint or were injected inadvertently into extra-articular structures, they caused the patient great pain. We discovered that the meglumine agents did not hurt the patient, and successfully substituted them. Having started with the knee, it seemed natural that the technique be applied to other joints, primarily the shoulder and the hip. In the earliest examinations of the shoulder, the patient was placed posterior oblique, a position that best showed the joint space on the fluoroscope but which made the injection difficult. Working with the procedure, modifying, and gingerly experimenting with positioning, we discovered that the injection became much easier with the patient flat supine. The later adoption of a double contrast technique—using both positive contrast agent and air—to the examination of the shoulder seemed to yield more information than the single positive contrast study.

For the hip there were different problems. Sticking the needle into the hip joint often proved to be technically difficult because feeling the tip impinge upon the femoral neck did not always confirm that the needle was within the joint. Using a more oblique approach seemed to insure greater success, but perseverence was necessary as it often required several tries at needle placement before an intra-articular position was achieved. Substitution of a 22-gauge needle for a larger one proved to be adequate for aspiration and examination, and was more pleasant for the patient.

In the early days, during simple aspiration for suspected infection of a total hip replacement, we stumbled on the fact that we could diagnose loosening. When positive contrast agent was injected after aspiration to confirm needle position, we could clearly see it in the bone-cement interface, because the cement used then was radiolucent. Contrast media there meant that the cement had become detached from the bone.

Slowly, other joints were added to the repertoire—elbow, ankle, wrist—as the need arose. None of them presented the anatomic complexities found in the knee, but we frequently went to the operating room to observe the surgery on a joint that we had examined arthrographically, in an attempt to strengthen our understanding of the anatomy and pathology.

Even as procedures for arthrographic examination of these other joints were being developed and the studies increasingly requested, the knee arthrogram remained a primary interest. The arrival of a fluoroscope unit with a fractional millimeter focal spot for spot filming induced us to try the double contrast technique described by Butt and McIntyre in Canada. Then, slowly, as we became more familiar with spot filming, the horizontal beam method was abandoned at the Hospital for Special Surgery.

Since its introduction, arthrography has burgeoned and blossomed; the techniques have become more refined, the equipment more sophisticated, and the examination more complete. The actual performance of an arthrogram, however, requires a moderate amount of skill. With this book in hand to illuminate the details of technique, pertinent anatomic structures, and their normal and abnormal arthrographic appearances, arthrography should be easier; and errors, pitfalls in procedure or interpretation, can be avoided. Arthrography is here to stay; let it be good arthrography.

RHF

Acknowledgments

Many people whose names do not appear in this book contributed to its existence and we wish to thank them for their efforts. Many physicians and surgeons supported our early efforts by sending us patients and helping us with anatomy, clinical examinations, surgical techniques, and pathology to allow us to become proficient in the interpretation of arthrograms. Dr. James A. Nicholas and Dr. William B. Arnold gave us the support in knee arthrography. Dr. Philip D. Wilson, Jr., supported us on hip arthrography, particularly on patients with total hip prostheses. Dr. Robert L. Patterson shared his knowledge on shoulder abnormalities with us and helped us with the shoulder arthrograms. Dr. Walter H. O. Bohne collaborated on the anatomic studies of the ankle joint which are illustrated in this book. Dr. Chitranjan Ranawat contributed to the study of the wrist and wrist arthrograms. A special thanks to Dr. Peter G. Bullough, the pathologist at the Hospital for Special Surgery, who made it possible for us to perform many dissections in his laboratory and to inspect and photograph excised specimens.

A second group of doctors who contributed to our arthrography program were former associates in the department of radiology. Dr. Paul J. Killoran was with us in 1963 when the arthrography program started. Without his interest and whole-hearted support this program might not have continued.

Similarly Dr. Margaret Harrison-Stubbs worked hard on making arthrography an acceptable diagnostic procedure and had a particular interest in wrist arthrography. While he was a fellow in Radiology at the Hospital for Special Surgery, Dr. William Spragge showed us the fluoroscopic spot-film knee arthrography method described by Butt and McIntyre.

For the anatomic drawings we wish to thank Mr. William Thackeray, and we extend special thanks to Ms. Dorothy Page and her staff for making and remaking the hundreds of photographs of X-rays and anatomic specimens for the illustrations. We should also mention our gratitude to Miss Shirley J. Kilfoyle, who allowed us to upset her laboratory routine by letting us use the band saw to cut frozen specimens and to inspect the surgical specimens.

Last but not least thanks go to the many secretaries who tirelessly typed and retyped the many versions of the manuscript. Most notable of these are Mrs. Barbara Schoenberg, who not only typed most of the manuscript but also took care of the many crises which arose in the preparation of the manuscript, and Mrs. Marie Melignano, who was similarly involved in the final stages of the book. Others who were instrumental in producing the typed manuscript include Ms. Arlene Briskin, Ms. Barbara Hunter, Ms. Linda Pigott, and Ms. Pamela Corley.

Finally and most importantly, the authors of this volume would like to acknowledge their debt to Ms. Jill Spiller. Without her encouragement, this work would probably never have come to fruition. Its comprehensibility and readability are ascribable largely to her editorial expertise.

Introduction

Arthrography is not a new procedure. The possibility that radiolucent intra-articular structures could be shown by a roentgenographic examination was thought of as soon as X-ray equipment became available for medical practice. In 1905, barely 10 years after the the discovery of the roentgen ray, a report on arthrography of the knee using gas as contrast medium was made by Werndorff and Robinson. Three years later Gocht was the first to perform an air contrast hip arthrogram on a cadaver. Positive contrast arthrograms were performed on cadavers in the early 1900s, but the available contrast media were too toxic for use on the living. When safe urographic positive contrast media had been developed, they were also used for arthrography both singly or combined with air to provide double contrast studies. Oberholzer appears to have been the first to perform double contrast studies of the elbow and shoulder in the 1930s. Ankle and wrist arthrography were developed rather late as clinical diagnostic procedures. Wolff was apparently the first to use ankle arthrograms in 1940, and Rosenthal may have been the first to perform wrist arthrograms late in the 1940s. Lindblom published his extensive experience with knee arthrography in the late 1930s and 1940s, but despite his reported high diagnostic accuracy with knee and shoulder arthrograms, arthrography did not become a widely accepted diagnostic procedure in the United States at that time. A setback for arthrography in the United States was a 1927 report by Kleinberg of a near-fatal gas embolism. That the injection of the knee was carried out by direct connection of the needle to a tank of oxygen—an unsafe method of injection—was not generally known.

A number of factors have made arthrography the widely accepted routine diagnostic procedure it is today. Water soluble contrast media have been improved and are noninjurious to synovium; they cause the patient no pain or discomfort even when inadvertently injected extra-articularly. The many technical developments, such as fractional millimeter focal spot X-ray tubes for radiography and fluoroscopy, powerful image amplifiers, and improvement of films and intensifying screens, have made it possible to obtain roentgenograms of consistent technical perfection. Commercially available sterile disposable arthrography sets have obviated the need for autoclaving injection equipment and have made it possible to perform arthrograms safely and expeditiously in office practice. Minor complications resulting from arthrography are exceedingly rare, and major complications practically nonexistent.

Arthrography is a technically simple procedure that can safely be performed on ambulatory patients. It has a high degree of diagnostic accuracy and it provides graphic documentation of intra-articular disease. This documentation is becoming increasingly desirable, particularly when surgical intervention is contemplated.

1
Introducing Arthrography

Robert H. Freiberger

Common to all arthrography are the materials used for joint puncture and for injection of contrast agents. Complications, too, may occur—however rarely—in any joint, and a description of such possible complications is given to the patient prior to the examination. These aspects of arthrography that precede any joint injection are described here.

THE ARTHROGRAM SET

The arthrogram set used at The Hospital for Special Surgery was developed by adding and subtracting items from an existing joint aspiration set (Fig. 1). It is somewhat more elaborate than absolutely necessary, but occasionally all the items in the set are used. If not, they may be resterilized. The set contains:

One 2-cc Luer-Lok tip glass syringe
One 10-cc Luer-Lok tip glass syringe
One 22-cc Luer-Lok tip glass syringe
One 16-gauge × 1½-in. sterile disposable needle
One 20-gauge × 1½-in. sterile disposable needle
One 19-gauge × 1½-in. sterile disposable needle
One 25-gauge × ⅝-in. sterile disposable needle
Five 4 × 3 in. gauze sponges
One thumb forcep
One medicine glass
One fabric drape with a 2 × 2 in. hole

Additional items available, but not on the sterile set, are:

Sterile surgical gloves
A disposable shaver
Povidone-iodine solution for skin preparation
1 percent lidocaine solution
1-cc ampule of 1:1000 epinephrine solution
60 percent diatrizoate meglumine (Reno-M-60), Squibb, or another meglumine-type contrast agent
Sterile plastic tubing (to permit fluoroscopic monitoring during contrast injection)
10-cc ampules of sterile saline solution without preservative
Sterile 22-gauge spinal needles (for shoulder and hip arthrograms)
Crushable ampules of spirits of ammonia (for patients who feel faint)
An emergency resuscitation set like those on hand for intravenous contrast injections. (Such a set has never been needed in the performance of over 25,000 arthrograms.)

Several commercially produced arthrogram trays are available and are entirely satisfactory for all types of arthrograms. The only difference between the commercial sets and the one described above is that disposable syringes rather than glass syringes with glass pistons are furnished. As disposable syringes usually have rubber pistons that do not move quite as freely as glass pistons, it is a little more difficult to determine, by gauging the resistance on the piston, whether the needle is intra-articular.

COMPLICATIONS OF ARTHROGRAPHY

Infection

Infection caused by needle puncture of a joint is possible, although experience indicates that with reasonable antiseptic skin preparation it is an extremely rare complication. In a series of over 25,000 arthrograms only one infection of a knee joint has occurred. It was a *Staphylococcus aureus* infection with symptoms of pain and swelling arising 48 hours after the performance of the arthrogram. The diagnosis was made by aspiration, smear, and culture. The patient was treated with antibiotics and the knee was immobilized. There was no residual damage to the joint. In another patient, cloudy fluid, suggesting infection, was obtained by aspiration from the knee prior to injection of contrast agent and was sent to the laboratory for smear and culture. The arthrogram was performed without difficulty. The laboratory report on the aspirated fluid indicated the presence of *Staphylococcus aureus* bacteria, confirming that the patient's symptoms had been caused by a septic arthritis. The patient was treated with appropriate antibiotics. The arthrogram did not affect the course of the disease or its treatment in any way.

Although it is reasonable to assume that an arthrogram should not be performed on a normal joint if a needle has to traverse infected soft tissue before it enters the joint, experience indicates that aspiration and arthrography of infected joints cause no harm and can provide important information. Hundreds of arthrograms on infected joints and joints clinically thought to be infected have been performed at The Hospital for Special Surgery without complications.

Allergic Reaction

Approximately 20·patients, or fewer than 1 per 1000 arthrograms, have experienced mild allergic reactions. The onset of urticaria—the only type of reaction encountered—was usually within 15 to 20 minutes of the injection of contrast media. These patients were still in the radiology department and were treated by oral antihistamines. One patient, whose urticaria began approximately one-half hour after the injection, had already left the hospital but returned for treatment.

Before the arthrogram is performed, the patient is asked about allergies, but only a history of previous serious allergic reaction to radiopaque contrast agent is considered pertinent, since other substances have no association with sensitivity to contrast agents. When a patient describes a serious reaction to an intravenous contrast agent, an arthrogram with water-soluble positive contrast agent is usually not performed, although in one case where the history indicated a serious reaction, the arthrogram was done and no complication of any kind was encountered.

Occasionally an arthrogram with air only as a contrast medium has been performed when a history of severe allergic reaction to injected contrast media was obtained. Such arthrograms are not satisfactory as double contrast studies for evaluation of the menisci.

Syncope following arthrocentesis and contrast and air injection into the knee occurs occasionally, particularly in teenage and athletic males. The patient should then be left lying on the table, with the knee manipulated manually. No major resuscitation measures have been necessary and patients recover quickly after inhaling spirits of ammonia.

Synovial Effusion

A rare complication occurring with the same or even lower frequency than systemic allergic reaction is a clinically significant sterile synovial effusion of the injected joint. When it occurs, the patient experiences pain and stiffness of the knee caused by the marked distention of the joint capsule within 12 hours of the arthrogram. The rapid onset of the synovial effusion is a clue that it is not caused by an infection; however, there have been too few incidences of either sterile effusions or septic arthritis to be able to differentiate clinically between the two conditions. When a patient complains about severe swelling and pain in the joint that had undergone arthrographic examination, he or she is asked to return to the radiology department. The effusion is aspirated as completely as possible and the fluid is sent to the laboratory for a smear and culture. The aspiration alleviates the patient's symptoms, and an immediate negative smear report and negative culture report obtained 24 hours later confirms that the reaction is a chemical or a local allergic synovitis. Although it is assumed that the positive contrast agent is responsible for the synovial effusion, this complication has been reported following arthrograms where only air was injected. Acute painful effusion has also occurred in a few patients who disregarded the advice to refrain from strenuous athletic activities immediately following the arthrogram. Such activity is best postponed for 24 to 48 hours, when most of the injected air will have been absorbed.

INFORMED CONSENT FOR ARTHROGRAPHY

Before an arthrogram is performed, the patient is asked to read an information sheet explaining the procedure, and to sign a consent form. If the patient is a minor, a parent or guardian must sign. Before the injection is made, the physician questions the patient about any previous reaction to injected radiographic contrast media. In the few instances where there was a history of a *severe* reaction, the arthrogram was not performed. Information on food, penicillin, or other drug allergies is irrelevant, and the patient is not asked about them.

Information Sheet

Purpose. An arthrogram is performed to allow roentgenographic visualization and evaluation of those parts of the joints that cannot be seen on ordinary X-ray pictures. Specifically, the arthrogram yields information about the cartilages, the supporting ligaments, and the joint linings as well as the presence and location of loose bodies. An arthrogram may also be performed to confirm the proper position of the needle tip within the joint cavity when joint fluid must be obtained for laboratory analysis.

Technique. After the skin over the joint to be examined has been scrubbed with antiseptic solution, a sterile needle is placed into the joint. Local anesthesia may or may not be used. Joint fluid may be withdrawn and may be sent to the laboratory for study. A solution that is visible on X-ray and that contains organically bound iodine is injected into the joint. Some air may also be injected. The needle is then removed and a series of X-ray pictures is made, usually under fluoroscopic control. The liquid contrast substance used is absorbed and eliminated by the body in a few hours. Injected air may take up to four days to absorb completely.

Possible complications. Serious complications are extremely rare, and most patients have no aftereffects. A sense of tightness of the joint may persist for about one day. Infection has occurred only once in more than 25,000 arthrograms performed at The Hospital for Special Surgery. Allergy to the contrast agent is a minor complication. Urticaria (hives) has occurred in only approximately 1 patient per 1000. No serious allergic reactions have resulted from this procedure.

A rare complication is rapid swelling and pain in the joint within hours following the arthrogram, apparently the result of an irritation of the joint lining caused by the contrast agent and/or the injected air. The swelling usually subsides within a day or two without treatment but can be relieved by withdrawing fluid from the joint with a needle.

Omission of the procedure. By not performing the arthrogram, the physician or surgeon is denied some information about the parts of the joint that cannot be visualized on ordinary X-ray pictures. If an operation is indicated, the information permits the surgeon to understand the abnormality in the joint and so plan the operative approach. Alternatives to the arthrogram are arthroscopy or surgical exploration, but the arthrogram is by far the simplest and least hazardous procedure.

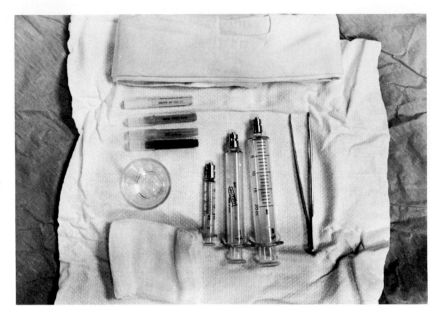

Figure 1
The arthrogram tray holds sponges, a medicine cup, several syringes, a forceps, a sterile drape sheet with a 2 × 2 in. hole, and an assortment of needles.

2
Technique of Knee Arthrography

Robert H. Freiberger

Knee arthrography is discussed first in this treatise because it is the most commonly requested arthrogram.

CHOICE OF ARTHROGRAPHIC METHOD

Prior to knee arthrography, preliminary plain radiographs are inspected for abnormalities. Although for most knee arthrograms, a double contrast study with the combination of a larger amount of air and smaller amount of liquid positive contrast agent is preferred, there are instances when air alone or liquid positive contrast alone are chosen. With the double contrast method, the intra-articular surfaces of the synovium and the articular and meniscal cartilages are coated with a thin dense layer of liquid positive contrast agent and are shadowed by adjacent radiolucent air. Very fine detail of the intra-articular surfaces, particularly those of the menisci, becomes visible.

Judicious use of distraction, flexion, and extension of the knee is necessary not only to provide tangential projections of the menisci but also to assure maximal envelopment of the menisci by air. Even if the meniscal cartilage adheres closely to the femoral condyle or to the tibial articular surface, blocking passage of air, a thin layer of positive contrast agent outlines the interface. With the double contrast method it is also possible to see the outline of the cruciate ligaments coated by a thin layer of positive contrast agent and shadowed by air. By placing the leg in a vertical position with the knee flexed, the positive contrast agent pools above the tibial pleateau and the air rises to the upper portions of the knee joint. The effect of a single positive contrast study of the cruciate ligaments is achieved at the same time as a double contrast study of the menisci—an ideal combination.

Under certain circumstances, a single contrast arthrogram should be selected. If the patient has a history of a severe reaction to positive contrast media, an arthrogram of air alone is indicated. There are often difficulties in the interpretation of an air study as there is only a moderate difference in density between the radiolucent meniscal cartilages and air. Additionally, residual synovial fluid often interferes with complete air shadowing of the intra-articular structures, particularly the menisci.

The single contrast study is preferred when intra-articular osteocartilaginous bodies are present, or cartilaginous bodies or synovial proliferative diseases are suspected, because in a double contrast study, contrast-coated air bubbles can mimic synovial nodules or small radiolucent cartilaginous bodies. Although better, in these circumstances, the single contrast study has limitations. With air alone, shadowing of all portions of the knee may not be adequate, and with solid positive contrast, the density of the contrast agent may be so great that small radiolucent bodies are totally obscured. A combination of single positive contrast agent and tomography helps delineate loose bodies.

If a double contrast arthrogram is being performed, and fluoroscopic observation or review of the films immediately afterward suggests that there is synovial proliferative disease or loose bodies, indicating that a single contrast study might have been a better choice, all is not lost. By switching from a vertical beam examination to a horizontal beam technique and by using a larger field to show the entire knee, including the suprapatellar pouch, the superior synovial surfaces can be sharply delineated by a thin film of contrast agent and shadowed by air. The liquid contrast agent, possibly with some air bubbles on the surface, pools in the dependent portion of the knee and does not interfere with synovial surface evaluation.

By turning the knee so that the positive contrast agent flows to a specific area, a partial positive contrast arthrogram can be achieved. The multiple filling defects caused by loose cartilaginous bodies of synovial chondromatosis are depicted in a partial solid contrast arthrogram that followed a conventional double contrast study of the menisci (Fig. 11B, Chapter 6).

INJECTION TECHNIQUE

The best place for needle puncture of the knee joint for the purpose of arthrography is beneath the center of the articular surface of the patella, either medially or laterally (Figs. 1–4). Some arthrographers prefer the lateral side, because the soft tissues of the lateral aspect of the knee are thinner and the needle does not traverse any muscles or other important structures. Others prefer the medial side because the medial facet of the patella is shorter and more steeply angulated. There appears to be somewhat more room for the needle between the articular surface of the medial femoral condyle and the medial facet of the patella. Medially, the needle will traverse a few fibers of the vastus medialis muscle but this seems to be of no clinical importance.

The patient is placed supine on the X-ray table with the medial side of the knee toward the examiner for medial needle placement (Fig. 3), or the lateral side toward the examiner for lateral needle placement (Fig. 4). A small, firm pillow is placed under the patient's knee. A sheet of absorbent paper backed with plastic is placed between the pillow and the knee to keep the pillow and table clean. The examiner puts on sterile surgical gloves. The arthrogram tray is opened and the medicine cup is filled with povidone-iodine solution. The knee is scrubbed three times with the povidone-

iodine solution and then draped. The syringes on the arthrogram tray are then assembled. If lidocaine is to be used, the 2-cc syringe is filled with 1 percent lidocaine solution and the 10-cc syringe is filled with 5 to 7 cc of a meglumine salt positive contrast agent. If epinephrine is to be used, 0.3 cc is aspirated from a 1-cc 1:1000 solution vial with the 10-cc syringe containing contrast agent. The 20-cc syringe is assembled and the piston is moved back and forth to ascertain that it is moving smoothly. The reason for delaying the assembly of the arthrogram tray and filling the syringes with the necessary solutions until after the knee has been scrubbed, is to allow the antiseptic solution to stay on the skin long enough to carry out its bacteriocidal action.

When the syringes are prepared, the patella is grasped with the left hand and the thumbnail is pushed into the space between the articular surface of the patella and opposing femoral condyle (Fig. 1). By pushing quite hard with the thumbnail, a pressure mark is left on the skin directly under the midportion of the patella. A 20-gauge 1½ in. needle held in the right hand is then inserted at the skin mark and pushed into the joint. Pushing the thumbnail under the patella is moderately painful, and if the needle quickly follows the release of thumbnail pressure the patient hardly feels the insertion of the needle. With practice, needle placement can be performed without the injection of local anesthesia and without causing more pain than the injection of anesthesia would have caused. If proper intra-articular needle placement is not achieved on the first try, 1 percent lidocaine solution is injected before the needle is moved. If the arthrographer does not have sufficient practice in placing needles into knee joints, an initial injection of 1 percent lidocaine using the small syringe and the 25-gauge hypodermic needle is suggested.

If the knee is distended with fluid, needle placement is easier because the patella is lifted by the fluid and the space between the patella and the femoral condyle is enlarged. Fluid will also drip from the needle as soon as it enters the knee joint, leaving no doubt about intra-articular placement of the needle tip. The fluid must first be aspirated as completely as possible. For thorough aspiration, the knee must be squeezed both above and below the patella, and the popliteal aspect of the knee must be pushed against the firm pillow beneath it so that the posterior compartment of the knee or a popliteal cyst, should one be present, is compressed. If fluid is cloudy and infection is suspected, a sample is sent for smear and culture.

If the knee contains no synovial fluid, the intra-articular placment of the needle tip will not be readily apparent. Occasionally in a young muscular patient, a faint hissing sound can be heard as air is drawn into the knee joint through the needle. Unfortunately, this does not occur frequently enough to be a reliable indicator. When it appears that the needle point has entered the knee joint, the 20-cc syringe filled with air is attached to the needle and the piston is gently pushed (Fig. 3). With intra-articular placement of the needle tip, air flows freely into the knee and there is practically no resistance on the piston. If the needle tip is extra-articular, there is resistance to pressure on the piston, and releasing pressure on the piston causes it to move outward. When the piston pushes back, the needle must be repositioned. Sometimes, if the needle has been pushed too deeply into the knee, pulling it back slightly allows the point to enter the intrasynovial space. When air is able to move freely into the knee, 20 cc of air is injected and the 20-cc syringe is disconnected. The syringe containing positive contrast agent is immediately connected to the needle (Fig. 4). If this is done quickly, only a minimal amount of the injected air is lost from the knee joint. Prior to injection of the positive contrast agent, the plunger of the syringe should be pulled back to see if air bubbles can be aspirated, indicating that the needle has not moved from its intra-articular position. The positive contrast is then injected, followed by injection of another 20 cc of air (Fig. 3), and the needle is withdrawn. The amount of positive contrast agent injected depends upon the size of the knee and whether or not a synovial effusion was present and aspirated. In a "dry" knee, 3 to 5 cc of positive contrast agent is injected. After aspiration of a synovial effusion, no more than 5 to 7 cc is injected. Sodium salt positive contrast agents are not recommended, as they cause great pain on inadvertant extra-articular injection.

Some variations of the technique are possible. After the injection of the first 20 cc of air, the needle can be connected to sterile plastic tubing and the injection of the positive contrast medium can be fluoroscopically observed to be certain that it is intra-articular. On intra-articular needle placement, the injected contrast agent immediately leaves the tip of the needle and runs into one of the recesses of the intrasynovial space that had already been partially distended with air. With extra-articular placement of the needle tip, the contrast agent hangs like a cloud at the tip of the needle and the injection of one or two drops of positive contrast agent is sufficient to indicate that the needle has to be repositioned.

Extra-articular contrast agent, which usually collects anterosuperiorly to the articular surfaces of the knee, does not usually interfere with a subsequent arthrogram if most of the contrast agent is injected intra-articularly. Even when all or most of the positive contrast agent is extra-articular (Fig. 5), its usual suprapatellar location does not interfere with the evalua-

tion of an arthrogram performed by immediately injecting more contrast agent intra-articularly.

At the end of the injection procedure, with a maximum of 40 cc of air and approximately 5 cc of positive contrast agent, the knee is not unduly distended and the patient remains comfortable. The patient is helped off the table and asked to walk a few steps to help distribute contrast agent between the articular surfaces and around the menisci. Alternatively, the knee can be moved passively with the patient sitting. Rapid motion of the knee should be avoided since the air, positive contrast agent, and retained synovial fluid can form bubbles which interfere with the evaluation of the arthrogram.

Air and positive contrast agent are normally not aspirated following the radiographic examination. Complete absorption of the injected air takes approximately four days, and the patient is so advised.

FLUOROSCOPIC SPOT-FILM EXAMINATION

Equipment

A fluoroscopic table equipped to take spot films on a fractional millimeter focal spot is mandatory. Most newer equipment is capable of doing this without modification of the control. On older fluoroscopic equipment, if equipped with a 0.3- to 0.6-mm focal spot for fluoroscopy and a larger focal spot for spot filming, the manufacturer can add circuits for spot filming on the smaller focal spot (Fig. 6). Tube rating charts need to be consulted to determine whether adequate exposure factors can be achieved. High rotation tubes are preferable, but with three-phase equipment high speed rotation may not be necessary for sufficient X-ray output. It is often not possible to exceed 100 mA on the fractional millimeter focal spot, but it is adequate for arthrograms using exposures of 1/20 to 1/10 of a second and kVp of 65 to 72 with High Plus (Dupont) screens. At exposures longer than 1/10 of a second, motion begins to interfere with the clarity of the roentgenograms. A reciprocating 6:1 or 8:1 grid in the fluoroscopic tower is ideal, but fine line stationary grids also can be used. By collimating the beam to a minimal area it is possible to obtain satisfactory roentgenograms without a grid, a technique that may be necessary on machines where radiation output is greatly limited. Although a 0.3-mm focal spot is ideal, 0.6-mm focal spot tubes are satisfactory. With larger focal spots, sharpness diminishes, and therefore, focal spots above 0.6 mm are not recommended.

The illustrated equipment is a relatively old three-phase fluoroscope (Figs. 6, 7). The 0.6-mm fluoroscopic focal spot has been made available for spot films, and separate protective circuits have been installed to prevent overloading. High target rotation is not available. The fluoroscopic tower contains a reciprocating grid, and by manually turning the spot film selector knob, six or nine exposures can be placed on a single 9½ × 9½ in. film. Exposure factors vary only slightly from patient to patient, so spot films are taken at 0.05 (1/20) second, 100 mA, and 65 to 72 kVp. During filming, the fluoroscopic tower should be kept close to the knee, since any increased tube-film distance markedly reduces the density of the resulting roentgenogram. A lead rubber curtain protects the arthrographer's arm from scattered radiation.

A device to fix the distal femur so that stress can be applied to distract the articular surfaces of the knee must be available. A cloth sling hooked to the edge of the table was improvised to provide this fixation (Fig. 3A, B). For the examination of the medial meniscus, the sling is passed under the opposite leg and fastened to the side of the table (Fig. 8A). To examine the lateral meniscus, the sling is switched to the ipsilateral side of the table (Fig. 8B). A small pillow placed under the distal thigh is frequently helpful in obtaining the proper projections and providing distraction of the anterior portion of the knee (Fig. 8B).

Recently, a knee-holding device (Fig. 9A, B) became available and has proved to be most useful. A large suction cup attaches the device to the table, and the distal thigh is cradled in it. It elevates the knee from the table top, so the small pillow is not needed for support. The holding device obviates the necessity of switching the sling attachment from one side of the table to the other, and speeds up the examination. By resting the fluoroscopic tower firmly atop the device, a constant tube-film distance can be maintained, a particularly important feature for exposures that are not photo-timed. Photo-timing of these severely collimated exposures can make the films vary in density because the amount of unabsorbed X-ray beam at the periphery of the knee varies from picture to picture. At The Hospital for Special Surgery the photo-timer is not used, although one is available.

Technique

In general, 9 to 18 exposures of each meniscus are made. The pictures are moderately small, and nine of them fit easily on a 9½ × 9½ in. film. A portion of the femoral condyle is always included, and the picture is made large enough so that the overlapping of the condyles in the most anterior and most posterior projection can be evaluated. This overlap is an indication that the examination has been carried as far anteriorly and posteriorly as is possible without obtaining a complete overlap of the medial and lateral menisci. Ideally, the most anterior and most posterior projections should show the margin of the opposite condyle immediately adjacent to the inner edge of the meniscus (Figs 8, 21B, Chapter 3). Collimation of the beam to postage stamp size, which would yield a picture only large enough to show the meniscal cartilage, is avoided.

Once the injection procedure has been completed, and the patient has walked or the knee has been passively moved to distribute the contrast agent, the examination begins. The examination of the cruciate ligaments with the patient sitting (Fig. 10), described in Chapter 5, may be made first. For the examination of the menisci, the patient is placed prone with the feet toward the examiner's right hand. A lead apron can be placed under the patient for further radiation protection. A left-handed examiner may prefer to reverse the patient's position and hold the foot with the left hand.

If the medial meniscus is to be examined first, as is usually the case, the restraining band is passed around the distal thigh and under the opposite leg and hooked to the edge of the table opposite the leg being examined (Fig. 11). The anterior or the posterior portion of the meniscus can be examined first. In either case, the patient is turned in an almost lateral position so that fluoroscopically there is nearly complete overlapping of the femoral condyles. The knee is then slightly rotated so that the margin of the opposite condyle clears the inner margin of the meniscus. The articular surfaces are distracted by extending or flexing the knee and pulling or pushing on the patient's foot or ankle. These manipulations are done under image-amplified fluoroscopy, and when the meniscus is seen tangentially with its articular surfaces maximally surrounded by air, a spot film is taken. Spot films are made sequentially, slightly turning the knee after each exposure. Usually, 9 to 12 exposures allow a complete examination; however, more are often made to document or clarify an abnormality seen on the television monitor (Figs. 11–15).

For examination of the lateral meniscus, the same procedure is used with the sling fastened to the ipsilateral side of the table (Fig. 16). For most of the exposures, the lateral side of the knee is examined with distraction in the extended position. The most anterior portions of the menisci are often seen best with the knee slightly flexed (Figs. 16–20).

HORIZONTAL BEAM EXAMINATION

The horizontal beam double contrast arthrography method described by Andren and Whelin in 1960 was used at The Hospital for Special Surgery for many years. The method permits the use of conventional radiographic equipment for filming and does not require a fractional millimeter focal spot X-ray tube since the target-film distance ranges between 48 and 52 in. (Fig. 23). A 1-mm focal spot, or even a 2-mm focal spot, yields excellent roentgenograms at that distance. The horizontal beam aimed at the superior aspect of the horizontally positioned knee produces good double contrast pictures because excess positive contrast agent falls to the lower portion of the knee and air rises to envelop the meniscus.

Compared with the fluoroscopic spot film method, the prime disadvantage of the horizontal beam method is that the tangential position of the X-ray beam cannot be checked under direct fluoroscopy at each exposure. Therefore, the optimal tangential view for visualization of the meniscus may not be obtained. Also, with the horizontal beam technique only six views per meniscus are routinely taken (Fig. 34). Twelve to 18 views are routine for the fluoroscopic method, and additional spot films can be made instantly when fluoroscopic observation indicates any abnormality. Supplemental views may be obtained by the horizontal beam method, but only after some delay.

In a report on a series of 225 cases of knee derangement investigated by the horizontal-beam double-contrast arthrography method, Nicholas, Freiberger, and Killoran reported an accuracy of 99.7 percent correct diagnosis in 143 lesions of the medial meniscus and a 93 percent accuracy in diagnosing 57 lesions of the lateral meniscus. There were no errors of reporting tears that were not found at operation; however, one medial meniscus tear and four tears of the lateral meniscus were not diagnosed on the arthrogram.

In another series of 2101 arthrograms and 623 operations, the diagnostic accuracy of meniscus tear was 95 percent for the medial meniscus and 93 percent for the lateral meniscus. Again, the major failure was not reporting tears of the lateral meniscus. These studies indicate that the horizontal beam double contrast arthrography method can provide very high diagnostic accuracy. No similar review of cases using the fluoroscopic spot film method of double contrast arthrography has been undertaken at The Hospital for Special Surgery, but it is the authors' impression that the fluoroscopic spot film method improves the accuracy of diagnosis of tears of the lateral meniscus.

Whether the horizontal beam method or the fluoroscopic spot film method should be used for arthrographic examination of the menisci can be resolved quite simply. If a modern fluoroscope with a fractional millimeter focal spot for spot filming is available, the fluoroscopic method is preferable. However, if only a 1 or 2 mm focal spot X-ray tube is available, the horizontal beam method is adequate.

Equipment

A lead-shielded filmholder with a 2½ × 7 in. (6.25 × 17.5 cm) window to permit six exposures on a 7 × 17 in. (17.5 × 42.5 cm) cassette is necessary, and two or three 7 × 17 in. cassettes must be marked to facilitate the positioning for six exposures. A wooden table 7¼ in. (18 cm) high with a radiolucent top 27 × 16 in. (68 × 40 cm) is utilized to support the leg during the filming of the lateral meniscus. A firm cylindrical pillow approximately 5 in. (12 cm) in diameter by 6 in. (15 cm) long is placed under the knee. The pillow can be made by covering a cut-off portion of a 1-lb roll of cotton. A 7-lb sandbag sits on the ankle to distract the knee joint during the examination (Figs. 21, 23).

Technique

Prior to the injection of the knee with air and contrast agent, the patient is placed in lateral position on a fluoroscopic table with the knee fully extended. With fluoroscopic guidance, (Fig. 22C) a metal ruler or rectangular piece of lead rubber is placed along the articular surface of the tibial plateau. The position and slope of the plateau is then marked on the skin of the medial aspect of the knee using a washable ink felt-tip marker (Fig. 22A). Placing the small cylindrical pillow under the ankle usually produces a better tangential view of the tibial plateau. The lateral aspect of the knee is marked in a similar manner by turning the patient and placing the leg on the low wooden table (Fig. 22B). Using the fluoroscope facilitates the marking (Fig. 22C) but is not essential. The margin of the tibial plateau can also be palpated and the lines placed by that method.

Arthrocentesis and injection of contrast media is then carried out.

Following the injection, the patient walks a few steps to distribute the contrast media and is then placed prone on the X-ray table. The symptomatic side of the knee—usually the medial—is examined first. The patient is placed in the prone position so that the posteromedial aspect of the knee joint is uppermost. The cylindrical pillow is placed under the knee and the sandbag is placed over the ankle to distract the posteromedial aspect of the knee joint. The foot should project beyond the edge of the table, as patients tend to alleviate the discomfort of the stress on the knee, produced by the sandbag, by placing the toes on the table top (Fig. 23).

The central ray of the X-ray beam is aimed at the line marking the tibial plateau, and the film holder is placed with its window centered on the X-ray beam. A target-film distance of approximately 52 in. is maintained throughout the filming. The patient and the knee are then rotated approximately 25°, and the same procedure is followed, aiming the central ray along the line marking the edge of the medial tibial plateau and moving the film cassette after each exposure (Figs. 24–28). At about the fifth exposure (Fig. 27), when the central ray becomes tangential to the anterior aspect of the meniscus, the knee flexes. The patient's opposite leg is arched over the cassette holder. If in short, fat patients the buttock interferes with the advancement of the cassette to the fifth and sixth positions, the cassette should be removed from the holder, turned 180°, and reinserted to take the last two projections.

In the anterior projection, when the knee is flexed, distraction of the joint is lost unless it is maintained by manual traction on the leg. The sixth exposure (Fig. 28) is tangential to the most anterior part of the medial meniscus. The cassette is then removed from the film holder and sent to the darkroom for processing.

The patient is turned for filming of the lateral meniscus. The leg is placed on the low, wooden table with the posterior aspect of the lateral side of the knee uppermost. The pillow is placed under the knee, with the sandbag over the ankle (Fig. 29). Filming proceeds as before, with the patient and knee rotated approximately 25° between each exposure until the sixth exposure is tangential to the most anterior portion of the lateral meniscus (Figs. 29–34).

When filming of the lateral meniscus has been completed, the cassette is immediately taken to the darkroom. The exposures of the medial meniscus should then be available for inspection. If further films of the medial meniscus are desired, they can be taken with only minimal loss of definition caused by the increased time interval between injection and filming. Similarly, a third set of exposures can be made of either the medial or the lateral meniscus; however, the increased time elapsed between injection and filming causes some loss of definition. The addition of 0.3 cc of 1:1000 epinephrine solution to the injected contrast agent slows its absorption and effectively extends the time available for obtaining sharply defined arthrograms.

Each of the two or more 7 × 17 in. films obtained has six projections of the arthrogram arranged sequentially from the back of the knee on the top of the film to the front of the knee on the bottom (Fig. 35).

The examination is completed by a lateral projection of the knee joint to show the cruciate ligaments and, if present, a popliteal cyst. Two methods are used to take these films. In the first, the patient is supine with the pillow placed beneath the calf and the sandbag over the dorsum of the ankle, causing forward traction of the tibia at the knee joint. A film is placed vertically on the inner aspect of the knee, and an exposure is made with the X-ray beam in horizontal position (Fig. 36).

The second method is identical to that used in the fluoroscopic spot film examination. The patient is seated on the edge of the X-ray table with the knee bent 90° over the firm pillow, which has been placed between the table edge and the tibia. A grid cassette is placed between the patient's knees, and a film is exposed with the horizontal X-ray beam at the appropriate distance, depending on the focus of the grid (Fig. 10).

Examination of the cruciate ligaments is described in greater detail in Chapter 5.

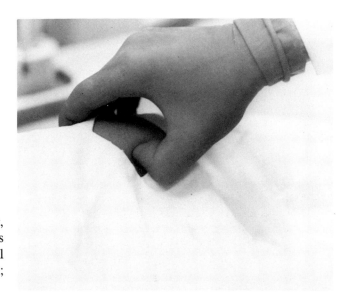

Figure 1

Having scrubbed and draped the knee, the arthrographer, wearing sterile gloves, grasps the patella. The thumbnail is pushed between the patella and medial or lateral femoral condyle hard enough to leave a pressure mark on the skin; the depression indicates the site of needle insertion.

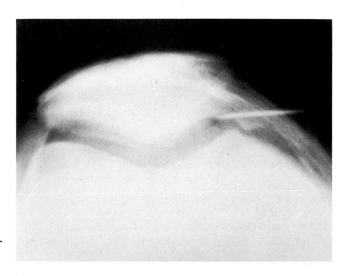

Figure 2

A tangential view of the patella shows a 20-gauge needle inserted into the knee joint from its medial aspect.

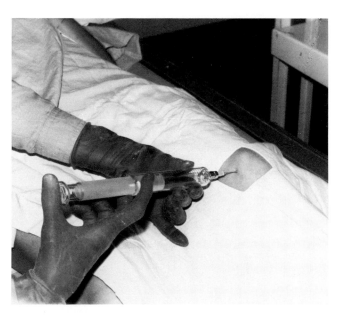

Figure 3

After aspiration of fluid, 20 cc of room air is injected.

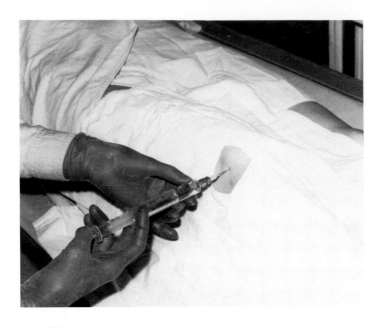

Figure 4
Approximately 5 cc of 60 percent meglumine positive contrast solution with epinephrine is injected, followed by another 20 cc of room air. Then the needle is withdrawn.

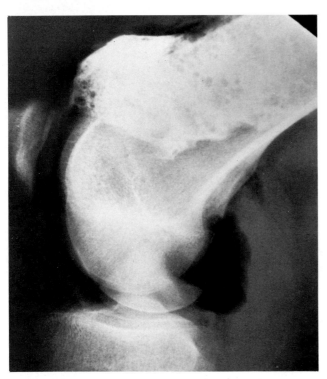

Figure 5
Extra-articularly injected positive contrast medium is located above the knee joint. If an intra-articular injection of positive contrast substance is made immediately, a satisfactory arthrogram can be obtained.

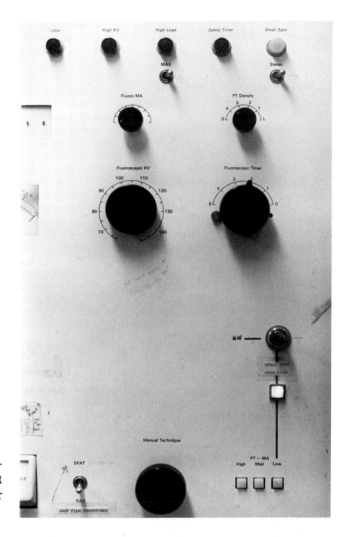

Figure 6
On a three-phase X-ray control unit, protective overload circuits and a key-operated switch permit fluoroscopic spot filming with the fractional millimeter focal spot used for fluoroscopy.

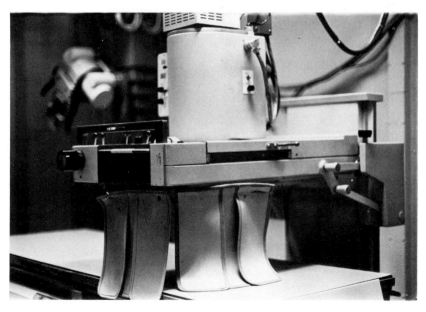

Figure 7
A lead apron has been added to the fluoroscopic tower to protect the radiologist's hand during manipulation of the patient's leg.

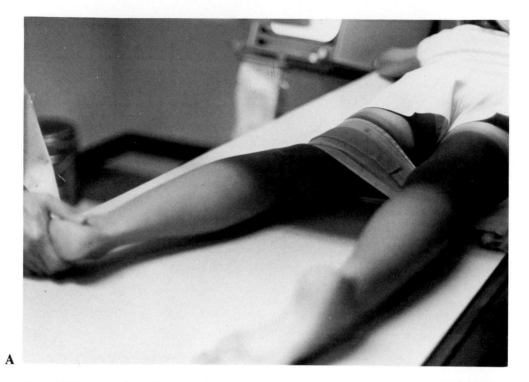

A

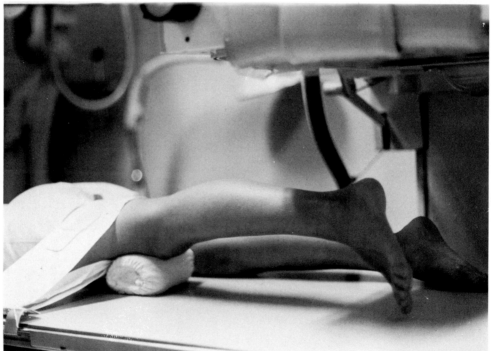

B

Figure 8
A. For examination of the medial meniscus, a sling placed around the distal portion of the thigh above the knee joint is passed under the opposite leg and fastened to the side of the X-ray table. The knee joint is distracted by having the examiner pull the patient's leg against the sling. The patient is in position for examination of the most posterior aspect of the medial meniscus.
B. For examination of the lateral meniscus, the sling is fastened to the ipsilateral side of the table. A small, firm pillow is placed under the distal thigh when the anterior portions of the menisci are examined.

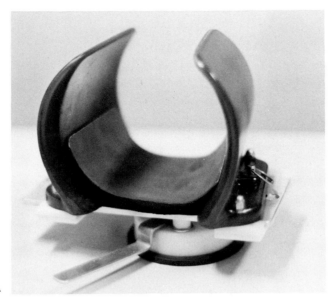

A

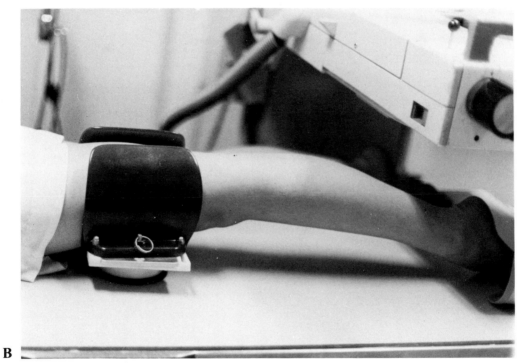

B

Figure 9
A, B. A recently developed and commercially available device to stabilize the distal
thigh eliminates switching the sling from one side of the table to the other. By resting
the fluoroscopic tower on top of it, a constant target-film distance is maintained, and
as the device slightly raises the knee, a pillow is not needed under the distal thigh.

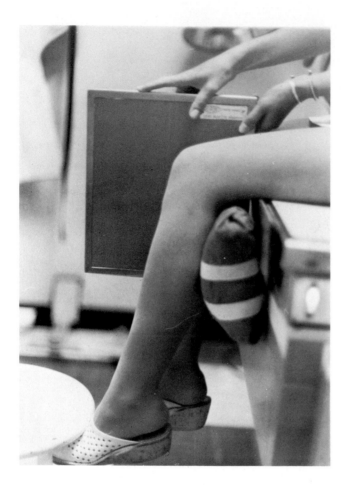

Figure 10
The cruciate ligaments are frequently examined first. The knee is forcibly bent over a pillow placed behind the calf. The patient holds a grid cassette for a horizontal X-ray beam projection.

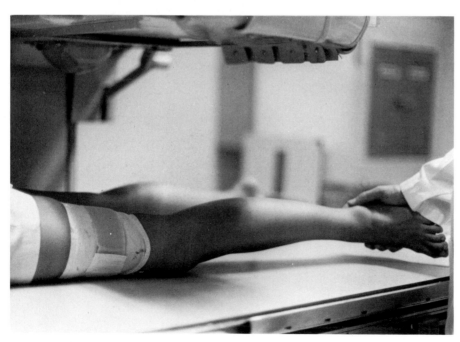

Figure 11
The leg is in position for examination of the posterior portion of the medial meniscus. Holding the foot rather than the ankle provides better control of rotation and causes the patient less discomfort.

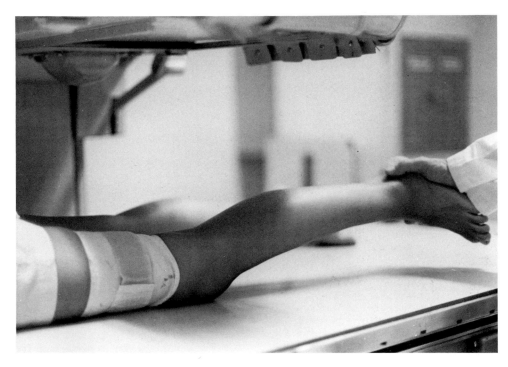

Figure 12
The leg has been turned to provide a projection that is slightly more anterior than
that of Fig. 11.

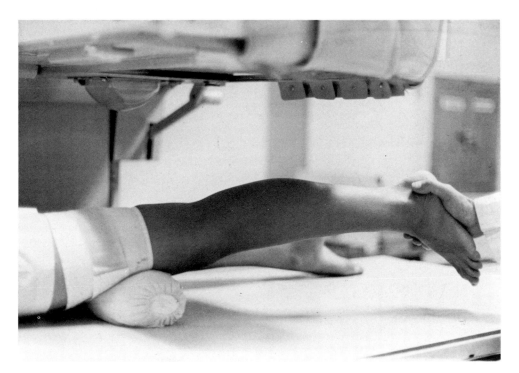

Figure 13
The patient's body and leg have been turned slightly to make a still more anterior
segment of the posterior portion of the medial meniscus tangential to the X-ray
beam. The pillow helps make the posteriorly downward slanting tibial plateau tangential to the X-ray beam.

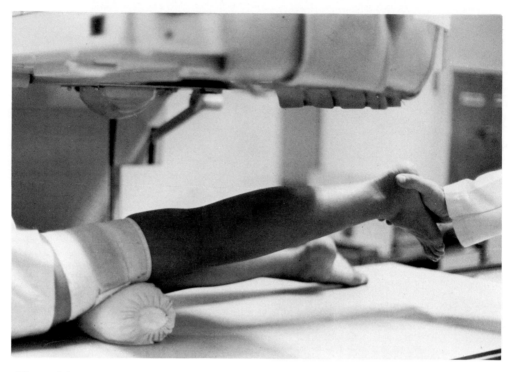

Figure 14
The midportion of the medial meniscus is tangential to the X-ray beam.

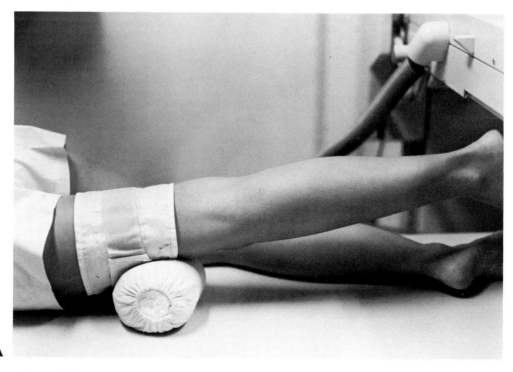

A

Figure 15
A. The anterior segment of the medial meniscus is being examined. Slight flexion of the knee is often necessary for best projection of the meniscus.

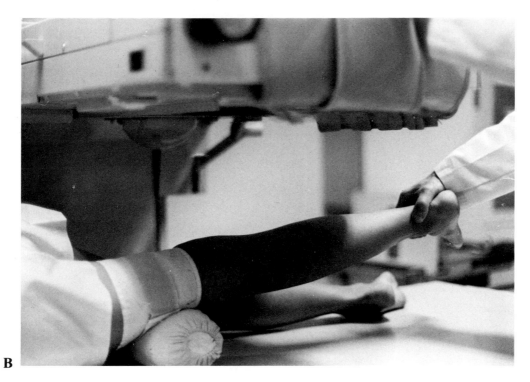

B

Figure 15
B. Downward pressure on the foot or ankle improves distraction.

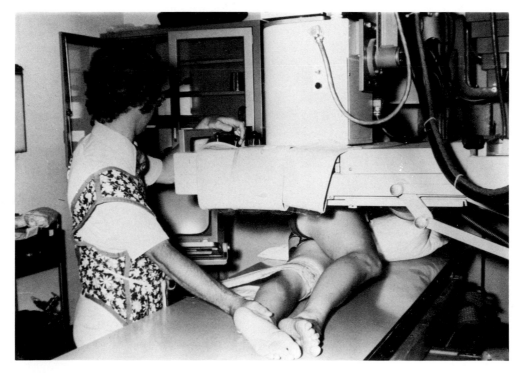

Figure 16
The patient is in position for filming the posterior aspect of the lateral meniscus. The sling around the distal thigh has been fastened to the ipsilateral side of the table. The posterior portion of the lateral meniscus is often seen best without a pillow under the distal thigh.

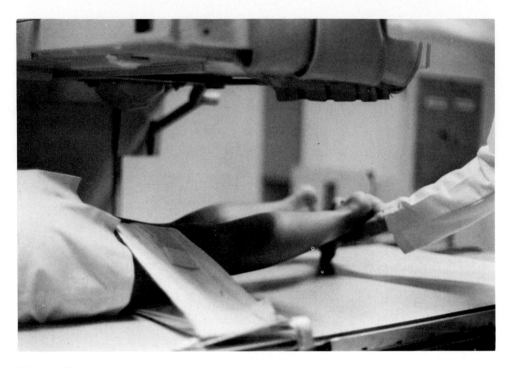

Figure 17
The position for filming the posterior portion of the lateral meniscus is seen from the side.

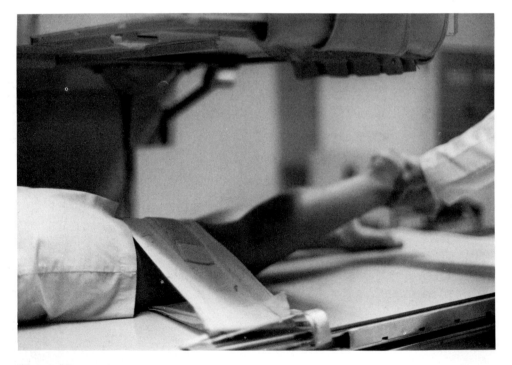

Figure 18
The postero-midportion of the lateral meniscus is tangential to the vertical X-ray beam. A pillow under the distal thigh may or may not improve the tangential projection of the meniscus in this position. Distraction is obtained by pushing on the foot or ankle against the stabilizing sling.

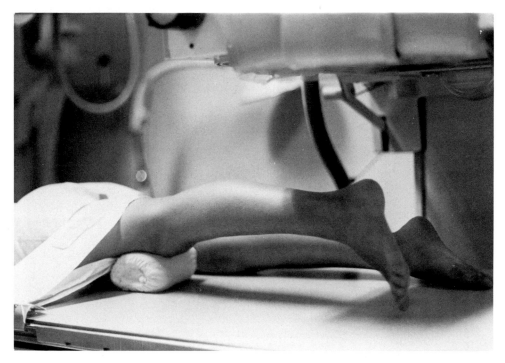

Figure 19
The patient is positioned for examination of the midportion of the lateral meniscus. The pillow under the distal thigh is used for this projection and projections of the anterior half of the lateral meniscus.

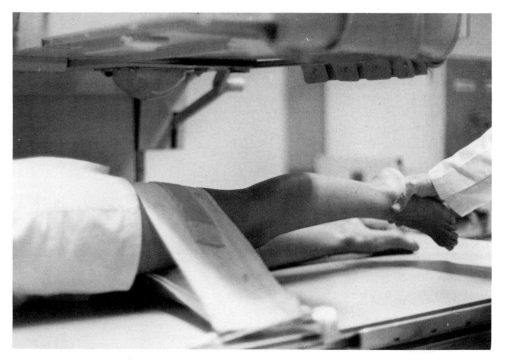

Figure 20
The anterior portion of the lateral meniscus is being examined. Downward pressure with flexion of the knee usually shows this portion of the meniscus to best advantage.

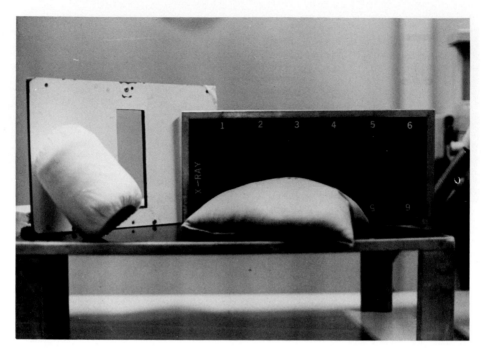

Figure 21
The equipment needed for the horizontal beam method includes a film holder with a rectangular cutout in a leaded plywood front to allow six exposures on a 7 × 17 in. cassette, a 7 × 17 in. cassette with six marked spaces corresponding to the cutout in the film holder, a cylindrical pillow, a 7-lb sandbag, and a low table to support the leg during the filming of the lateral meniscus.

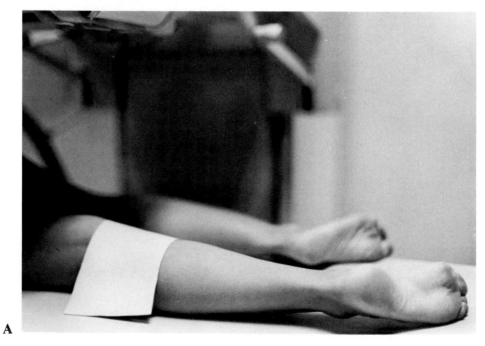

A

Figure 22
A. The straight edge of a piece of lead rubber has been placed over the leg at the level of, and parallel to, the tibial plateau. A line is then drawn on the skin of the medial side of the knee at the margin of the tibial plateau.

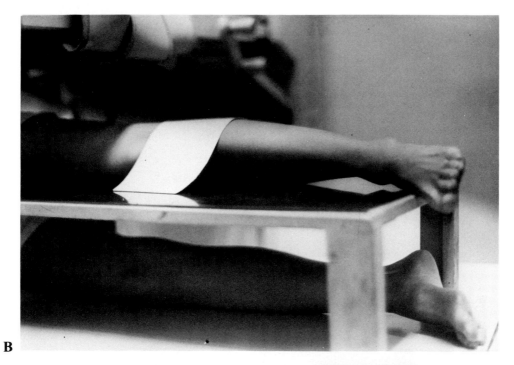

B

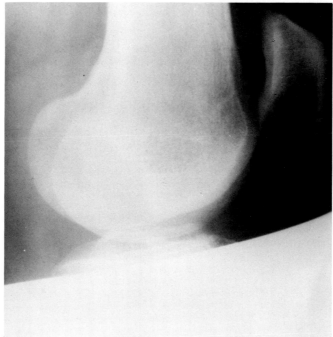

C

Figure 22
B. The leg is placed on the low table, the lead rubber is placed on the lateral side of the knee at the level of the tibial plateau, and a line is drawn on the skin.
C. Under fluoroscopy, the upper edge of the lead rubber is seen parallel to the edge of the tibial plateau which normally has a posteriorly downward slant.

Figures 23–28
The following six illustrations show the positions for filming of the medial meniscus by the horizontal beam method.

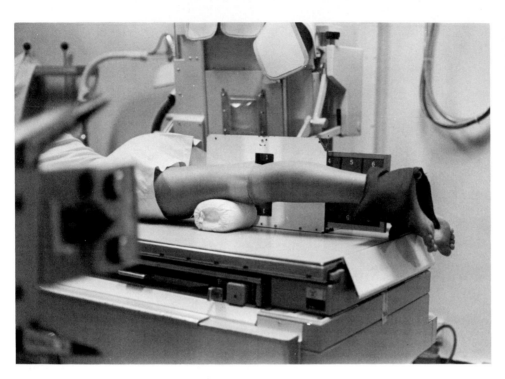

Figure 23
For the first exposure, the patient is placed prone, very slightly obliqued so that the most posterior portion of the medial meniscus is uppermost. The pillow is positioned below the distal thigh, and the 7-lb sandbag is placed over the ankle to distract the knee. The patient's toes project beyond the lower edge of the table so that the patient cannot relieve the pressure of the sandbag by placing the toes on the table. The film holder and the cassette are in position for the first exposure. The X-ray tube is placed 48 to 52 in. from the film, and the central ray is aimed along the line drawn on the patient's skin.

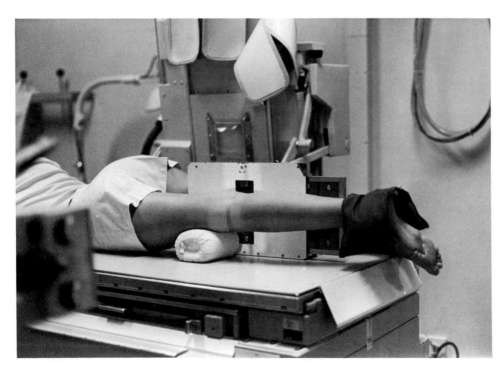

Figure 24
For the second exposure, the cassette is advanced to position two, and the knee is turned approximately 25° to place a slightly more anterior portion of the medial meniscus uppermost.

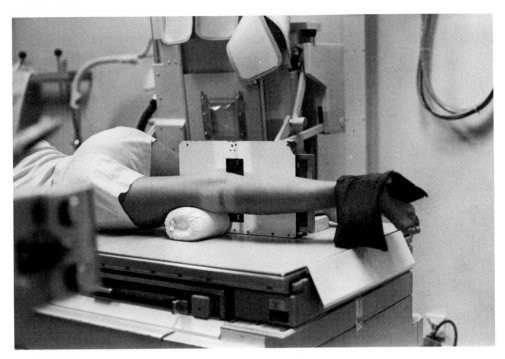

Figure 25
For the third exposure, the cassette is advanced to position three, and the patient is turned approximately 25° to examine the meniscus slightly more anteriorly than the previous position.

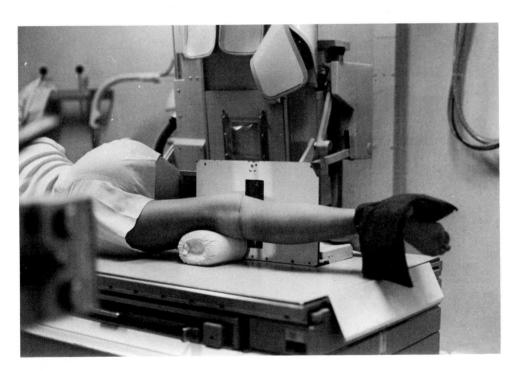

Figure 26
For the fourth exposure, the cassette is advanced to position four, and the patient is turned to bring the midportion of the medial meniscus uppermost. The X-ray beam is adjusted to fall along the line drawn on the skin.

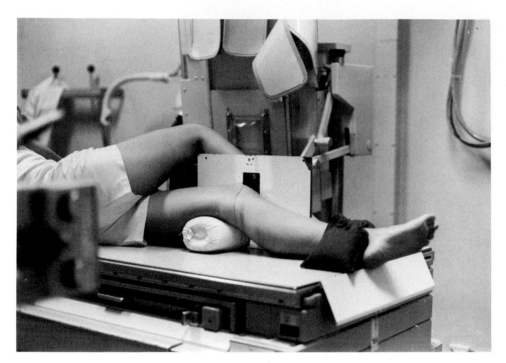

Figure 27
For the fifth exposure, the cassette is advanced to position five. The patient is turned into a supine oblique position for examination of the antero-midportion of the medial meniscus. The knee is slightly flexed and the patient's foot and ankle rest on the table so that distraction of the knee has been lost. The other leg arches over the film holder and cassette.

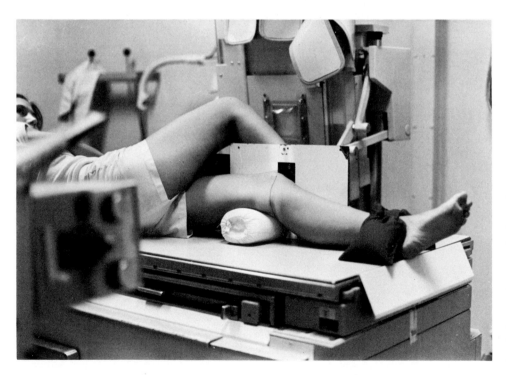

Figure 28
For the sixth exposure, the cassette is advanced to the sixth position. The patient is turned more supine to bring the anterior portion of the medial meniscus uppermost and tangential to the X-ray beam. The other leg arches over the film holder and cassette. On completing the sixth exposure, the cassette is sent to the darkroom for developing.

Figures 29–34
The following six photographs demonstrate the filming of the lateral meniscus by the horizontal beam method.

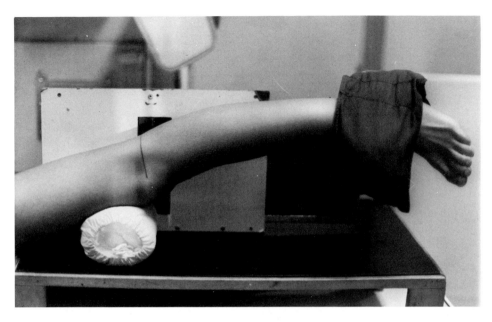

Figure 29
For the first exposure of the lateral meniscus, the patient is in the prone oblique position. The leg to be examined has been placed on the low table and the opposite leg is beneath it. The pillow is under the distal thigh, and the film holder with the cassette in the number one position is placed behind the patient's knee. The central ray of the X-ray beam is aimed along the skin line representing the position and slope of the tibial plateau. The sandbag has been placed over the ankle to provide distraction of the knee joint.

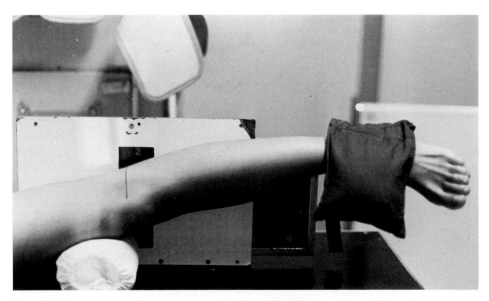

Figure 30
For the second exposure, the cassette is advanced to the number two position, and the patient is turned approximately 25° to bring a slightly more anterior portion of the lateral meniscus tangential to the X-ray beam.

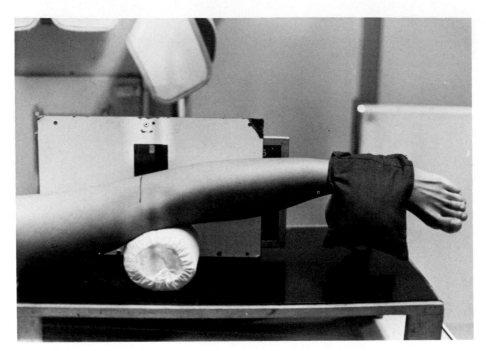

Figure 31
For the third exposure, the cassette is advanced to the number three position, and the patient is turned to bring the X-ray beam tangential to a portion of the lateral meniscus that lies slightly posterior to its midportion. With each change in the patient's position, the sandbag over the ankle is adjusted to provide distraction, and the X-ray beam is moved to follow the skin line on the patient's knee.

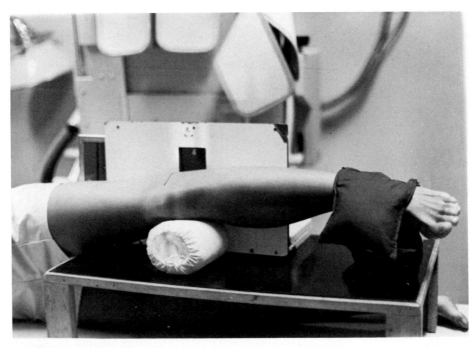

Figure 32
For the fourth exposure, the cassette is advanced to the number four position, and the patient is turned so that the midportion of the lateral meniscus is uppermost and tangential to the X-ray beam.

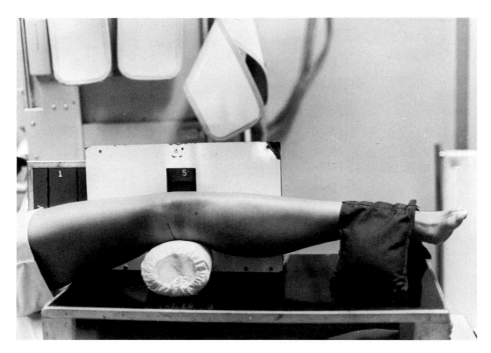

Figure 33
For the fifth exposure, the cassette is advanced to the number five position, and the patient is turned to be supine oblique, to position the antero-midportion of the lateral meniscus tangential to the X-ray beam. The knee flexes slightly.

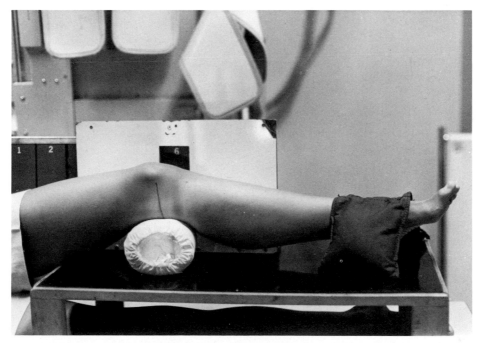

Figure 34
For the sixth exposure, the cassette is moved to the number six position, the most anterior portion of the lateral meniscus tangential to the X-ray beam, and the knee is flexed over the pillow. The film is sent to the darkroom for developing.

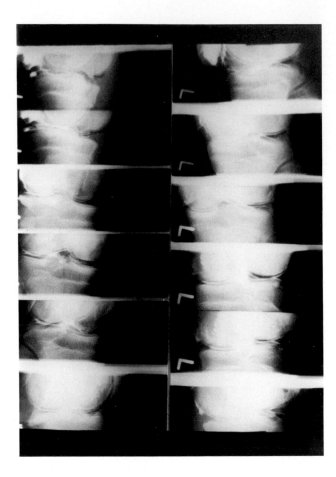

Figure 35

The two 7 × 17 in. films of the medial and lateral menisci each show from top to bottom the sequence of six exposures from posterior to anterior. The views of the medial meniscus examination show air in the medial aspect of the knee joint. The views of the lateral meniscus show air in the lateral compartment of the knee. Air rises to the superior distracted portion of the knee.

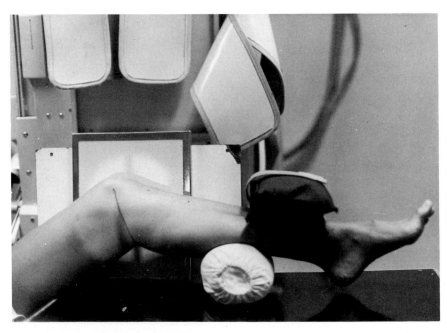

Figure 36

A double contrast evaluation of the cruciate ligaments is made with the patient supine. The pillow under the calf, and the sandbag on top of the ankle provide a forward pressure on the tibia at the knee joint. A second roentgenogram with the patient sitting on the table (Fig. 10) completes the examination.

3
Anatomy and Arthrography of the Normal Menisci

Jeremy J. Kaye

Because the anatomy of the entire knee is so complex, only those parts that are essential to the evaluation of the menisci are described.

The normal structures that are directly visualized by knee arthrography and that can affect the evaluation of the menisci are the synovium and its extensions, including the suprapatellar pouch or bursa, and occasionally a very small gastrocnemius-semimembranous bursa located posteromedially. Intrasynovial structures are the articular cartilages of the patella, femur, and tibia. Extrasynovial but intra-articular structures are the anterior and posterior cruciate ligaments and, most importantly, the anterior fat pad.

THE MEDIAL MENISCUS

The medial meniscus as seen from above is a C-shaped fibrocartilaginous structure, narrower in its anterior than in its posterior portion (Fig. 1). Viewed microscopically in vertical section it is triangular in shape and has a fibrocartilaginous pattern (Fig. 2). At its periphery, the medial meniscus has a complete attachment to the capsule (Figs. 3–5). This capsular attachment is reinforced by the medial collateral ligament. A synovial-lined portion of the capsule attaches the inferior peripheral margin of the medial meniscus

to the margin of the tibial plateau (Figs. 3–5). Another synovial-lined capsular attachment extends from the superior margin of the meniscus to the medial femoral condyle (Fig. 4). Since the medial meniscus has a gliding motion between the hyaline cartilages of the articular surfaces of the tibia and femoral condyles, the peripheral capsular attachments of the medial meniscus are somewhat lax (Figs. 3, 4B, 6). A vertical section through the anterior portion of the medial meniscus shows it as a triangular structure (Fig. 3B) in the same way that it is seen on an arthrogram, with the radiographic beam tangential to the margin of the tibial plateau (Figs. 5, 6). The base of the triangle is formed by the capsular attachment of the meniscus, and the sides of the triangle are formed by the articular surfaces of the meniscus. On the arthrogram, a thin layer of positive contrast material coats the meniscus, which is partially surrounded by air (Figs. 5, 6). Since the medial meniscus has a complete peripheral attachment to the capsule, no air or positive contrast material injected into the knee during arthrography enters the meniscus.

The lax capsular attachments of the meniscus, starting at the meniscosynovial junctions, form shallow troughs or slightly irregular indentations (Figs. 4, 5, 7–9). On the arthrogram these are called recesses. The normal recesses are readily identified on the anatomic

31

vertical sections (Figs. 3, 4), and also on arthrographic projections tangential to the meniscus that resemble the anatomic vertical sections (Figs. 5–9). Although it may appear that the anatomic vertical section and the tangential arthrographic projection of the meniscus are identical, this is not entirely true. On the anatomic vertical section only a small part of the meniscus is seen, whereas on the arthrogram the entire meniscus is projected. Structures lying in front or in back of the area tangential to the radiographic beam are included on the radiograph (Fig. 8). Contrast material at the meniscosynovial junction or capsular attachment recesses of the meniscus can therefore be projected through the meniscus (Figs. 7–9). These contrast-coated recesses appear as wavy radiopaque lines that must not be mistaken for oblique or horizontal meniscal tears.

There are two reliable signs that allow the differentiation between contrast-coated meniscosynovial junctions projected through the meniscus and contrast within a meniscal tear. The first of these is the choppy sea sign. The meniscosynovial junction is slightly irregular; therefore, when coated by positive contrast on the arthrogram, it looks wavy, like a choppy sea (Fig. 8). The second sign is the end sign. Since the meniscosynovial junction is continuous from front to back of the meniscus, that contrast-coated part projected through the meniscus, whether in front or back, must *end* at the apex of the recess seen in tangent (Figs. 7–9).

It is essential to recognize the difference between contrast at the recesses projected *through* the meniscus and contrast *within* the meniscus, which indicates a tear. That distinction eliminates the possible false positive diagnoses of a horizontal or oblique meniscal tear.

THE LATERAL MENISCUS

The lateral meniscus is more circular than the medial meniscus and is nearly as wide anteriorly as it is posteriorly (Fig. 10). Its anterior and posterior attachments, owing to its circular shape, are deep within the knee and cannot be evaluated on an arthrogram. The lateral meniscus has a greater excursion on the tibial plateau during knee motion than the medial meniscus. The capsular attachments of the lateral meniscus are more lax than those of the medial meniscus, and the capsular recesses seen on arthrography are larger (Figs. 11A, B). Anterior to the popliteus tendon, the capsular attachments of the lateral meniscus are complete, similar to those of the medial meniscus (Figs. 10, 11).

The projection of the contrast-coated meniscal attachment through the meniscus, called the choppy sea sign and described with the anatomy of the medial meniscus, also occurs at the lateral meniscus (Fig. 11B).

In the arthrographic projection of the anterior portions of the normal lateral meniscus, one to three small radiopaque dots are often seen near the periphery of the meniscus (Fig. 11A). They are probably small venules or lymphatics containing absorbed contrast material and should not be mistaken for a meniscal tear or opacification of a meniscal cyst.

The posterior attachments of the lateral meniscus are complex and have normal defects. One consistent defect is in the superior capsular attachment, where the popliteus tendon descends into its bursa and crosses the lateral meniscus (Figs. 12, 13).

The popliteus muscle takes its origin from the groove in the lateral femoral condyle and passes downward and posteriorly, becoming partially intra-articular. It has a second, less prominent origin from the posterior aspect of the capsule with a muscular insertion on the posterior aspect of the proximal tibia. The tendinous portion of the popliteus attaches to the capsule and within its bursa crosses the periphery of the lateral meniscus (Figs. 13, 17). The superior and inferior meniscal attachments form the roof and floor respectively of the popliteus bursa (Figs. 17, 18). In the superior attachment, there is always a defect where the popliteus tendon enters the bursa (Figs. 12, 13). The lack of a superior attachment of the lateral meniscus at this location is evident on arthrograms and is *normal* (Figs. 14–16, 18). Injected contrast media pass through this defect, filling the bursa that partially surrounds the popliteus tendon. Contrast media within the popliteus bursa are normally seen at the periphery of the lateral meniscus when the bursa is tangential to the radiographic beam (Figs. 14–16, 18, 21, 22). Contrast media are projected through the meniscus when areas in front or in back of the popliteus tendon are examined and are tangential to the X-ray beam (Figs. 15, 16).

Where there is a defect in the superior attachment of the lateral meniscus, an inferior attachment is present and usually seen on the arthrogram (Figs. 13, 14). Posterior to its normal defect, the superior attachment of the lateral meniscus is intact and becomes thicker as it extends posteriorly (Figs. 17, 18). The inferior attachment tends to become thinner and often incomplete far posteriorly. Vertical radial anatomic sections and arthrograms show the popliteus bursa defined above by the superior capsular attachment, below by the inferior or tibial attachment, medially by the lateral meniscus, and laterally by the capsule to which the popliteus tendon is attached (Figs. 17, 18).

In most dissected knees, the inferior attachment of the lateral meniscus is defective or incomplete. This occurs far posteriorly where the popliteus tendon crosses the level of the tibial plateau (Figs. 19–22). Because of this defect, a second communication exists between the popliteal bursa and the knee joint at the under-surface of the lateral meniscus. The defect in the inferior attachment of the lateral meniscus is demonstrated on vertical radial anatomic sections (Figs. 19, 20) and can be seen on arthrograms (Figs. 21, 22, 26).

The normal defect in the inferior attachment of the lateral meniscus can be demonstrated on dissected specimens. A probe passed into the popliteus bursa can be seen from beneath the elevated lateral meniscus (Fig. 23), or a probe passed beneath the posterior portion of the lateral meniscus can be seen through the popliteus bursa (Fig. 24). The margin of the inferior attachments of the defect can also be visualized by looking directly into the opening of the popliteus bursa (Fig. 25).

In a few specimens, the inferior attachment of the lateral meniscus remains intact posteriorly and the popliteus bursa ends in a blind pouch at the level of the tibial plateau.

The normal defects in both superior and inferior attachments of the posterior portion of the lateral meniscus should not be mistaken for a peripheral detachment of the lateral meniscus. Usually, when a defect in one attachment is visualized on an arthrogram, the other attachment of the meniscus can be seen to be intact. Since the superior and inferior attachment defects are close to each other, both attachment defects can occasionally be seen on a single arthrographic projection (Fig. 26). Other projections demonstrate that the inferior attachment is intact where the defect for the popliteus tendon in the superior attachment is seen best, and also that the superior attachment is intact far posteriorly where the defect in the inferior attachment is seen best.

Awareness of the superior and inferior attachment defects of the lateral meniscus is of importance to both the arthrographer and the surgeon. The arthrographer should not mistakenly make a diagnosis of traumatic meniscal detachment or peripheral tear. The surgeon, who at arthrotomy may catch the periphery of the meniscus by passing a hook-probe over or under the posterior part of the lateral meniscus, should not misinterpret this as an indication of a meniscal tear or peripheral separation.

ARTICULAR CARTILAGES

The hyaline articular cartilages of the femur, tibia, and patella, which are seen completely on anatomic specimen, can be examined in part on arthrograms. Coated by positive contrast agent, those parts of the articular cartilage that can be made tangential to the radiographic beam during arthrography can be evaluated. Those areas not seen tangentially cannot be evaluated.

EXTRASYNOVIAL STRUCTURES

The only extrasynovial structure that is pertinent to evaluation of the menisci is the anterior fat pad. The contrast-coated surface of the anterior fat pad (Figs. 27A, B) is frequently seen superimposed over the anterior portion of the menisci, particularly the lateral meniscus (Fig. 28). Its rounded, lobulated contour overlaps and may obscure the sharp inner wedge of the meniscus and could lead to a misdiagnosis of meniscal tear.

The normal and abnormal extrasynovial, intracapsular cruciate ligaments are described in Chapter 5.

The capsule, medially reinforced by the collateral ligaments, is a watertight structure; therefore, only the smooth synovial surface is seen on the normal arthrogram. Synovial, capsular, and extracapsular abnormalities are described in Chapter 6.

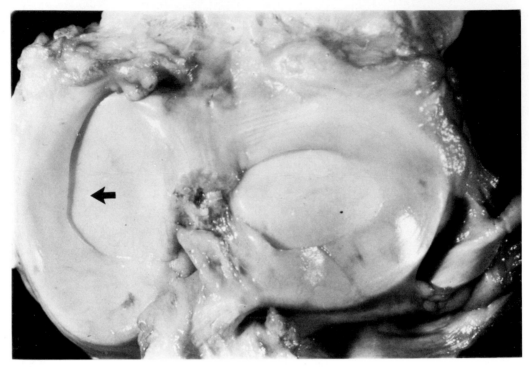

Figure 1
The normal medial meniscus (arrow), when viewed from above, is a C-shaped structure, somewhat narrower anteriorly than posteriorly. It has a complete peripheral capsular attachment.

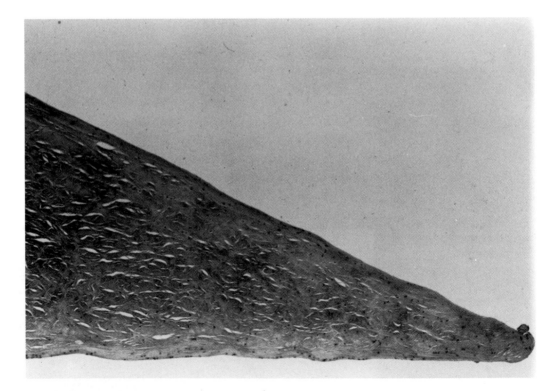

Figure 2
The menisci are fibrocartilaginous and in vertical sections are triangular.

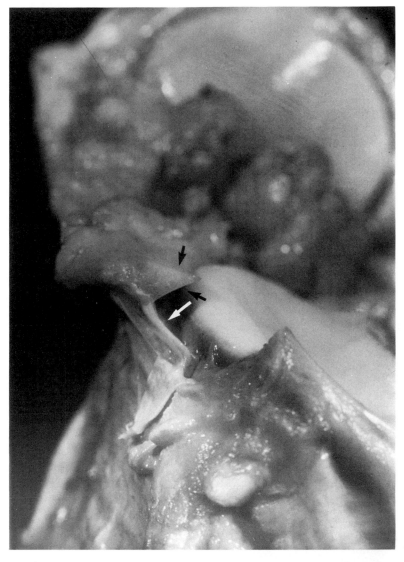

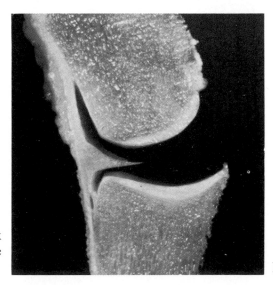

Figure 3
A, B. The medial meniscus cut vertically is triangular (black arrows). The normal laxity of the capsular attachment of the medial meniscus is demonstrated (white arrow).

A

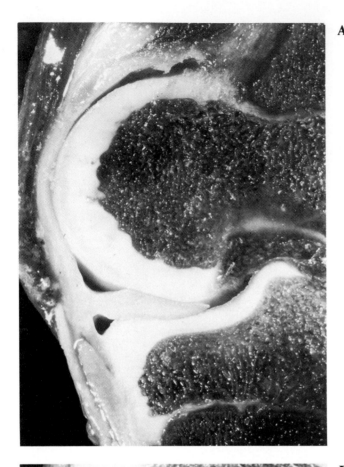

B

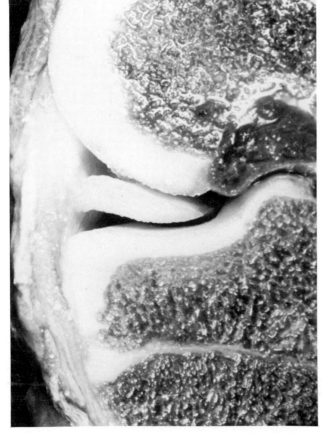

Figure 4
A. Normally, the medial meniscus is in contact with the articular cartilage of the femoral condyle and the tibial plateau. It is completely attached to the capsule at its periphery.
B. During arthrography, the femoral condyle is distracted from the tibial plateau, which allows the meniscus to float freely. The meniscus remains attached to the capsule peripherally.

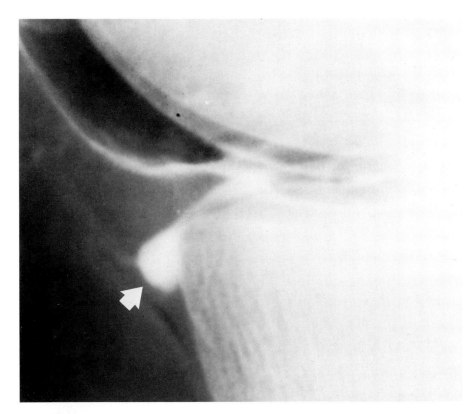

A

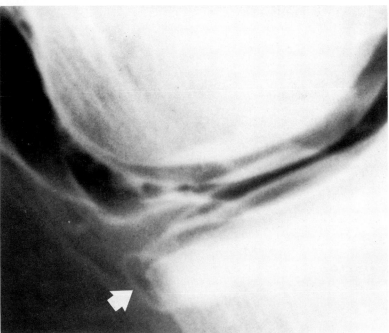

B

Figure 5
A. A normal double-contrast arthrogram of the anterior segment of the medial meniscus shows the meniscus coated by a thin layer of positive contrast material and surrounded by air. No air or contrast material is seen within the substance of the meniscus. The tibial attachment recess is filled with positive contrast substance (arrow).
B. The tibial attachment recess is filled with air (arrow).

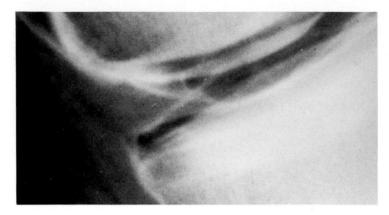

Figure 6
On an arthrogram tangential to the antero-midportion of a normal medial meniscus, the meniscus is somewhat narrower than it is further posteriorly, as seen in Figure 7.

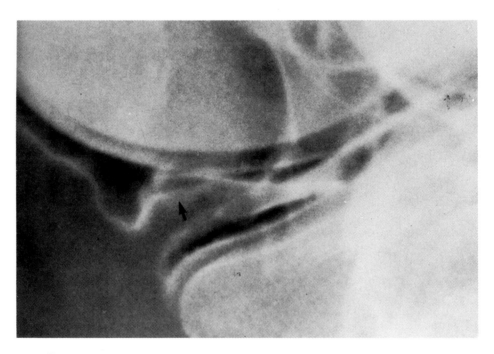

Figure 7
The posterior segment of the medial meniscus seen on a double contrast arthrogram is wider than the anterior segment. The superior attachment recess is lax, and a wavy line (arrow) is seen extending horizontally across the meniscus from the apex of the recess. The wavy line represents opaque contrast agent at the meniscosynovial junction either in front or in back of the region seen tangentially. It is not a horizontal meniscal tear.

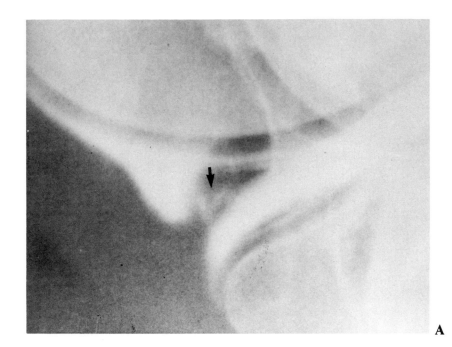

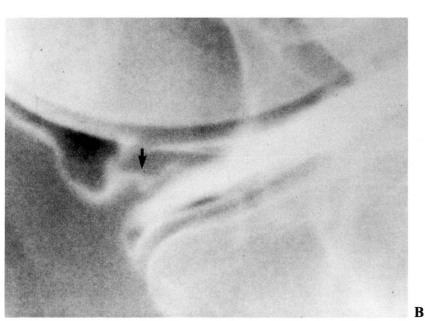

Figure 8
A. On a double contrast arthrogram, the posterior segment of the medial meniscus is surrounded almost entirely by positive contrast substance. An oblique line of positive contrast agent is seen through the meniscus.
B. By manipulating the knee, some of the positive contrast has been displaced by air. On both projections, a wavy horizontal line (arrows) extends across the meniscus, ending at the apex of the superior recess. This is called the choppy sea sign. The termination of the line at the apex of the attachment recess is called the end sign. The end sign indicates that positive contrast substance is in the attachment recess and not in a meniscal tear.

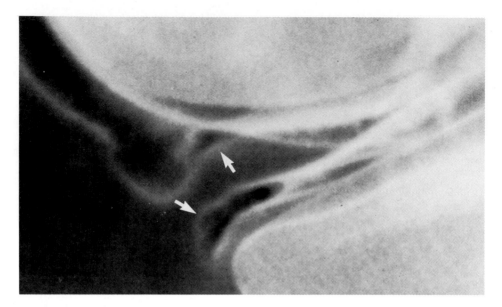

Figure 9
Air- and positive contrast-coated recesses cast shadows over the medial meniscus both superiorly and inferiorly (arrows). On all normal arthrograms the tibial attachment of the meniscus is around the corner of the tibial plateau. Contrast agent extends to the peripheral edge of the tibial articular cartilage.

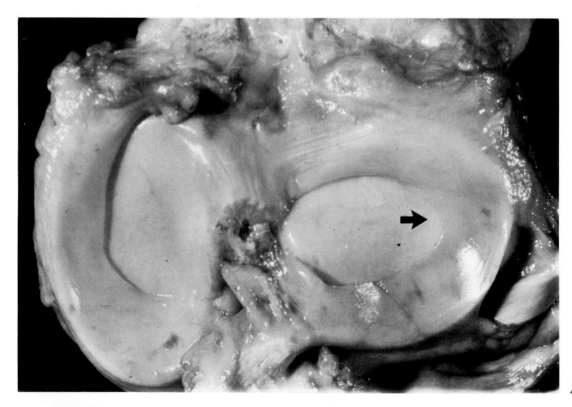

A

Figure 10
A. The normal lateral meniscus (arrow), with its central attachments deep within the joint, is more circular than the medial meniscus. It is about the same width anteriorly as posteriorly.

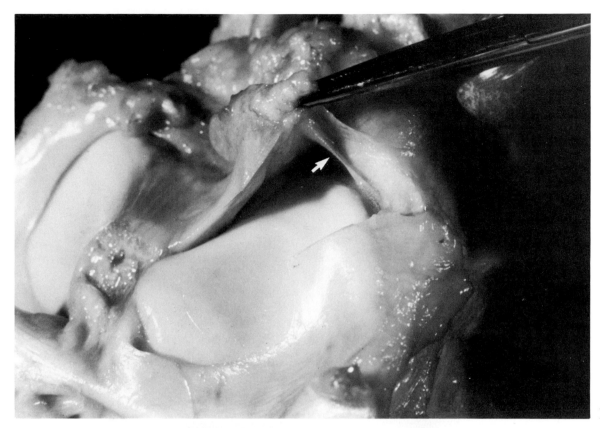

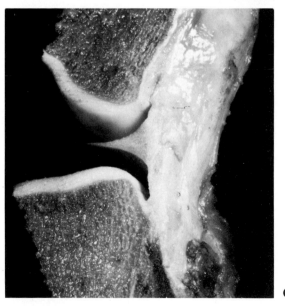

Figure 10
B. The lateral meniscus has greater mobility than the medial meniscus and its capsular attachments are lax. The femur and femoral attachments of the lateral meniscus have been excised from the specimen. The meniscus has been transected and forceps elevate its anterior portion to demonstrate the laxity of the tibial attachment (arrow).
C. In an anatomic vertical radial section, the lateral meniscus, suspended by its normally lax capsular attachments, appears to float between the femoral condyle and tibial plateau.

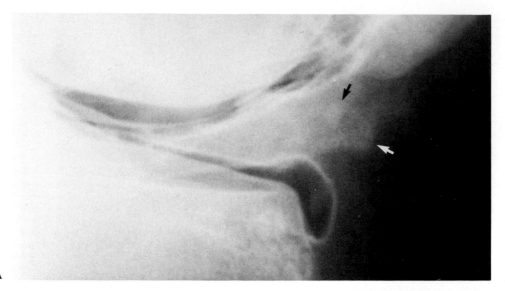

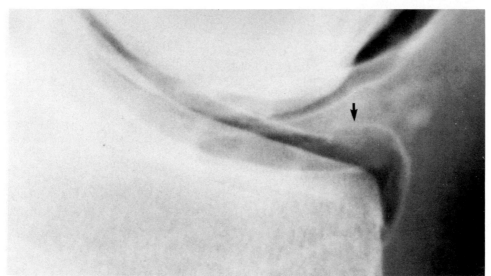

Figure 11
A. On a double-contrast arthrogram, the anterior segment of a normal lateral meniscus is seen with its large, lax, folded capsular attachments. One to three small radiopaque dots or short streaks (arrows) are visible near the periphery of the meniscus. They represent contrast material in small venules or lymphatics.
B. A slightly less anterior projection shows the lax capsular attachments and small radiopaque dots and streaks near the periphery of the meniscus. A choppy sea sign and an end sign are seen inferiorly (arrow).

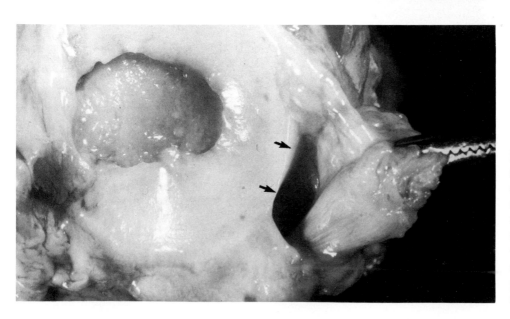

Figure 12
Seen from above, the hole (arrows) in the superior attachment of the lateral meniscus represents the normal defect in the superior attachment where the popliteus tendon enters its bursa and crosses the peripheral aspect of the meniscus.

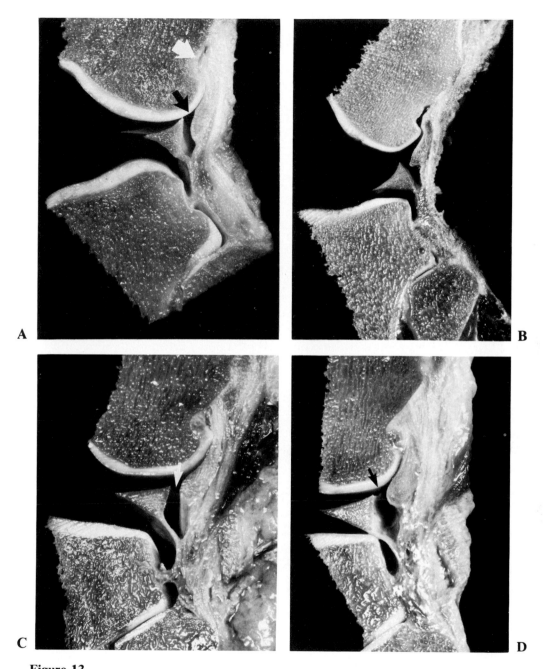

Figure 13

A–D. A series of vertical anatomic sections taken through the defect in the superior attachment of the lateral meniscus shows the origin of the popliteus at the groove of the lateral femoral condyle (big white arrow). The tendon, attached to the capsule, descends in a slightly posterior direction. It enters the popliteus bursa through the superior attachment defect (arrows). The superior attachment of the meniscus is absent, although on the two posterior sections (C, D) the beginning of the superior attachment posterior to the defect is faintly seen (arrows). The inferior meniscal attachment is intact.

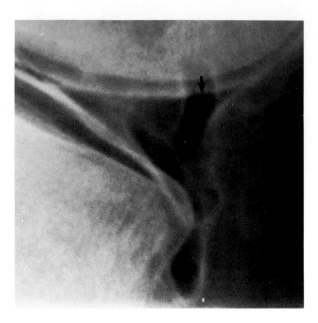

Figure 14
A normal arthrogram with the beam tangential to the defect in the superior attachment of the lateral meniscus shows that the superior meniscal attachment is absent (arrow).

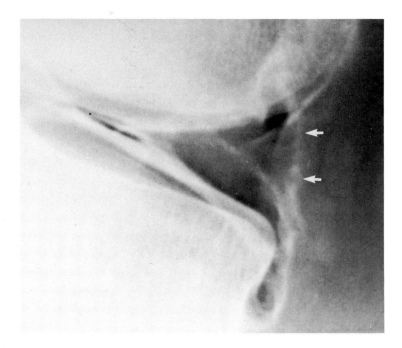

Figure 15
The X-ray beam is tangential to the area of the defect in the superior attachment of the lateral meniscus. The defect in the superior attachment is apparent on the arthrogram. A vertical line of opaque contrast agent extends downward from the peripheral margin of the defect in the superior attachment (arrows). The line represents the contrast-coated lateral surface of the popliteal tendon sheath projected through the meniscus. It should not be mistaken for a peripheral tear or detachment.

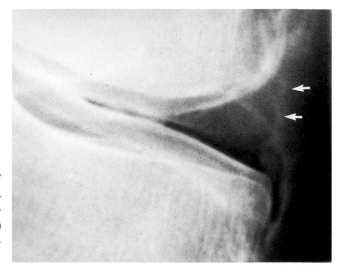

Figure 16
An arthrogram with the beam tangential to an area slightly anterior to the defect in the superior attachment shows a complete peripheral attachment of the meniscus. The contrast-coated surfaces of the popliteus tendon sleeve (arrows) are projected through the meniscus and must not be mistaken for a tear. Compare with Figure 15.

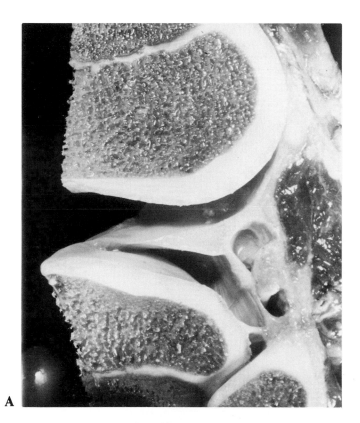

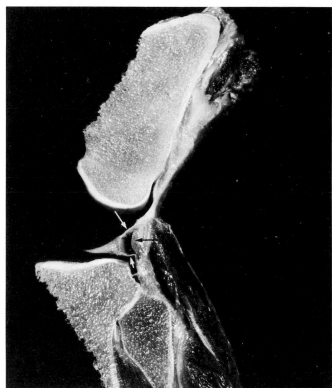

A   B

Figure 17
A. A vertical radial anatomic section posterior to the defect in the superior attachment of the lateral meniscus shows a thick, intact, superior attachment forming the roof of the popliteal bursa. The meniscus and inferior meniscal attachment form the medial inferior wall of the bursa, and the capsule with the attached popliteus tendon forms the lateral wall. In this region, immediately behind the defect of the superior meniscal attachment, both the superior and inferior attachments are intact. **B.** An anatomic section posterior to the superior attachment defect of the popliteus tendon shows the intact superior and inferior meniscal attachments (white arrows), the popliteal bursa, and the popliteus tendon (black arrow) closely adhering to the capsule.

A

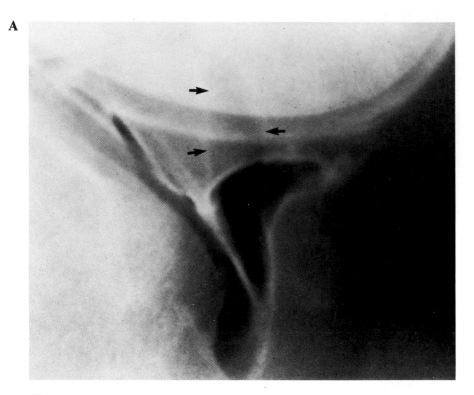

B

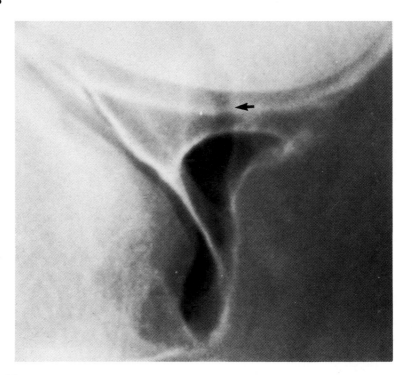

Figure 18
A, B. Arthrograms with the X-ray beam tangential to the region posterior to the superior attachment defect shows the intact superior and inferior attachments of the lateral meniscus. The bulge in the lateral wall of the popliteus bursa is the popliteus tendon. The more anterior portion of the air-filled and contrast-coated popliteal bursa (arrows) is projected faintly through the meniscus superiorly and somewhat medially to the bursa seen in tangent.

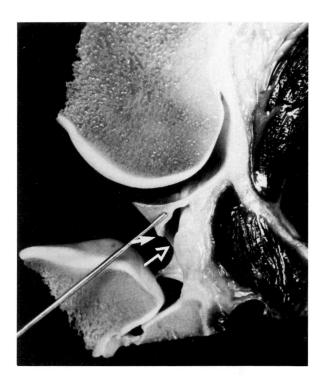

Figure 19
A vertical radial anatomic section through the posterior segment of the lateral meniscus seen from its posterior cut surface shows an intact superior meniscal attachment and the beginnings of a defect in the inferior attachment (arrow). The intact portion of the inferior attachment is visible more anteriorly (open arrow).

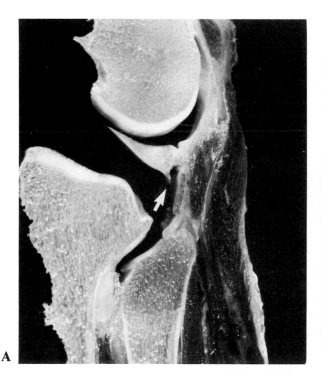

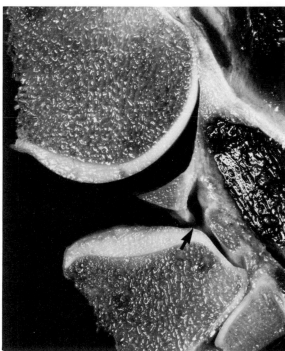

A

B

Figure 20
A, B. Vertical radial anatomic sections through the posterior part of the lateral meniscus show a thick intact superior attachment and a defect in the inferior attachment (arrows). The popliteus tendon has descended to the level of the inferior attachment defect at the posterior margin of the lateral tibial plateau.

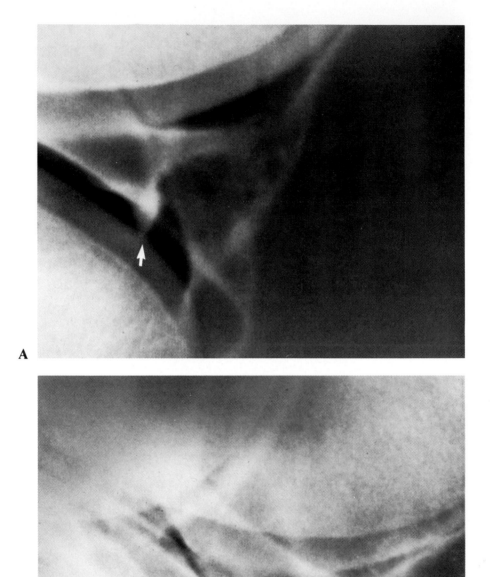

Figure 21
A, B. Arthrograms of two patients show the posterior segment of the lateral meniscus in tangent. The normal inferior attachment defect (arrows) is seen. The superior attachment is thick and intact.

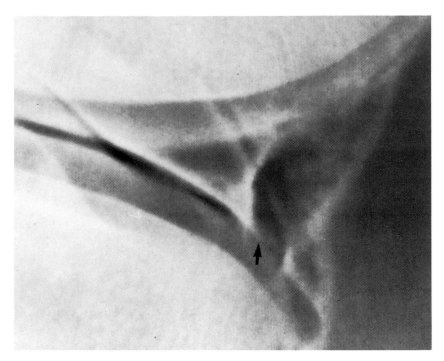

Figure 22
On an arthrogram of the posterior segment of the lateral meniscus, the normal defect in the inferior attachment is apparent (arrow). For technical reasons, the intact superior attachment is not seen as well as in Figure 21 and should not be mistaken for a complete detachment of the lateral meniscus.

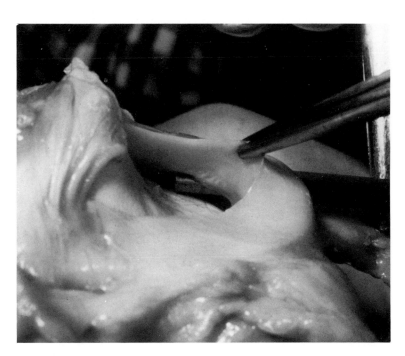

Figure 23
A probe has been inserted into the popliteus tendon sleeve and can be seen through the inferior attachment defect of the posterior portion of the lateral meniscus, which is raised by a forceps.

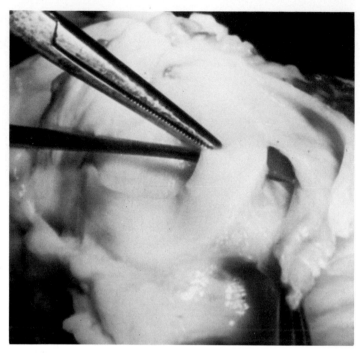

Figure 24
In the specimen of a child's knee, a probe inserted under the posterior segment of the lateral meniscus extends through the normal inferior attachment defect into the popliteal bursa. The tip of the probe in the popliteal bursa is seen from above. The proximity of the superior and inferior attachment defects is apparent.

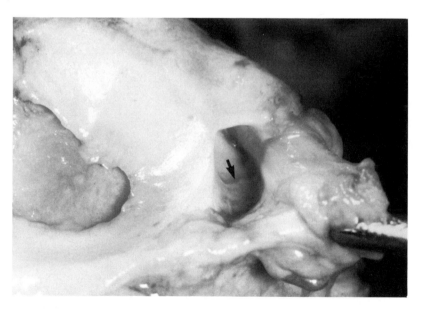

Figure 25
Looking into the popliteal bursa, from above and anteriorly, the margin of the inferior attachment defect is visualized (arrow). A clamp holds the popliteus tendon to the side for better visualization. The proximity of the superior and inferior attachment defects is apparent.

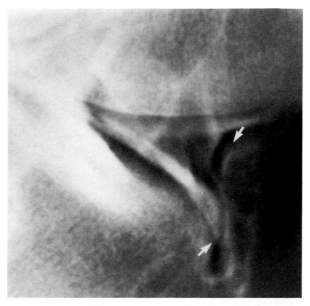

A

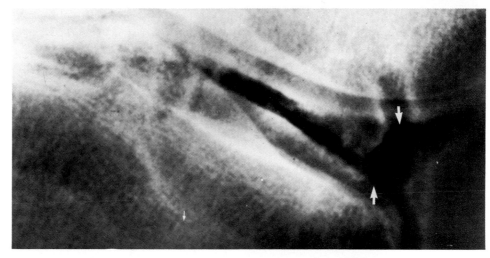

B

Figure 26
A, B. Because of the proximity of the superior and inferior attachment defects, an arthrogram with the beam tangential to the posterior portion of the lateral meniscus may show both defects (arrows) on a single projection. This must not be misinterpreted as a lateral tear or detachment of the posterior portion of the lateral meniscus. Projections in front of this region will show the superior attachment defect with the inferior attachment intact. **C.** A projection posterior to this region shows the intact superior attachment (black arrow) with an inferior attachment defect (white arrow).

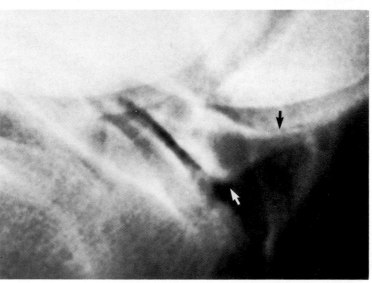

C

A

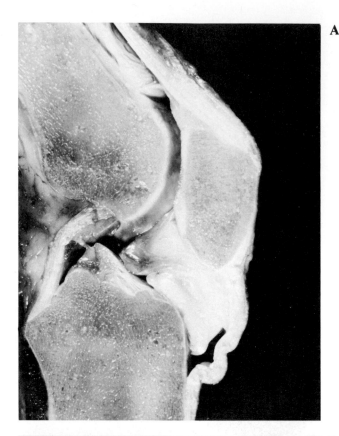

B

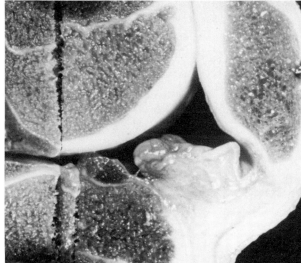

Figure 27
Sagittal anatomic sections through the knees of (**A**) an adult and (**B**) a child show the intra-articular, extrasynovial fat pad. The irregular lobulated contour of the fat pad overlies the anterior portion of the menisci.

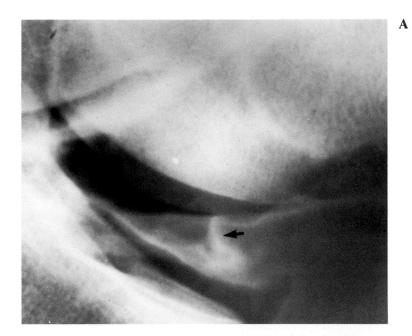

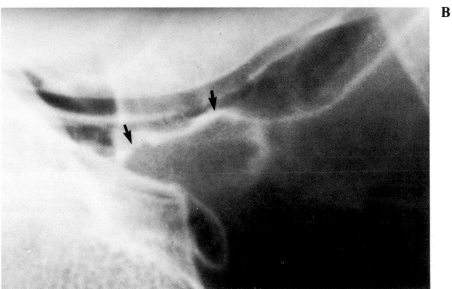

Figure 28
The contrast-coated lobulated margins of the fat pad are projected through the anterior segment of the lateral meniscus.

A. The contour of the lateral meniscus is normal. The irregular radiopaque line (arrow) representing the contrast-coated fat pad is projected through the meniscus and should not be mistaken for a meniscal tear.

B. The lobulated contour of the fat pad (arrows) is superimposed on the articular surface of the lateral meniscus. The inner margin of the lateral meniscus is apparent. Other arthrographic projections of this area made with the knee flexed, extended, or slightly rotated shifts the lobulated margin of the fat pad and allows adequate evaluation of the meniscus.

4

Meniscal Abnormalities

Robert H. Freiberger

TEARS

A meniscal tear is a disruption or a fracture that splits the meniscal cartilage into two or more parts. The double contrast arthrogram is particularly suitable for detection of meniscal tears since the surface of the meniscus and the edges of the tear are coated by a thin layer of positive contrast agent and shadowed by air, permitting visualization of fine detail. Tears can be vertical, oblique, horizontal, or radial, or they can be complex, combining several compontents (Fig. 1). The configuration of the tear on the double contrast arthrogram depends on the degree of separation of fragments which is, in turn, influenced by the amount of distraction applied to the knee.

The vertical concentric tear splits the meniscus into an inner and outer portion (Figs. 1A–C, 2, 3). If the anterior and posterior portions of the inner fragment remain attached to the outer fragment it is called a bucket handle tear (Figs. 1A–C). One or both ends of the inner fragment may be detached from the outer fragment. If the fragments remain in close apposition at the time of arthrography, positive contrast agent seeps into the tear. When the tear curves, following the shape of the meniscus, a tangential beam traverses the radiopaque contrast agent and produces a roentgenogram showing opacification of the inner fragment (Fig. 2).

With separation of the fragments, the edges of the tear become coated by positive contrast agent and shadowed by a small amount of air in the gap between the fragments (Figs. 3, 6, 8–10). Occasionally the inner fragment displaces completely into the intercondylar notch and either cannot be seen or is seen very indistinctly on the arthrogram. The diagnosis of tear is then made by appreciating the deformity of the peripheral fragment of the meniscus, which is short with an irregular, often blunted or squared-off inner contour (Figs. 7, 8).

If the tear is oblique and the inner fragment is displaced, the tear can be difficult to detect because the wedge shape of the meniscus is maintained. The tear is recognized by noting that the meniscus is less wide than normal (Figs. 10, 11).

A slightly different type vertical tear occurs at the inner margin of the meniscus (Fig. 12). It produces a small attached cartilage fragment (Figs. 12A, C). When the fragments of the tear are close together, a small area of opacification of the inner meniscal wedge appears on the arthrogram (Fig. 12B). If the fragments are separated, the abnormal contour of the apex of the meniscus is apparent. The inner fragment, separated from the main portion of the meniscus by a short, curved vertical tear, resembles the curved beak of a parrot and is known as a parrot beak tear. Although small, these tears can produce symptoms of intermittent locking because the small fragment slides in and out of the space between the articular surfaces of the femoral and tibial condyles.

A vertical radial tear is roughly at right angles to the tangent of the meniscus (Figs. 13A, B). A roentgenogram tangent to the tear shows opacification of the inner portion of the meniscus because positive contrast agent has been trapped in the tear (Fig. 13C). Radial tears can be produced during menisectomy if the surgeon pulls hard on the clamp attached to the anterior horn of the meniscus. By examining the edges of the tear of the excised specimen, it is possible to tell whether the meniscus was torn prior to or during the surgical procedure. Horizontal tears are clefts extending into the meniscus either from the superior or inferior articular surface or occasionally from the apex of the meniscus, splitting it into superior or inferior portions (Figs. 14–17). These tears are often caused by degenerative changes in the meniscus and may be associated with osteoarthritic changes in the knee or may be seen in conjunction with meniscal cysts. (Figs. 34–37.)

Complex tears are analagous to comminuted fractures (Figs. 18–21). Tears within the meniscus have different orientations, in part vertical, oblique, and horizontal. Fragments of cartilage may be completely torn from the major fragment and be loose within the knee joint. At times the meniscus is deformed, but the type of tear cannot be determined by arthrogram (Fig. 22).

Tears of the meniscal cartilages are uncommon in children except when an abnormally formed meniscus, a discoid lateral meniscus, is present. When a child presents with symptoms of internal derangement of the knee, it is advisable to begin the arthrogram with an examination of the lateral meniscus (Figs. 25–32).

An arthrographic finding that can indicate a small meniscal tear, is incomplete contrast filling of the space between the undersurface of the meniscus and the articular surface of the tibial plateau (Fig. 23A). This space normally fills to the peripheral attachment of the meniscus. When fluoroscopic observation during the arthrogram, or review of films immediately following it, indicates that the periphery of the space between the meniscus and the tibial plateau is *not* filled with contrast agent, the arthrographic examination must be continued. The patient should exercise the knee for a minute or two, and a second set of roentgenograms should be made with a special effort to obtain maximal distraction on the involved side of the knee. It is then often possible to demonstrate a small tear on the undersurface of the meniscus in the area where there was lack of contrast filling (Fig. 23B). Unfortunately, a tear cannot always be seen on the delayed postexercise examination. In that case, the arthrographic report should mention the lack of filling, describing it as an

abnormality. Diagnosis of a meniscal tear cannot be made unless a tear is actually visualized.

The cause of lack of opacification at the undersurface of the meniscus is not fully understood. The space may be filled with tenacious synovial fluid that is trapped in the region of the tear and prevents the spread of contrast agent at the initial examination. It is also possible that inflammatory adhesions between the periphery of the meniscus and the tibial plateau prevent filling of the periphery of the inframeniscal space, persisting even after exercise.

An arthrographic finding indicating an abnormality of the meniscus but applicable only to the posterior segment of the lateral meniscus is the compression of the popliteal tendon sleeve (Figs. 19–22). The popliteal tendon sleeve is normally rectangular to oval on its tangential projection. Its surfaces are coated with positive contrast agent, and its lumen is filled with air (Fig. 18). When the popliteal tendon sleeve is reduced to a narrow slit—particularly when its contrast-filled margins are bowed posterolaterally—an abnormality, usually a tear of the lateral meniscus, should be suspected. A meticulous re-examination of the posterior segment of the lateral meniscus after a period of exercise may reveal the tear. If a tear cannot be demonstrated, the abnormality should be described on the arthrogram report, even though the etiology of the finding is not fully established.

When it is possible to classify a tear as vertical, horizontal, or radial, it should be done on the arthrogram report; however, the precise description of a tear that is seen only on tangential views is not always possible since many are complex in their configuration. The description of the type of tear is less important than an accurate description of the location of the tear. That a tear is located in the far posterior segment of the meniscus (Figs. 24A, B) can be of considerable importance to the surgeon, since a posterior approach or second posterior incision may be necessary to insure complete excision of the torn portion of the meniscus.

The criteria described for the arthrographic diagnosis of meniscal tears apply to the medial as well as lateral meniscus. When applied to the lateral meniscus, certain anatomic features must be kept in mind to avoid an erroneous diagnosis of tear. Because of the popliteal tendon sheath, which partially separates the posterior aspect of the lateral meniscus from the capsule, it is normal to see contrast agent at the periphery of this segment of the meniscus. If contrast agent is seen at the periphery of the medial meniscus it is always an indication of a tear. The projection of a thin, wavy, horizontal line of positive contrast agent overlying the tangential projection of the meniscus must not be mistaken for a horizontal tear. This normal finding, described in Chapter 3, represents positive contrast agent trapped in the meniscal attachment fold. These wavy radiopaque lines always end peripherally at the apex of the synovial attachment fold, which differentiates them from horizontal tears. Other dense lines of positive contrast are seen in the anterior segment of the menisci, usually the lateral, due to superimposition of the positive contrast-coated synovial surface of the fat pad over the meniscus. These lines change their position relative to the meniscus when the knee is flexed and extended and thus can be differentiated from tears by fluoroscopic observation and on spot films.

When there is considerable laxity of the ligamentous structures of the knee and the articular surfaces can be widely separated by distraction, a segment of the meniscus anterior or posterior to the area seen in tangent will become visible (Fig. 32). This segment appears somewhat rectangular, representing an *en face* projection of the meniscus shadowed by air superiorly as well as inferiorly. On careful examination of the arthrogram, it will be noted that the superior and inferior surfaces of this apparent fragment are continuous with the superior and inferior peripheral margins of the meniscus, a feature which differentiates it from a separated fragment.

THE POSTMENISCECTOMY ARTHROGRAM

The postmeniscectomy arthrogram can present problems in interpretation. Usually the anterior and midportion of the meniscus is completely excised and a portion of the posterior horn is left. The retained posterior portion of the meniscus is normally smooth, and when intact, is not clinically significant. Occasionally a tear in the retained posterior fragment can be demonstrated (Fig. 24), but whether it is an unexcised torn fragment or a new tear cannot be determined arthrographically.

DISCOID MENISCUS

A discoid meniscus, as the name implies, is either completely or partially disk-shaped rather than crescent-shaped (Fig. 25). It interposes itself between the articular cartilages of the femoral and tibial condyles whose central portions are normally in contact. Discoid menisci are commonly torn because their abnormal shape subjects them to excessive stresses. The discoid deformity is fairly common in the lateral meniscus (Figs. 25–30) but rare in the medial meniscus (Fig. 31). The origin of the discoid meniscus is disputed. Some believe that it is a congenital abnormality, but others believe that it develops because the posterior peripheral attachments of the meniscus are abnormal.

Some discoid menisci never give a person significant clinical symptoms, however, the majority produce symptoms in childhood. Since tears of normal menisci are very rare in children under the age of 10, it is reasonable to assume that a child with signs and symptoms of internal derangement of the knee has a discoid or torn discoid lateral meniscus. For this reason, when performing an arthrogram on a child, the lateral side of the knee is examined first, whereas in an older patient, unless there are definite localizing symptoms, the examination begins with the medial meniscus.

On the arthrogram a discoid meniscus appears abnormally wide and lacks a normal sharp inner edge. It is very thick, particularly in its posterior portion. The interposition of a discoid meniscus between the articular condyles can be confirmed by compressing the affected side instead of distracting it, showing that the articular surfaces are separated by the width of the meniscus.

Tears of a discoid meniscus can present difficulties for arthrographic interpretation. If the inner fragment of a discoid or partially discoid meniscus is displaced, the abnormal width of the meniscus may not be appreciated and a diagnosis of torn meniscus, rather than torn *discoid* meniscus can be made (Figs. 29, 30). Conversely, if the tear cannot be seen clearly, but the discoid shape of the meniscus is appreciated, only a diagnosis of discoid meniscus may be made from the arthrogram (Fig. 26). The decision to excise a discoid or torn discoid lateral meniscus depends primarily on the patient's symptoms.

In a knee with lax ligaments where articular surfaces can be widely distracted, the menisci are often seen *en face*. The rectangular projection of the meniscal cartilage should not be mistaken for a discoid meniscus (Fig. 32). Usually the triangular vertical section of the meniscus can be identified to prove that it is not a discoid meniscus.

MENISCAL CYSTS

A meniscal cyst is a ganglion-like cystic lesion located at the periphery of the meniscus (Fig. 33). It is often palpable on clinical examination and may be visible as a subcutaneous soft tissue mass on conventional roentgenograms if the radiographic beam falls tangential to the location of the cyst. The lesion commonly occurs in the anterior half of the lateral meniscus, and is rare in the medial meniscus where it tends to be located in the posterior portion.

Meniscal cysts can often be diagnosed by arthrography because they are associated with degenerative horizontal tears extending from the cyst cavity to one of the articular surfaces of the meniscus. The characteristic arthrographic appearance is opacification of the tear, with the tear extending beyond the margin of the tibial plateau. Contrast agent partially opacifies the peripherally located cyst (Figs. 34–37). The initial arthrographic pictures may show the horizontal tear but not the opacification of the cyst. When such tears are encountered, particularly when located in the anterior portion of the lateral meniscus, or when a cyst of the meniscus is suspected, a second or third set of roentgenograms should be made. After the arthrographic study of the knee has been completed for the first time, and the films are reviewed, the patient should be asked to walk and exercise the knee. A second set of films should then be taken in the area of the tear. Following exercise, extension of contrast agent into the cyst is often demonstrated. When no tear is present, or when the tear is present but contrast agent does not extend beyond the periphery of the tibial plateau, the diagnosis of cystic lateral meniscus cannot be made with certainty by the arthrogram.

MENISCAL OSSICLES

Small ossicles can occasionally be seen within the substance of the meniscus. These ossicles are visible on routine roentgenograms but their intrameniscal location is confirmed by an arthrogram (Figs. 38, 39). A meniscal ossicle may or may not be associated with a tear of the meniscus.

These ossicles occur in the menisci of rodents and therefore there is the possibility that they represent a normal variant in humans. However there is also evidence to suggest that they represent heterotopic bone formation caused by trauma.

CALCIFICATIONS OF THE MENISCI

Calcifications within the menisci are common in older persons, and the condition is known as chondrocalcinosis. These calcifications can be seen on routine radiographs (Fig. 40A), and they may occasionally be associated with calcification within the articular cartilages of the tibia and femoral condyles and other joints. The clinical significance of most calcifications is uncertain except where there is a clear clinical picture of the pseudogout syndrome. Rarely, metabolic systemic disease such as hyperparathyroidism or hemochromatosis and other still rarer conditions can cause cartilage calcifications.

If a patient has calcified menisci, it does not preclude the possibility of a coexisting tear of the meniscus or a cruciate ligament injury. When clinical evidence of internal derangement is present an arthrogram may be indicated. However, the calcifications, which are most often in a horizontal location, can interfere with the evaluation of the arthrogram, particularly in discerning a horizontal meniscal tear without displacement of the fragments (Fig. 40B). The calcifications pose no special problems in the diagnosis of vertical tears or horizontal tears with displaced fragments.

PITFALLS

In the normal knee contrast agent in the peripheral attachment folds of the menisci can produce wavy, horizontal lines—choppy sea signs—which can be mistaken for horizontal tears. These radiopaque lines always touch the apex of the recess, when seen tangentially (Chap. 3, Figs. 7, 8).

The contrast-coated synovial surface of the fat pad may be superimposed upon the anterior portion of the meniscus, usually the lateral, causing a misdiagnosis of meniscus tear (Chap. 3, Figs. 27, 28).

Variations exist in the very far posteroinferior attachment of the lateral meniscus and a defect at this site is not clinically significant (Chap. 3, Figs. 21A, B).

Calcifications in the menisci (chondrocalcinosis), seen as radiopaque horizontal streaks, can mimic a horizontal tear. Therefore, always carefully examine the routine films for these calcifications.

One or two very small radiopaque dots can often be seen superimposed upon the anterior portion of the meniscus, usually the lateral. The dots tend to turn to streaks as the more mid portion of the meniscus is tangential to the beam. This finding is of no known clinical significance, and the dots and streaks most probably represent opacified vessels, probably lymphatics (Chap. 3, Fig. 11A). They should not be mistaken for meniscal cysts.

Loosely attached menisci can be seen *en face* and must not be mistaken for either discoid menisci or torn menisci with displaced fragments (Fig. 32).

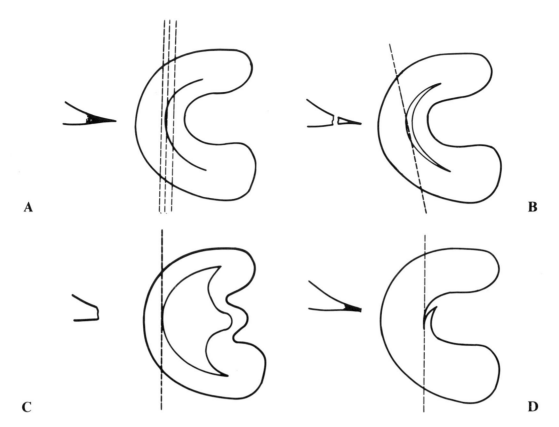

Figure 1
A. A vertical concentric tear splits the meniscus into an inner and outer fragment. When fragments remain in close apposition, positive contrast agent but not air enters the tear. In tangential projection, the inner portion of the meniscus appears denser than the outer portion because the X-ray beam (dotted lines) traverses the contrast agent-filled tear.
B. When the fragments of a vertical concentric tear are slightly separated, the edges of the tear are enhanced by positive contrast agent and the space between the fragments fills with air.
C. When the fragments of a vertical concentric tear are widely separated (bucket handle tear), the inner fragment may be displaced into the intercondylar notch and not seen on the arthrogram. The diagnosis of tear is made by recognizing the absence of the normally sharp inner wedge of the meniscus.
D. A small flap-like tear on the inner margin of the meniscus (parrot beak tear) traps positive contrast agent, and the inner wedge of the meniscus is opacified. The arthrographic appearance is similar to a vertical radial tear.

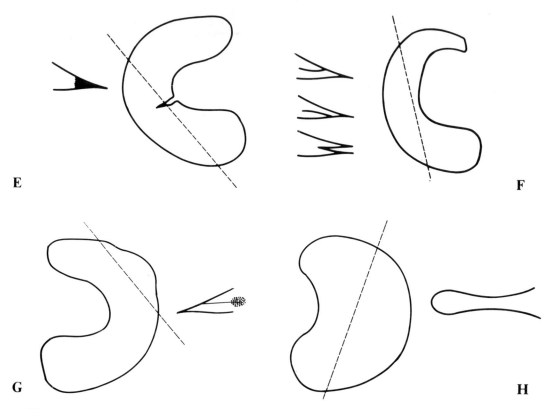

Figure 1

E. A vertical radial tear traps positive contrast agent and the inner portion of the meniscus is opacified.

F. Horizontal tears can extend into the meniscus from its superior or inferior surface or from the apex.

G. The bulge on the periphery of the meniscus represents the ganglion-like cyst of a cystic meniscus. It is often associated with a horizontal tear. When there is a tear, the peripheral cyst may partially opacify, particularly on exposures made after exercise. Cysts are common in the lateral meniscus but rare in the medial meniscus.

H. A discoid meniscus is completely or partially disk-shaped. It lacks the large central hole of the normal meniscus and is susceptible to tears. On tangential projection, a discoid meniscus is wide and lacks the normal wedge shape. The condition affects the lateral meniscus almost exclusively.

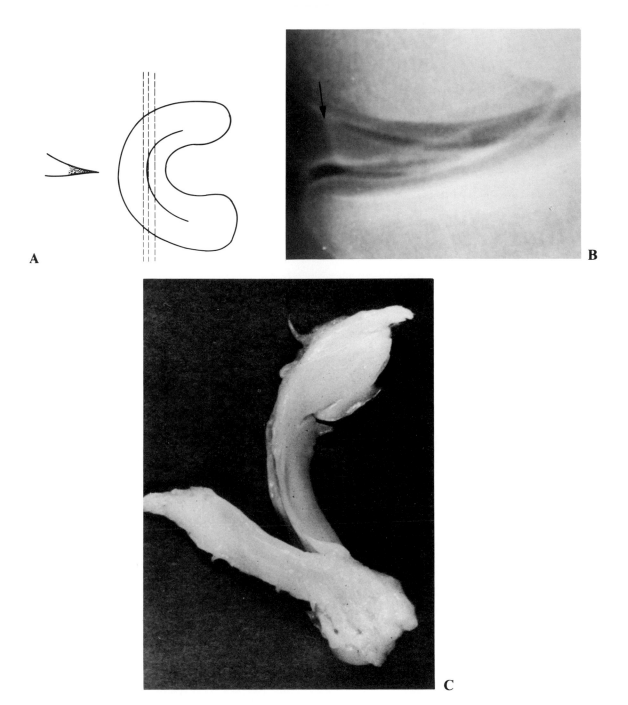

Figure 2
A. A line drawing shows a vertical concentric tear with the fragments in close apposition. The tangential X-ray beam (dotted lines) passes through the opacified tear, and on the vertical cross section the inner fragment is more opaque than the outer fragment.
B. The inner two-thirds of the meniscus appear moderately opaque because the X-ray beam passes through contrast agent trapped in a vertical tear (arrow) with fragments in close apposition.
C. The excised torn meniscus is shown with the fragments separated.

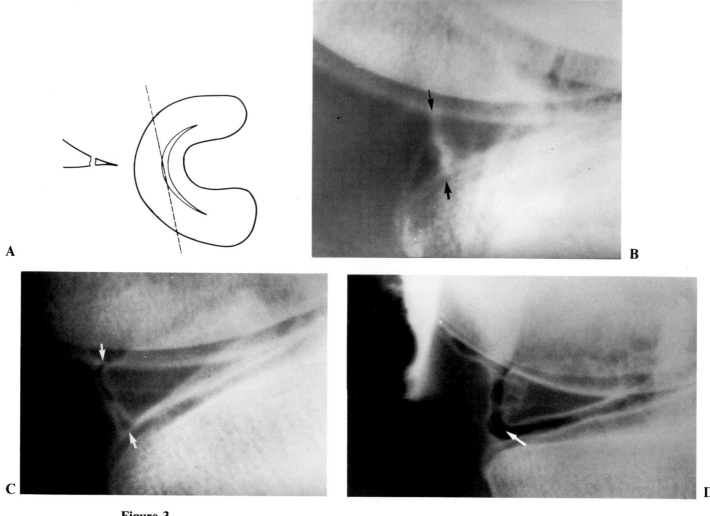

Figure 3
A. A drawing illustrates a vertical concentric tear with separated fragments.
B. Far posteriorly, the fragments of a vertical tear are close together and a layer of positive contrast agent is seen between them (arrows).
C. In a more anterior view, the fragments are slightly separated. The surfaces of the tear (arrows) are coated by positive contrast agent and separated by air.
D. In a still more anterior projection with greater distraction of the joint surfaces, separation of the fragments has increased (arrow).

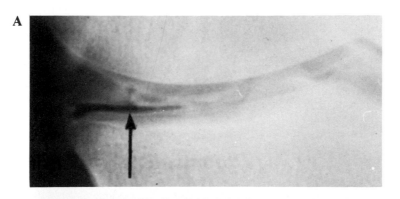

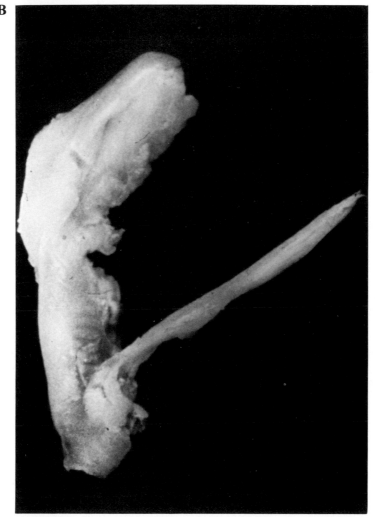

Figure 4
A. The arthrogram shows the slightly separated fragments of a vertical tear (arrow). The irregular margins of the tear are opacified by positive contrast agent. There is a small amount of air between the fragments.
B. On the excised meniscus, the fragments are separated more widely than they were at the time of arthrography.

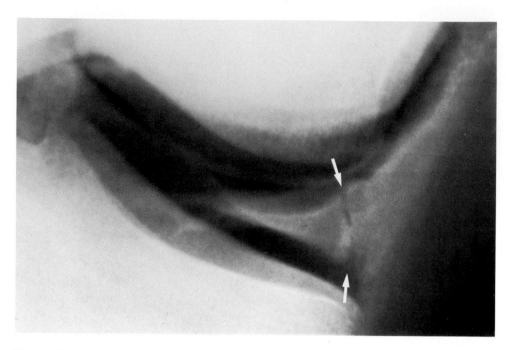

Figure 5

A vertical tear in the lateral meniscus anterior to the popliteus tendon is demonstrated (arrows). The lateral meniscus has a complete but lax peripheral capsular attachment.

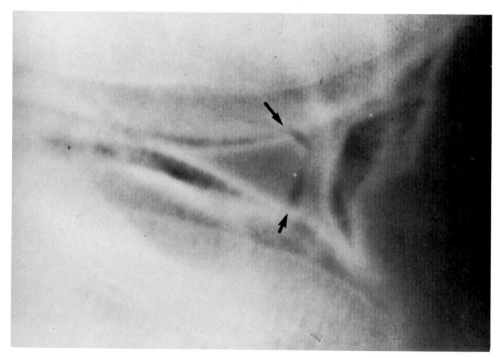

Figure 6

A vertical tear with slight separation of fragments is medial to the popliteal tendon bursa. The surfaces of the tear are coated by positive contrast agent and the space between the fragments is filled with air. The tear (arrows) is easily distinguished from the air-filled popliteus bursa.

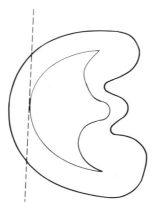

A

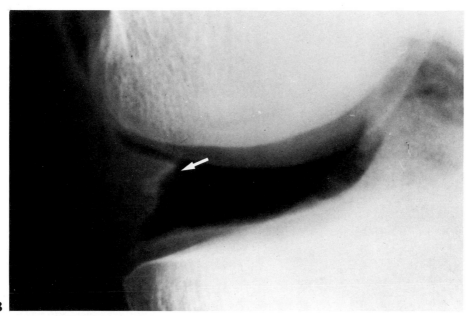

B

Figure 7
A. A line drawing of a vertical concentric (bucket handle) tear demonstrates the wide displacement of the inner fragment.
B. On the arthrogram, the meniscus is abnormally narrow and its inner margin is deformed (arrow). The normally sharp inner wedge is absent, an indication that the inner fragment has displaced into the intercondylar notch.

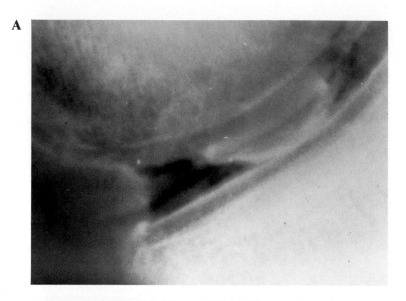

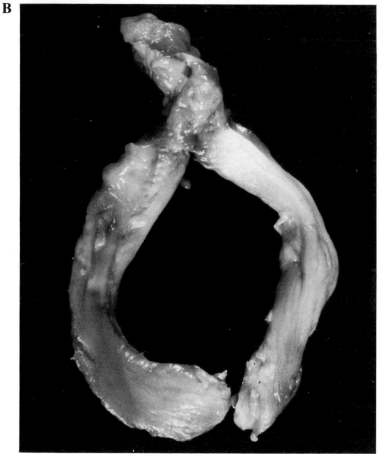

Figure 8
A. An irregular vertical tear is present with considerable separation of fragments. The inner fragment is interposed between the articular surfaces. The outer fragment is narrow and has a blunt rounded inner margin. Positive contrast agent seeping into the irregular surface of the tear produces a thick, slightly irregular zone of opacification.
B. The excised specimen shows the extensive tear and massive inner fragment.

A

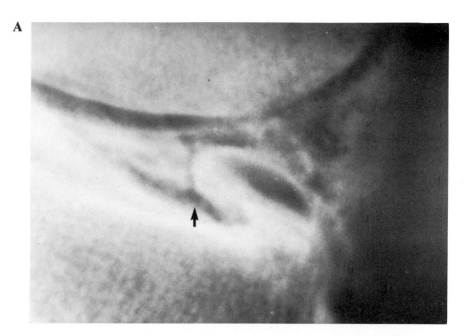

B

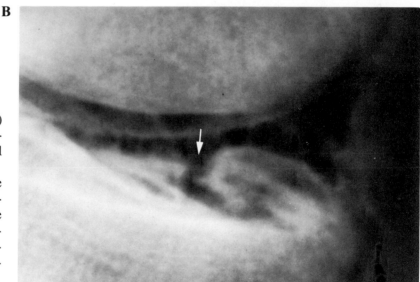

Figure 9
A. A vertical tear (arrow) splits the midportion of the lateral meniscus with minimal separation of fragments.
B. Greater separation of the fragments (arrow) was obtained by manipulating the knee during fluoroscopic observation and taking appropriate spot films. Note the distortion of the popliteal bursa.

Figure 10
An oblique tear (arrows) slightly separates the meniscal fragments. If the inner fragments were displaced further into the intercondylar notch, the tear would be difficult to recognize since the visible outer fragment appears narrow but has not lost the wedge shape of a normal meniscus.

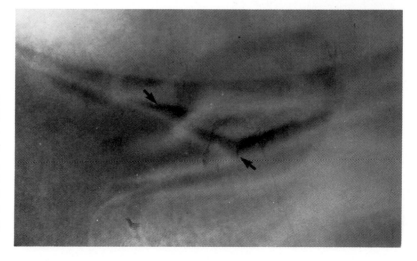

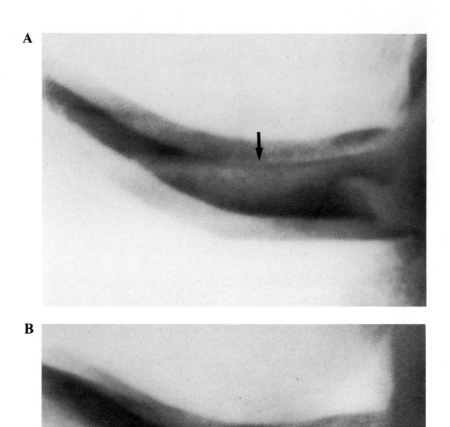

Figure 11
A, B. The midportion of the lateral meniscus is abnormally narrow and its inner edge, although wedge-shaped, is deformed. A fragment of meniscus (arrows) that is displaced medially can be identified.

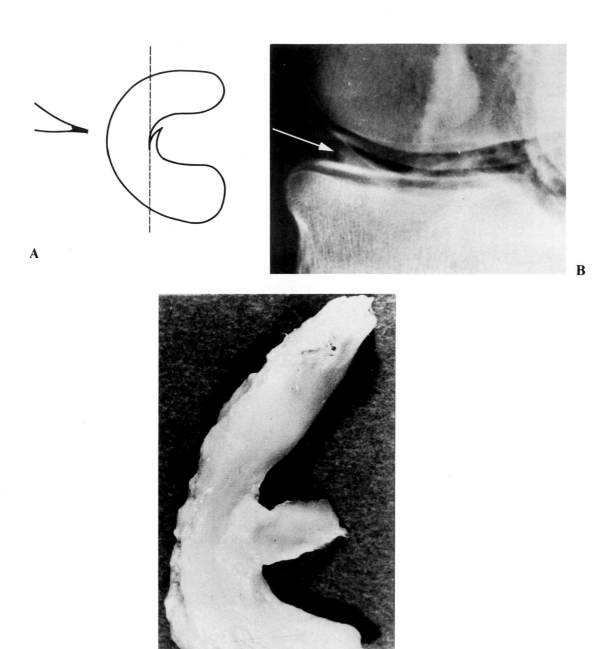

A

B

C

Figure 12
A. A drawing shows a parrot beak tear seen from above, and the opacification of the apex of the meniscus seen by arthrography. The small vertical or oblique tear at the apex of the meniscus resembles the beak of a parrot.
B. The arthrogram shows opacification of the inner half of the medial meniscus (arrow) because positive contrast agent is trapped between the fragments of the tear, permitting the diagnosis of a torn meniscus. However, the type of tear cannot be accurately determined.
C. The excised meniscus demonstrates a small, flap-like parrot beak tear on the inner margin of the medial meniscus.

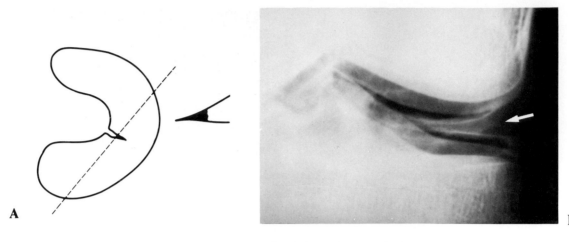

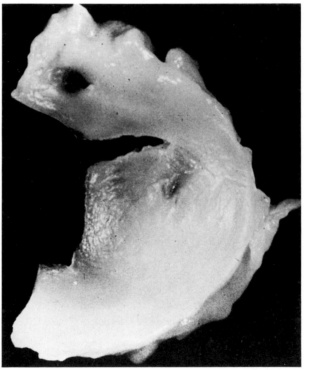

Figure 13
A. A line drawing shows a vertical radial meniscus tear with opacification of the apex of the meniscus.
B. The lateral meniscus of an 18-year-old male is wedge-shaped but unusually wide. Opacification of the inner aspect (arrow) indicates a tear.
C. The excised meniscus shows its abnormal width and its partially discoid shape. A vertical radial tear is present.

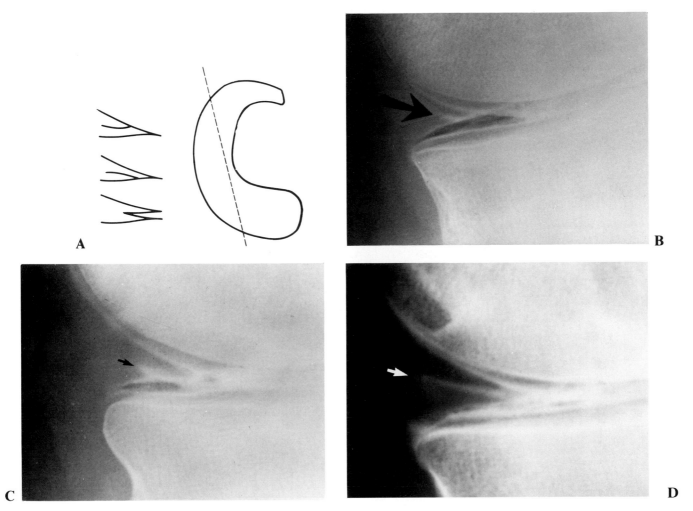

Figure 14
A. The line drawing shows horizontal tears extending into the meniscus from its superior surface, inferior surface, and apex.
B-D. Arthrograms of medial menisci with horizontal tears (arrows).

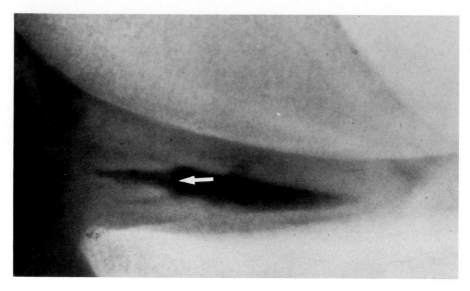

Figure 15
A horizontal tear (arrow) is far posterior in the medial meniscus. The degree of
overlap of the femoral condyles indicates the posterior location.

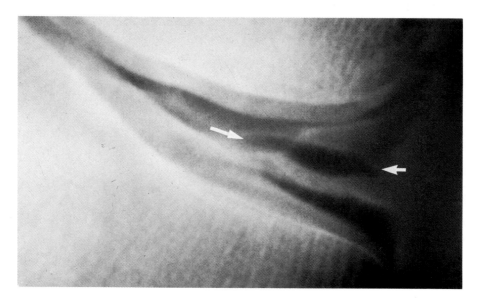

Figure 16
A horizontal tear with slight separation of fragments (arrows) of the anterior segment
of a lateral meniscus.

A

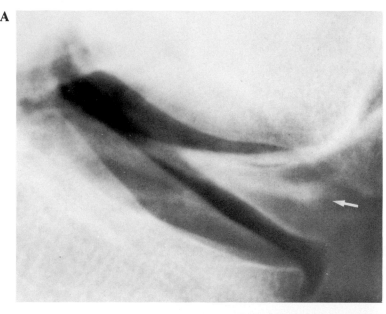

C

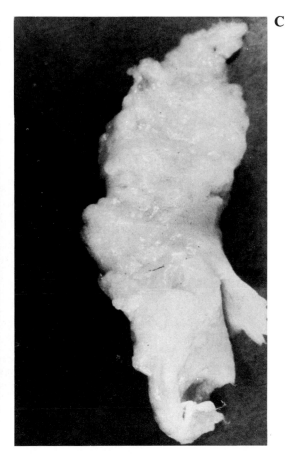

B

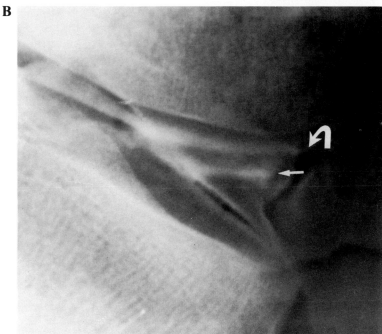

Figure 17
A. A horizontal tear (arrow) with its fragments in close apposition bisects the anterior portion of the lateral meniscus.
B. The same extensive tear (arrow) is seen in the projection of the posterior portion of the lateral meniscus (note the popliteus tendon sleeve). The X-ray beam is tangential to the superior attachment defect forming the opening of the popliteal bursa. The absence of the superior meniscal attachment (curved arrow) is normal and is not indicative of a tear.
C. A specimen of a lateral meniscus has been photographed to show the horizontal tear on its inferior surface.

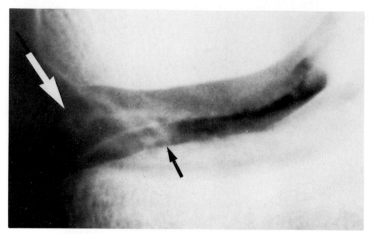

A

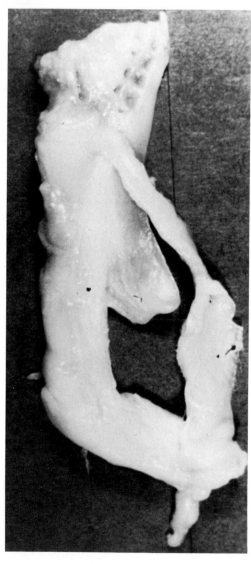

B

Figure 18
A. A complex tear of the medial meniscus shows deformity of the contours of the meniscus and streaks of contrast agent within it (arrow). Although a tear is indicated, its exact configuration is not apparent from the arthrogram.
B. The excised meniscus shows a complex tear with vertical, oblique, and horizontal components.

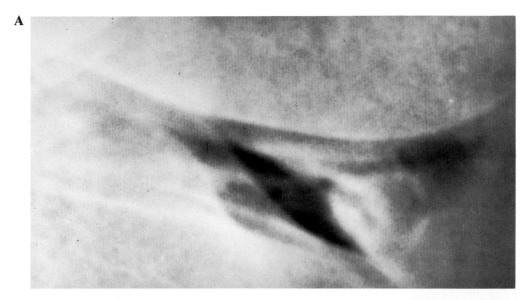

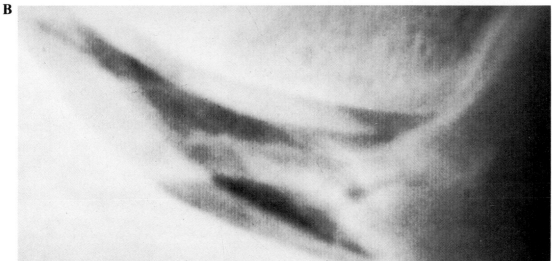

Figure 19

A complex tear having vertical, oblique, and horizontal fissures in the posterolateral portion of the lateral meniscus is shown in two projections.

A. In the posterior segment of the lateral meniscus, the inner fragment is displaced. The inner margin of the outer fragment is deformed and lacks a sharp inner wedge. Opacification of the meniscus indicates the presence of positive contrast agent within a tear; air is seen in a horizontal aspect of the tear. The popliteal bursa is compressed.

B. Slightly more anteriorly, several tears can be seen with less displacement of the inner fragment than posteriorly. On the multiple exposures taken using the fluoroscopic spot film method of examination, tears are seen on more than one projection.

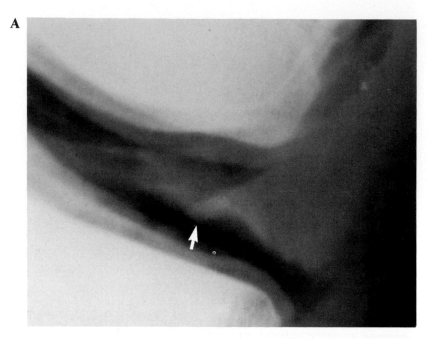

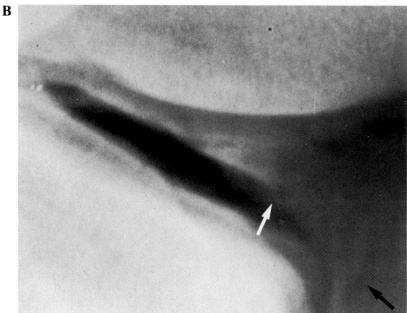

Figure 20
A. The midsegment of the lateral meniscus is abnormally narrow. The inner margin of the meniscus is deformed although the wedge shape is not completely lost (arrow). The inner portion of the meniscus is abnormally dense, indicating that contrast agent has entered the meniscus through a tear.
B. More posteriorly, the opacified inner fragment is slightly separated from the peripheral fragment of the meniscus by a vertical component of a complex tear (white arrow). The popliteus bursa is compressed and barely visible (black arrow).

A 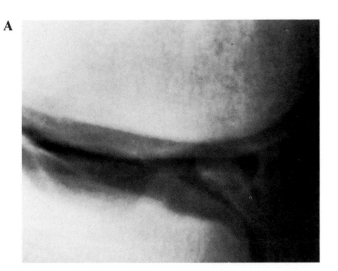 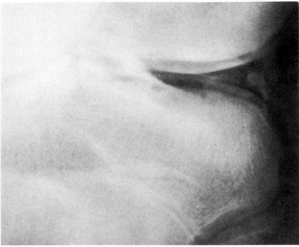 B

Figure 21
A, B. Two slightly different projections show an extensive complex tear of the lateral meniscus of a child. The peripheral fragment is narrow and deformed. The possibility that this is a torn discoid lateral meniscus can neither be confirmed nor excluded by this study since the size of the displaced fragments cannot be evaluated.

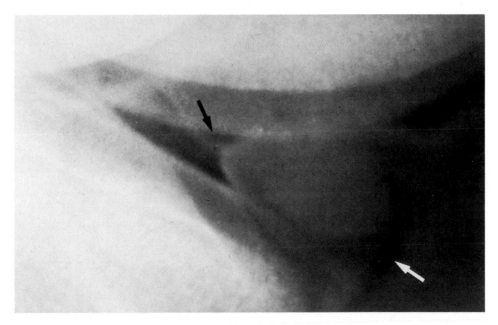

Figure 22
The contour of the posterior portion of the lateral meniscus is grossly abnormal. Its inner wedge is blunted (black arrow) and its peripheral portion thickened. The popliteus tendon sleeve is compressed (white arrow). An old meniscus tear with displacement of fragments and thickening of the meniscus was found at surgery.

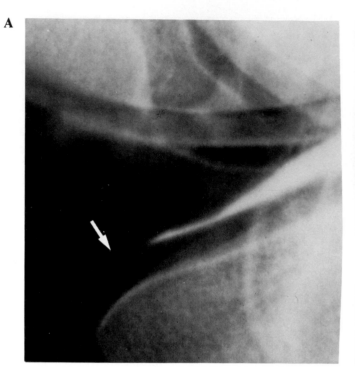
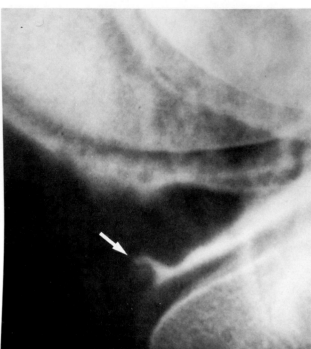

Figure 23
A. Lack of contrast coating at the undersurface of the posterior segment of the medial meniscus (arrow) suggests a tear and indicates the need for a post-exercise examination.
B. An exposure after the patient had walked for a few minutes still shows incomplete filling of the space beneath the meniscus, but a tear extending upward from the undersurface of the meniscus is now opacified (arrow).

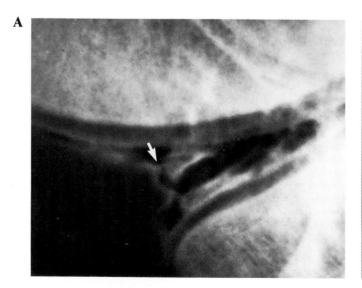
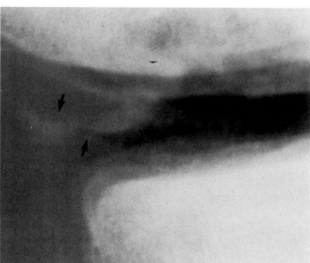

Figure 24
A. On a postmenisectomy arthrogram the posterior horn of the medial meniscus is torn (arrow). It is impossible to determine from the arthrogram whether this is a new tear or whether the torn posterior horn was not excised. A portion of the posterior horn is commonly seen after menisectomy through an anterior incision.
B. An opacified horizontal tear (arrows) can be seen in the irregular residual medial meniscus of a patient who had a medial menisectomy.

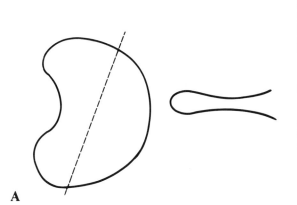

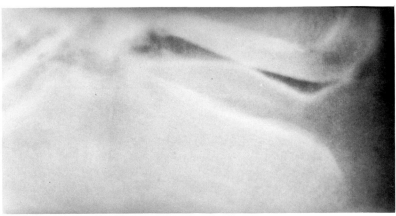

A

B

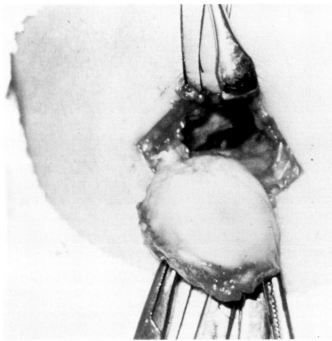

C

Figure 25
A. A line drawing of a discoid lateral meniscus with its arthrographic projection.
B. An arthrogram of the lateral meniscus of a child shows an abnormally wide and thick lateral meniscus.
C. A photograph taken in the operating room shows an excised discoid lateral meniscus of a child's knee.

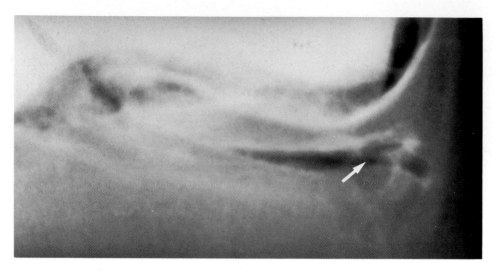

Figure 26
A. A tear (arrow) is seen at the periphery of the undersurface of this abnormally wide meniscus which has the typical arthrographic appearance of a discoid meniscus.

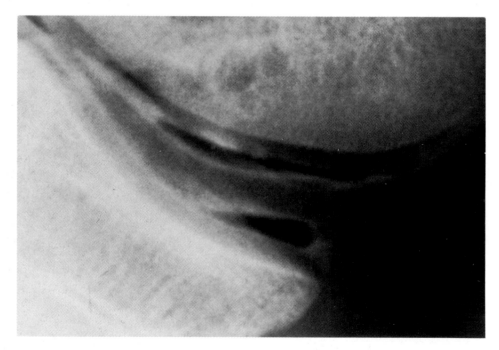

Figure 27
The lateral meniscus of a child's knee is abnormally wide and the normal, sharply wedged, inner margin is not seen. The findings are those of a discoid meniscus.

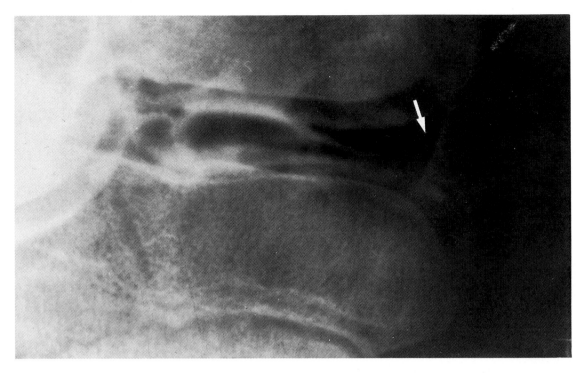

Figure 28
The club-shaped thickening of the posterior horn of a lateral meniscus is typical of a discoid lateral meniscus. A peripheral tear is present (arrow).

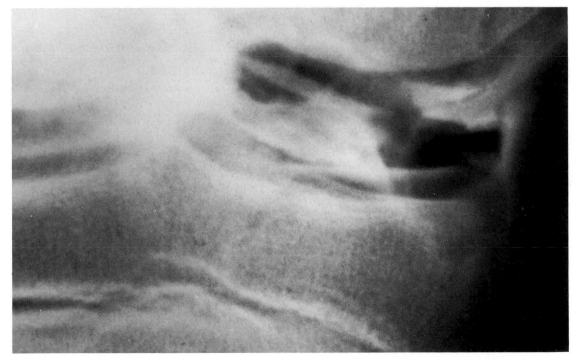

Figure 29
In the torn lateral meniscus of a child, the width of the inner fragment and its abnormal thickness indicates that it is a torn discoid meniscus, which was confirmed at surgery.

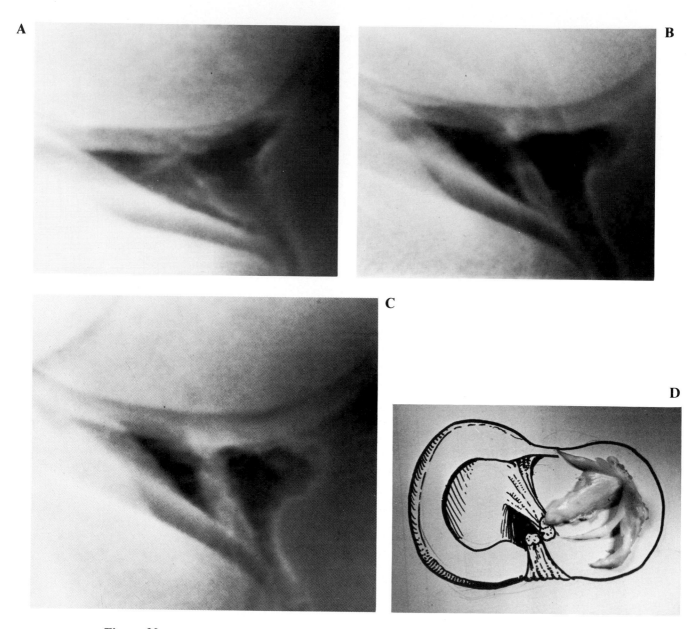

Figure 30
A–C. The arthrogram of a 10-year-old boy shows a markedly distorted, fragmented lateral meniscus on three projections. Since tears of normally-formed menisci are rare in children, the findings suggested a torn discoid lateral meniscus.
D. A photograph of the excised specimen shows a complex tear in a thickened and partially discoid lateral meniscus. (Courtesy of Dr. R. Goldstone)

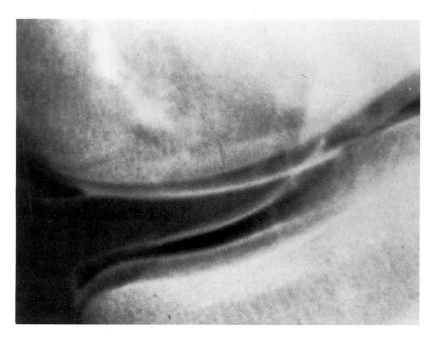

Figure 31
An abnormally wide, partially discoid *medial* meniscus is a very uncommon abnormality.

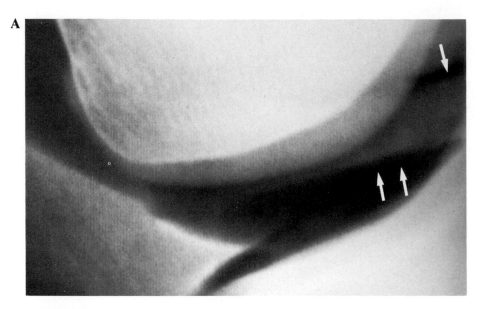

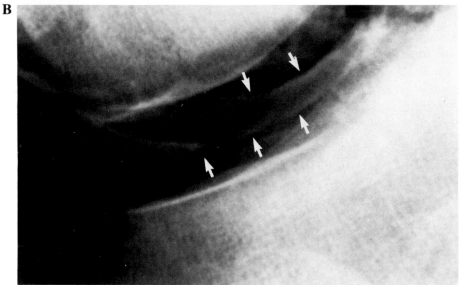

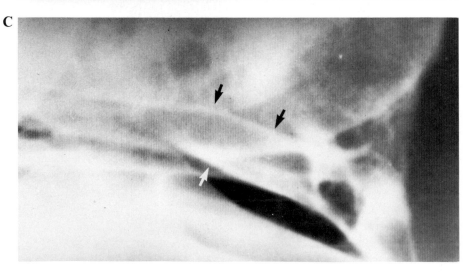

Figure 32
When the knee ligaments are lax and the articular surfaces of the knee can separate widely, the meniscus, shadowed by air, can be seen *en face* (arrows) as well as in triangular vertical section. It occasionally occurs at the medial meniscus (A,B) and, more commonly, because of laxer attachments, at the lateral meniscus (C,D).

D.

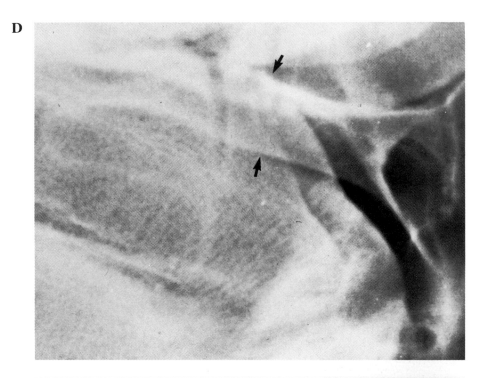

E.

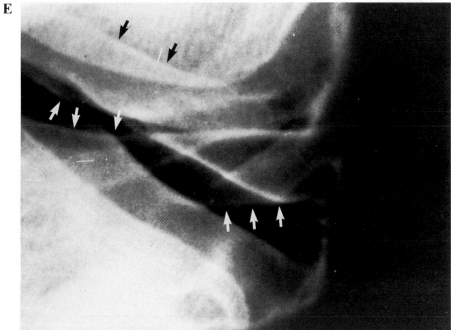

Figure 32
D. The posterior segment of the lateral meniscus is seen *en face* (arrows).
E. Occasionally both the segments anterior (white arrows) and posterior (black arrows) to the tangential projection are seen *en face*. Such ribbon-like *en face* projections of the menisci should not be mistaken for discoid menisci or separated fragments.

A
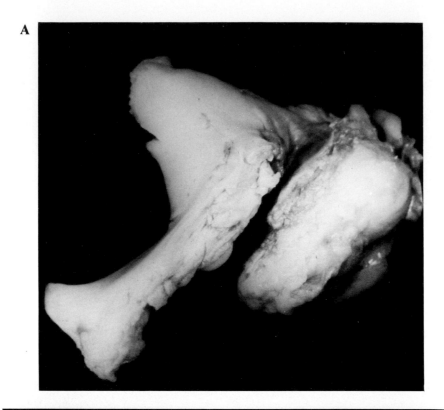

B
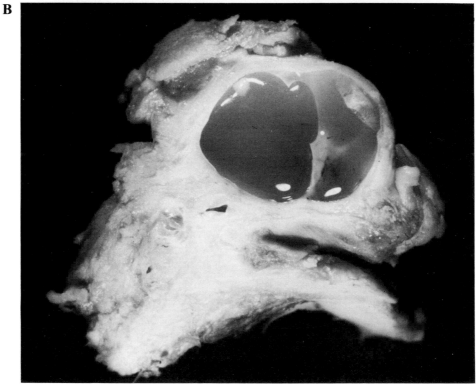

Figure 33
A. An unusually large cyst is located at the periphery of an excised lateral meniscus.
B. The ganglion-like nature of the cyst is evident on the cut specimen. (Courtesy of
Dr. R. L. Patterson.)

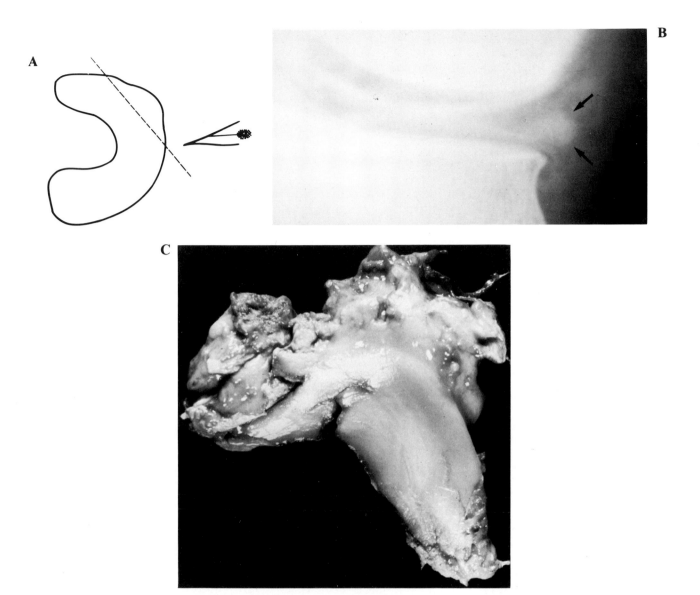

Figure 34
A. A line drawing shows the peripheral contour deformity of the meniscus caused by a cyst. The vertical section shows a horizontal tear extending into the cyst, with the tear and cyst opacified by positive contrast medium.
B. This exposure was made after delay and exercise of the knee, after the initial arthrogram showed a small irregular horizontal tear in the antero-midportion of the lateral meniscus. The opacification of the tear extends into a meniscal cyst, partially opacifying the cyst at the periphery of the lateral meniscus (arrows).
C. The excised meniscus shows the cystic expansion at its periphery.

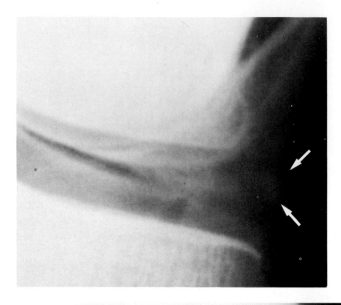

Figure 35
A horizontal tear extends through the antero-midportion of a lateral meniscus. A faintly visible collection of contrast agent on the periphery of the meniscus represents partial opacification of a meniscal cyst (arrows).

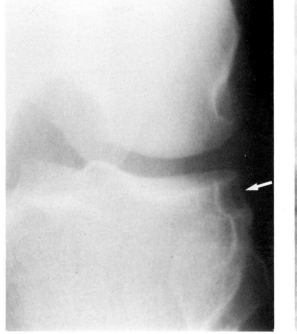

A

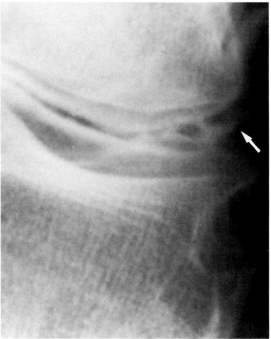

B

Figure 36
A. A pressure erosion on the lateral aspect of the tibial plateau (arrow) plus an overlying soft tissue mass are indicative of a long-term cystic lateral meniscus.
B. The arthrogram demonstrates an irregular, predominantly horizontal tear extending to the periphery of the meniscus (arrow). The cyst opacifies only minimally.

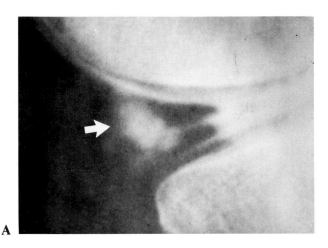

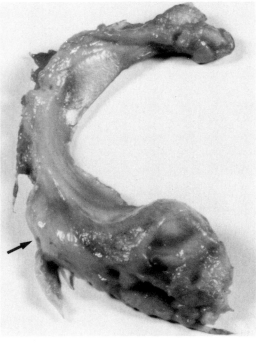

Figure 37
A. The arthrogram shows a torn cystic medial meniscus with positive contrast agent extending into the cyst (arrow) through a horizontal tear.
B. The excised specimen shows the bulge (arrow) caused by the cyst at the periphery of the meniscus. Cysts of the medial meniscus are rare.

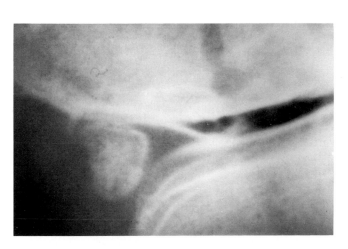

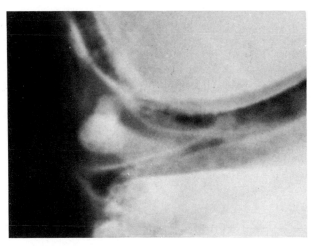

Figure 38
A. An ossicle is apparent within the posterior segment of the medial meniscus.
B. The same ossicle, seen on a more anterior projection, appears elongated since it is no longer tangential to the X-ray beam.

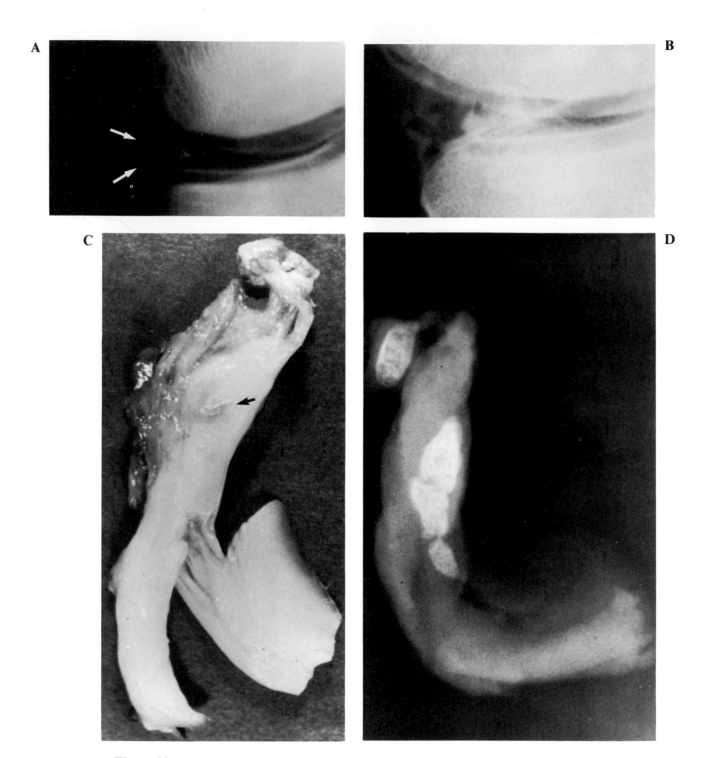

Figure 39
A. An ossification (ossicle) (arrows) within the remaining portion of the medial meniscus of a patient with a history of a menisectomy is visible on the arthrogram.
B. On a more posterior projection, a tear of the meniscus with a very irregular inner margin of the outer fragment is demonstrated.
C. The excised meniscus shows the posterior tear seen on the arthrogram. A depression and roughening of the superior surface of the meniscus anterior to the tear (arrow) is the site of the meniscal ossicles.
D. The ossicles are seen clearly on a roentgenogram of the specimen.

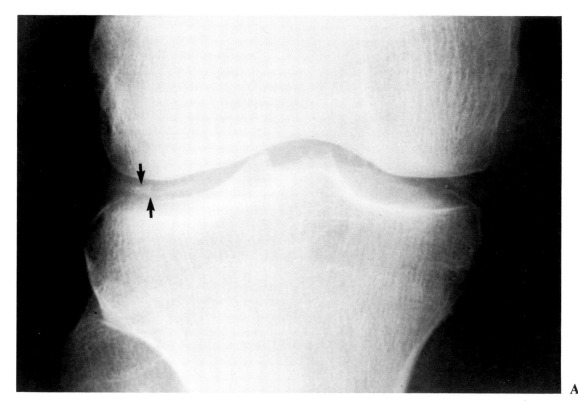

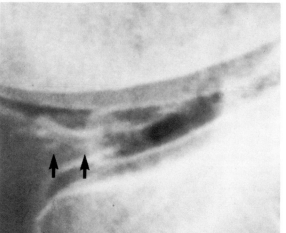

Figure 40
A. Linear radiopaque streaks (arrows) caused by chondrocalcinosis are seen in the meniscus.
B. On the arthrogram these radiopaque streaks of calcium (arrows) can be mistaken for an opaque contrast agent in a horizontal tear.

5

The Cruciate Ligaments

Helene Pavlov

The cruciate ligaments are recognized as the prime stabilizing ligaments of the knee. Isolated tears of the anterior cruciate ligaments occur on occasion, although the majority are associated with meniscal or collateral ligament tears. The cruciate ligaments can be examined with a high degree of accuracy by the double contrast arthrographic method used for evaluation of the menisci. Since the combination of cruciate ligament tears and meniscal tears is common, it is important that the same examination procedure be applicable.

The cruciate ligaments should be examined radiographically twice in each patient: first, using a horizontal X-ray beam with the patient sitting at the edge of the table, and second, using a vertical X-ray or fluoroscopic beam with the patient lying on the side with the knee to be examined on the table. The horizontal beam study is usually done immediately following the intra-articular injection, before the meniscal examination, whereas the vertical beam study is done after the meniscal examination. The diagnostic criteria are identical, but having two different views of the cruciate ligaments available for comparison and evaluation improves diagnostic accuracy (Figs. 2, 4). The demonstration of an intact ligament on just one view is interpreted as normal.

TECHNIQUE

To achieve a technically adequate examination of the cruciate ligaments, it is important to understand and apply the following examination techniques common to both horizonal and vertical beam methods:

1. The anterior cruciate ligament must be tensed, which is accomplished by flexing the knee 60° to 80° from full extension and applying pressure to the posterior aspect of the proximal tibia in an attempt to displace the tibia forward under the femoral condyles.
2. The contour of the posterior cruciate ligament must be delineated. Visualization of the posterior cruciate ligament assures the optimum position for an accurate evaluation of the anterior cruciate ligament.
3. There must be sufficient contrast agent anteriorly to coat the surface of the anterior cruciate ligament, and sufficient distraction of the knee to separate the anterior fat pad from the surface of the anterior cruciate ligament.

The injection procedure described in Chapter 2 is followed. Contrast medium with 0.3cc of a 1:1000 solution of epinephrine is used to delay contrast absorption and to permit longer visualization of sharp contrast edges. The patient should be placed prone after the intra-articular injection to enable the contrast to flow anteriorly within the joint.

The Horizontal Beam Method

Following the injection of contrast and air the cruciate study is begun. A horizontal beam radiograph is taken with the patient sitting at the edge of the X-ray table, with legs hanging over the side. The knee to be examined is closest to the X-ray tube and a grid cassette is placed against the medial aspect of the involved knee. A firm pillow is placed between the edge of the table and the posterior aspect of the proximal calf, to push the tibia anteriorly and to simulate an anterior "drawer maneuver." A chair is placed against the foot to block extension of the knee and increase forward pressure on the upper leg (Figs. 1A, B). With the patient in this position, positive contrast agent pools in the dependent portion of the joint above the tibial plateau and coats the synovial surfaces of the cruciate ligaments. The cruciate ligaments, shadowed by the radiopaque contrast, appear as radiolucent bands (Figs. 2A, B). An intact cruciate ligament presents as a straight contrast-lucent interface over the anterior aspect of the anterior cruciate ligament and the posterior aspect of the posterior cruciate ligament.

Technical Factors. A grid cassette (100-plus lines 8:1 ratio with Dupont High Plus screens) is carefully positioned at right angles to the central ray and held by the patient. Exposure factors range from 54 to 64 kVp and 30 mAs at a 40-in. distance using a three phase unit. The films should be overpenetrated. The sharply collimated X-ray beam approximately 5 in. in diameter should be centered just posterior to the middle of the knee (Figs. 1A, B).

The Vertical Beam Method

The study is ordinarily performed after the menisci have been examined. It is mandatory that the anterior cruciate ligament be stretched, and this can be accomplished in a number of ways. The patient is placed on the side to be examined, the hip and knee are flexed. A sling is placed around the distal femur and anchored to the table anteriorly. The knee is flexed 60° to 80°, and a mechanical block is placed in front of a dorsiflexed foot to maintain both distal pull on the leg and knee flexion (Figs. 3A, B). Another method of tensing the cruciate ligaments, particularly the anterior cruciate

ligament, is to place the sling or other restraining device around the posterior aspect of the calf, flexing the knee and firmly pushing the ankle posteriorly and inferiorly. Lying on one side, the contrast agent becomes layered in the dependent portion of the knee and the positive contrast-coated synovial surface of the cruciate ligaments is shadowed by air. Contrasted by air, the anterior edge of the intact anterior cruciate ligament and the posterior edge of the intact posterior cruciate ligament appear as radiopaque lines (Figs. 4A, B).

Fluoroscopy is beneficial because the knee can be manipulated until the contour of a normal anterior cruciate ligament can be optimally delineated. It is important to maintain sufficient distraction of the knee to elevate a large fat pad from the surface of the anterior cruciate ligament (Fig. 4B). Also, occasionally, slight internal rotation is necessary to obtain a true lateral projection of the anterior cruciate ligament. When a definite anterior cruciate ligament contour cannot be identified, spot films should be obtained in the position that best visualizes the contour of the posterior cruciate ligament. Visualization of the posterior cruciate ligament, which is less commonly injured, confirms proper knee position and provides the assurance that the nonvisualization of the anterior cruciate ligament is not caused by incorrect positioning.

Technical Factors. Filming can be performed with the fluoroscopic spot film device using a grid and by increasing 8 kVp from the setting used for the examination of the menisci. Alternatively, a standard overhead vertical X-ray exposure can be made by placing the film into the table bucky tray. The roentgenogram should be more penetrated than a routine lateral film of the knee.

ANATOMY

The cruciate ligaments are located within the intercondylar notch of the knee. The anterior cruciate ligament extends from the inner surface of the lateral femoral condyle to the anteromedial aspect of the tibial plateau (Fig. 5). Seen from the side, the ligament forms a straight band attaching inferiorly on the tibial plateau just anterior to the tibial spines, approximately 8 mm posterior to the anterior margin of the tibial plateau (Fig. 6). The posterior cruciate ligament extends from the inner surface of the medial femoral condyle to the posterior margin of the tibial plateau, inserting on its posterior aspect inferior to the plateau surface (Fig. 7). The intra-articular surfaces of the cruciate ligaments are covered by synovium, making them intracapsular, extrasynovial structures.

THE NORMAL ARTHROGRAM

On the lateral arthrogram of the knee, with either the horizontal or the vertical beam, the anterior cruciate ligament is seen as a straight line, its contrast-coated anterosuperior surface touching the tibial plateau approximately 8 mm posterior to the anterior margin of the tibia. The intact posterior cruciate ligament is a straight line extending posteriorly to the posterior margin of the tibial plateau (the following table). With the horizontal beam technique, the positive contrast-shadowed cruciate ligaments appear radiolucent (Figs. 2A, B). With the vertical beam technique, the air-shadowed cruciate ligaments appear slightly radiopaque (Figs. 4A, B). Various conditions of the anterior cruciate ligament and its investing synovium are defined in Table 1.

Status of the Anterior Cruciate Ligament and Its Investing Synovium

1. INTACT: Synovium intact
2. ATTENUATED, intact but lax: Synovium intact or disrupted
3. PARTIALLY TORN: Synovium intact or disrupted
4. TORN: Synovium intact or disrupted
   a. Tattered and shredded
   b. Free-floating or incarcerated in the intercondylar notch
   c. Persistent nubbin remaining on the tibia
5. ABSENT: Synovium disrupted
6. ABSENT: Thick fibrotic band of synovium

THE ABNORMAL ARTHROGRAM

A combination of abnormalities can be present, depending upon whether the cruciate ligament is completely torn or absent, or if it is partially torn, attenuated or lax. Since the anterior cruciate ligament is partially invested by synovium, the overlying synovial membrane may be intact or completely disrupted. Even with a complete ligament tear, the overlying synovium may be intact.

The most common presentation of an anterior cruciate ligament tear with disruption of the investing synovium is an acutely angulated or completely absent anterior contrast band (Figs. 8A–D). An acutely torn anterior cruciate ligament or an old disruption, in which the ligament is absent at surgical exploration, has the same radiographic pattern. Following surgical removal (Fig. 9) or traumatic avulsion of the entire ligament (Figs. 10A, B), the arthrographic appearance is that of a disrupted anterior cruciate ligament.

Partial tears in which the ligament and the synovium are not completely disrupted but are stretched and incompetent are recognized by the decreased slope or a wavy appearance of the anterior edge of the anterior cruciate ligament (Figs. 11A–C).

Occasionally, more specific abnormalities such as a partial tear (Fig. 12), a grossly shredded ligament (Fig. 13), or a nubbin of ligament remaining attached at its tibial insertion (Fig. 14) can be demonstrated.

In longstanding injuries, the previously torn synovium may form a thick fibrotic band. This band attaches to the tibial plateau in a more anterior position than the normal cruciate ligament and should not be mistaken for an intact cruciate ligament (Fig. 15).

On rare occasions, only the posterior cruciate ligament is injured. The arthrographic diagnosis of rupture of the posterior cruciate ligament is more certain when the intact anterior cruciate ligament can be seen, but not the posterior cruciate ligament (Fig. 16A). Failure to demonstrate either ligament can occur when both ligaments have been damaged (Fig. 16B). In such rare instances, it is important to exclude faulty technique as the cause for nonvisualization. The overall accuracy of arthrographically diagnosing the status of the cruciate ligaments in two hundred cases is 91 percent.

Surgical correlation requires careful evaluation of the anterior cruciate ligament by both direct vision and palpation. Such a double examination is necessary because in old anterior cruciate ligament injuries the investing synovium may become a fibrotic band, which visually mimics an intact anterior cruciate ligament, while an underlying ligament tear is detected only by palpation.

INCIDENCE OF INJURY

The incidence of injuries of the anterior cruciate ligament is high. Surgical exploration of knees in 100 amateur athletes with a medial or lateral meniscus tear revealed that only 29 had a normal anterior cruciate ligament. There were 71 surgically documented abnormal anterior cruciate ligaments, ranging from attenuation to complete absence. In a study of 50 patients who presented with acute knee injuries with significant hemarthroses, arthrograms followed by surgery and/or arthroscopy revealed that 42 of the 50 had torn anterior cruciate ligaments. The presence of hemarthrosis after acute trauma to the knee is therefore strongly suggestive of an anterior cruciate ligament tear. A double contrast arthrogram can accurately determine the status of the cruciate ligaments and the menisci so that definitive management can be planned, based on accurate analysis of all the damaged structures in the injured knee.

PITFALLS

Improper positioning can be responsible for nonvisualization of the normal cruciate ligaments.

Insufficient traction on the cruciate ligaments, particularly the anterior cruciate ligament, allows a normal ligament to bow and can lead to a misdiagnosis of tear or abnormal laxity.

Overlapping of the fat pad contour over the anterior cruciate ligament can also lead to a mistaken diagnosis of ligament tear—proper traction and knee flexion eliminate this problem.

Blurring of synovial interfaces should be avoided by adding epinephrine to the contrast medium, and by taking the horizontal beam view first, before the menisci are examined. This film must be more penetrated than routine knee exposures, otherwise the laterally and medially pooled positive contrast medium may hide the cruciate ligaments and cause a misdiagnosis of a tear.

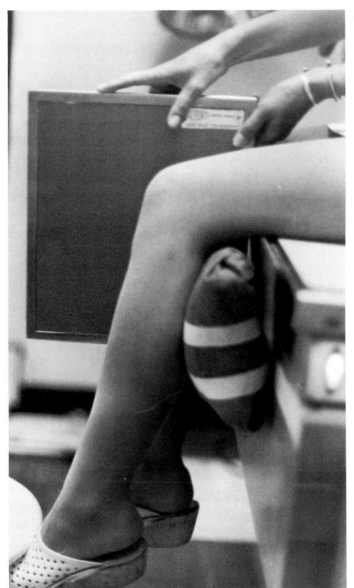

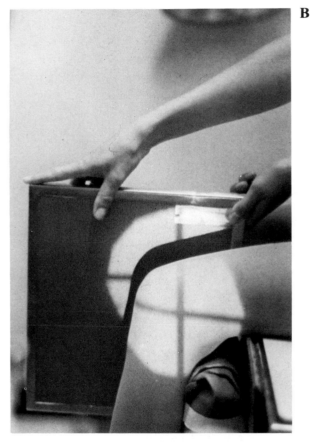

Figure 1
A. For the horizontal beam method, the patient sits on the edge of the radiography table with the knees bent approximately 60° to 80° from full extension. A firm bolus is placed behind the proximal calf to push the tibia anteriorly. A chair mechanically blocks the forward motion of the distal tibia.
B. The patient holds a grid cassette parallel to the face of the X-ray tube. The collimated X-ray beam is directed just posterior to the midpoint of the knee.

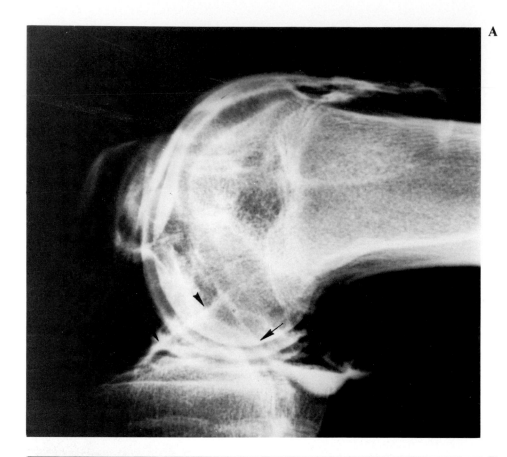

A

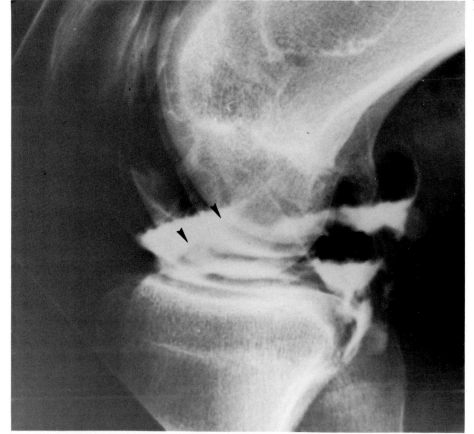

B

Figure 2
The cruciate ligaments are lucent on an overpenetrated lateral view of the knee with the horizontal beam method. The anterior surface of the anterior cruciate ligament is perfectly straight and coated with contrast (arrowheads) as is the posterior surface of the posterior cruciate ligament (arrow).
A. The amount of contrast is not critical as long as the anterior surface is coated.
B. A large amount of contrast anteriorly layers on the intact anterior cruciate ligament (arrowheads).

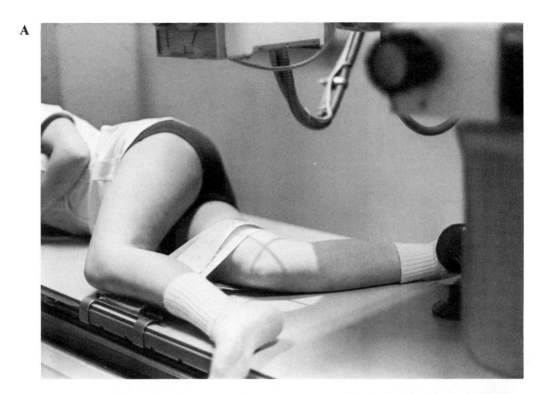

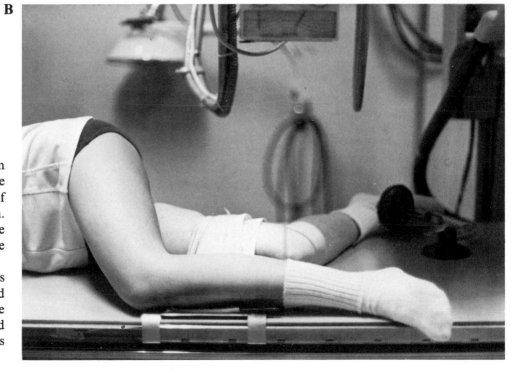

Figure 3
A. For the vertical beam method, the patient lies on the table with the lateral aspect of the knee closest to the film. The hip is relaxed and the knee is flexed 60° to 80°. The X-ray beam is collimated.
B. A mechanical block fixes the tibia distally and is placed anterior to the ankle with the foot dorsiflexed. The band around the distal femur pulls anteriorly.

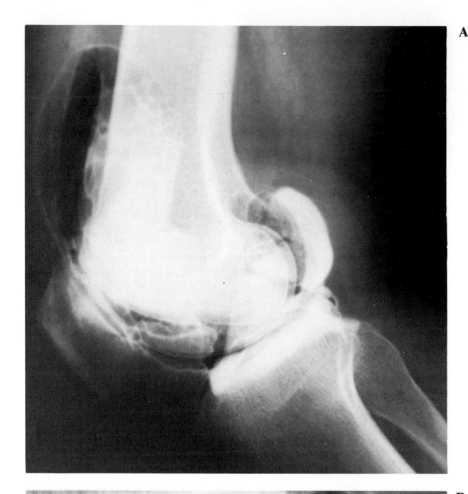

A

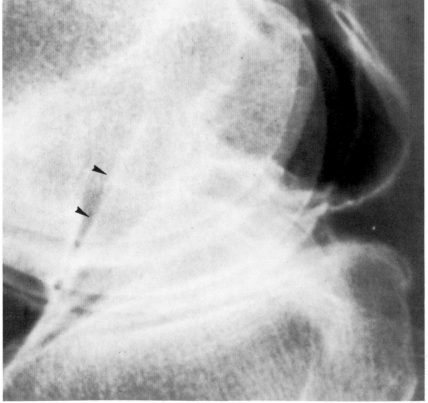

B

Figure 4
A. In the overhead vertical beam method, the anterior and posterior cruciate ligaments are straight with contrast edges that form a tent.
B. The fat pad can be in close proximity to the anterior cruciate ligament. Fluoroscopy is helpful to adequately distract the knee and elevate the fat pad from the surface of the anterior cruciate ligament (arrowheads).

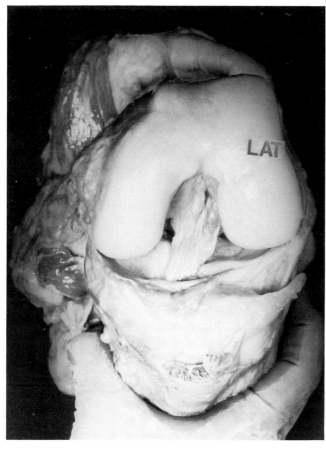

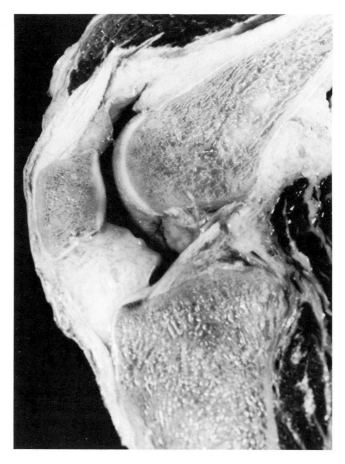

Figure 5
The anterior cruciate ligament extends from the inter-condylar aspect of the lateral femoral condyle to the tibial plateau, anterior and medial to the tibial spines. The posterior cruciate ligament extends from the intercondylar aspect of the medial femoral condyle to the posterior aspect of the proximal tibia.

Figure 6
A sagittal slice of the knee demonstrates the anterior cruciate ligament as a straight band. The insertion point is approximately 8 mm posterior to the anterior tibial margin.

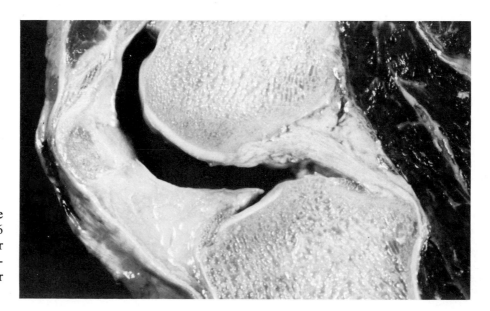

Figure 7
A sagittal slice of the knee more medial than Figure 6 demonstrates the posterior cruciate ligament. This ligament inserts over the posterior surface of the tibial plateau.

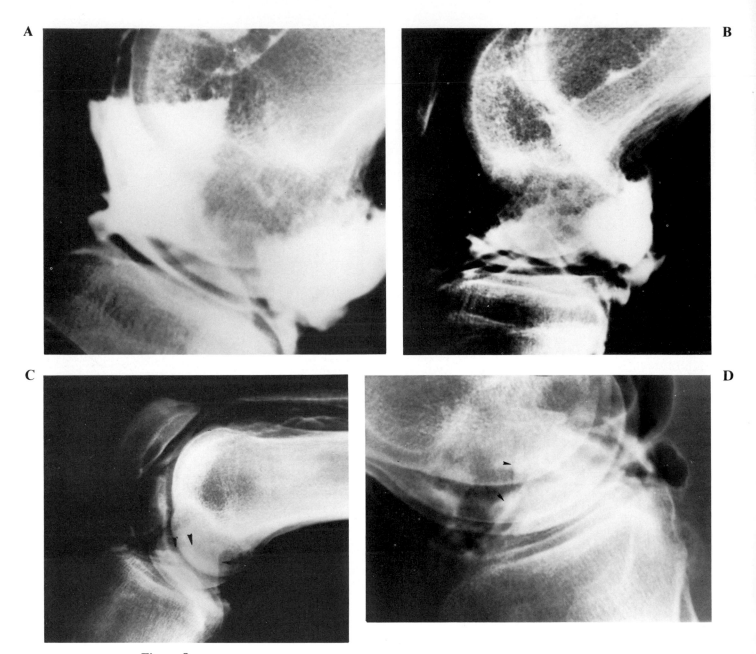

Figure 8
A–D. Acute or chronic disruption of the anterior cruciate ligament and the investing synovium gives several roentgen patterns. The posterior cruciate ligament is well delineated in all figures.
A,B. Using the horizontal beam there is pooling of positive contrast in the location of the anterior cruciate ligament.
C,D. Using the vertical beam and the fluoroscopic spot film method, there is an angulated contrast edge instead of a straight edge for the anterior cruciate ligament (arrowheads).

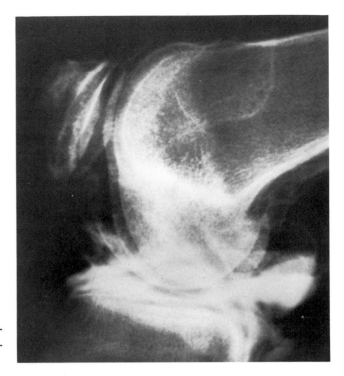

Figure 9
In a patient whose anterior cruciate ligament has been surgically removed, no anterior edge is seen. The posterior cruciate ligament is demonstrated.

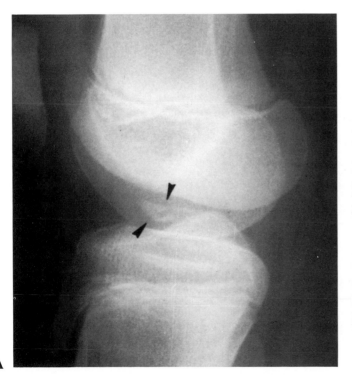

A

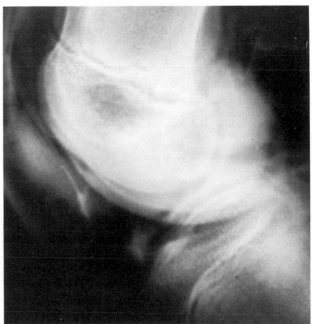

B

Figure 10
A. Plain films of a child demonstrate avulsion of a bone chip in the anterior aspect of the joint (arrowheads).
B. The arthrogram demonstrated the posterior cruciate ligament, but there was no visualization of the anterior cruciate ligament. At surgery, the patient had a completely avulsed, although intact, anterior cruciate ligament.

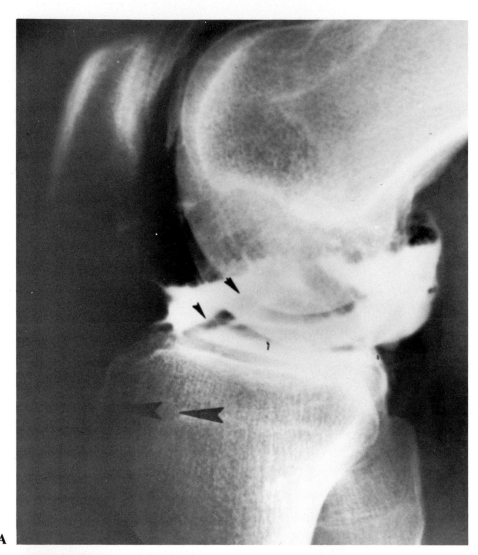

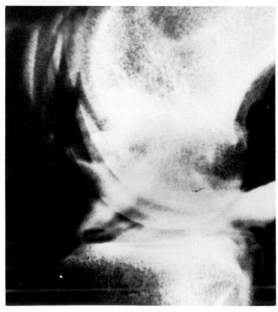

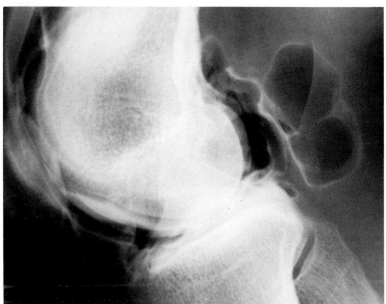

Figure 11

A. With the horizontal beam method, the slope of the anterior cruciate ligament is not as sharp as the normal, and the contrast-lucent interface is slightly irregular. This demonstrates an attenuated, partially torn ligament (arrowheads). (Large arrowheads indicate the anterior tibial displacement.)

B. The anterior surface of the anterior cruciate ligament is wavy and somewhat lumpy, indicating an abnormality. The ligament was attenuated and stretched upon surgical exploration.

C. On this vertical beam film, the posterior cruciate ligament has a well-defined straight posterior edge. The anterior edge of the anterior cruciate ligament is wavy, "S" shaped, and appears interrupted. At surgery, the anterior cruciate ligament was torn, but its investing synovium was intact.

A

B

C

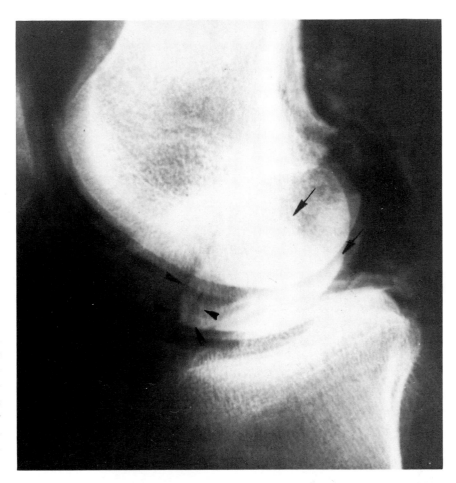

Figure 12
There is a "flap" demonstrated along the distal aspect of the anterior cruciate ligament (arrowheads). At surgery, the patient had a partial tear of the anterior portion of the anterior cruciate ligament. The posterior cruciate ligament is delineated (arrows).

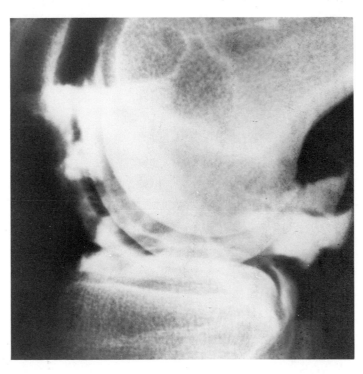

Figure 13
A straight anterior cruciate ligament contrast edge could not be demonstrated by multiple attempts. At surgery, the ligament and its investing synovium were torn and were described as being "shredded like spaghetti."

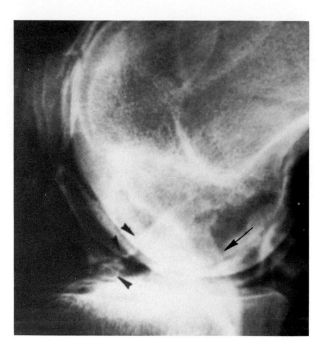

Figure 14
The posterior cruciate ligament is well delineated (arrow) and the inferior portion of the anterior cruciate ligament is not. A remnant of the torn anterior cruciate ligament is outlined by contrast at its tibial insertion (arrowheads). At surgery, the patient had a torn anterior cruciate ligament with a residual nubbin attached to the tibia.

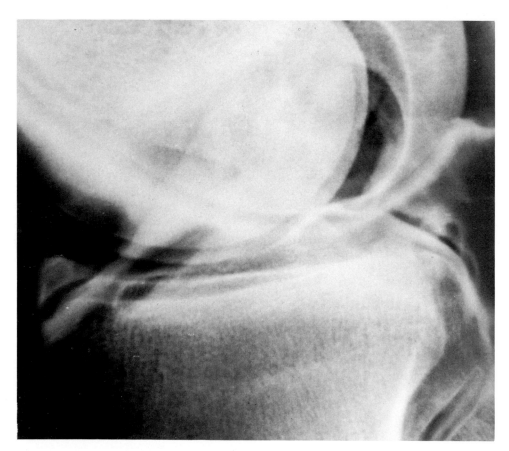

Figure 15
A straight edge is visible in the approximate region of the anterior cruciate ligament; however, its inferior attachment is anterior to the normal location. At surgery, the anterior cruciate ligament was torn and a thick fibrotic band had formed.

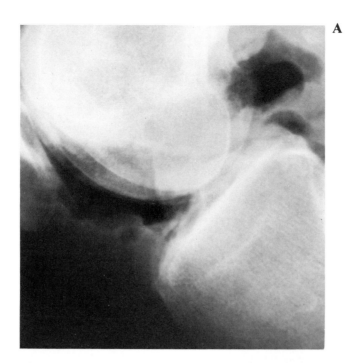

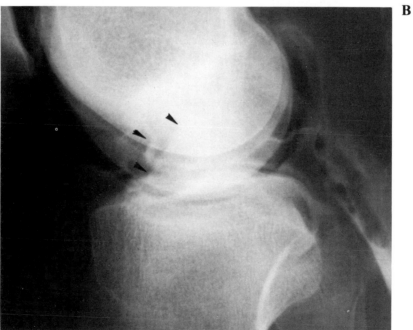

Figure 16
A. The anterior cruciate ligament is sharply demonstrated. The posterior cruciate ligament could not be demonstrated despite multiple attempts. The posterior cruciate ligament was found torn at surgery.
B. The anterior cruciate ligament is visualized as a wavy line (arrowheads) and no posterior cruciate ligament is seen. At surgery, there was a rupture of the posterior capsule and disruption of both cruciate ligaments.

6
Extrameniscal Abnormalities

Robert Schneider
Robert H. Freiberger

Since most arthrograms are performed for the verification of a clinically suspected meniscal tear, some extrameniscal lesions are found serendipitously on the conventional double contrast studies. Specific problems may require single contrast arthrographic techniques, special views, and sometimes tomography for adequate evaluations. Fractures and erosions of the articular cartilages can be seen on the spot films taken for examination of the menisci, and popliteal cysts are apparent on the lateral films taken for the examination for cruciate ligaments. Ruptures of the capsule with leakage of contrast agent are visible on the small spot films of the menisci and can be shown more completely on larger films taken immediately after the initial examination is finished. Although loose bodies and proliferative lesions of the synovium, like pigmented villonodular synovitis, synovial chondromatosis, or rheumatoid arthritis, can be seen on the routine double contrast study, air bubbles may interfere with interpretation. When an arthrogram is requested for diagnosis of synovial disease or for loose bodies, a choice must be made whether to use only air or only positive contrast, or double contrast with larger fields and a horizontal X-ray beam.

POPLITEAL CYSTS

A popliteal cyst is usually a distended gastrocnemius semimembranosus bursa that communicates with the knee joint through a small opening in the posteromedial aspect of the joint capsule (Fig. 1). The bursa lies between the medial head of the gastrocnemius and the semimembranosus muscle, posterior and slightly medial to the midline of the knee joint. A popliteal cyst is usually caused by chronic synovial effusion which opens the communication between the knee joint and the gastrocnemius semimembranosus bursa and distends the bursa. Some popliteal cysts may present clinically as palpable swellings behind the knee, but others are not apparent on clinical examination.

On the lateral projection of the arthrogram taken with the knee in flexion, a well-distended capsule may show considerable bulging of the posterior capsular recesses of the knee joint, which should not be mistaken for a popliteal cyst (Fig. 2).

In adults a popliteal cyst usually indicates that some abnormality is producing synovial effusion. It might be a torn meniscal cartilage, but it could also be osteoarthritis, chondromalacia, or an inflammatory disease of the knee joint. In children, popliteal cysts may appear and spontaneously disappear for no apparent reason. Opacified popliteal cysts sometimes interfere with adequate evaluation of the posterior horn of the medial meniscus but rarely with the posterior horn of the lateral meniscus. If the cause for synovial effusion of the knee can be corrected, popliteal cysts usually disappear.

Occasionally—especially in patients with rheumatoid arthritis—a popliteal cyst may become very large and descend into the calf between the gastrocnemius and soleus muscles (Figs. 3, 8). The cyst causes swelling of the calf and localized tenderness that can be clinically mistaken for thrombophlebitis. The arthrogram clearly differentiates between these two conditions and can prevent unnecessary treatment with anticoagulants.

With overdistention of the knee joint or when exercise raises the pressure of injected air and contrast substance, the capsule may rupture. This usually occurs either at the posterior capsular recess (Fig. 4A), at the suprapatellar bursa (Fig. 4B), or at a popliteal cyst (Fig. 4C). If meglumine contrast agents have been used, such ruptures with leakage of contrast agent from the knee joint cause no symptoms and have no clinical significance.

PIGMENTED VILLONODULAR SYNOVITIS

Pigmented villonodular synovitis is a disease of the synovium that primarily affects young adults. It is a monarticular arthritis that occurs most commonly at the knee joint, but also appears at other joints and in synovial tendon sheaths. The usual presentation at the knee joint is chronic swelling with minimal pain. Routine X-ray examination can demonstrate distention of the knee joint, but rarely shows any intra-articular bone erosion. Osteoporosis is normally absent. Aspiration of the knee joint produces bloody or xanthochromic fluid.

When the history, clinical findings, and aspiration of xanthochromic fluid prior to the arthrogram suggest the diagnosis of pigmented villonodular synovitis, a single contrast arthrographic technique, using only positive contrast or only air, may be preferable. Fluid in the knee, which usually cannot be completely aspirated, interferes less with the solid positive contrast arthrogram than with the others (Fig. 5). The usual double contrast arthrogram with 5 cc of positive contrast and 40 cc of air may produce air bubbles that can be confused with the small nodular synovial lesions of this disease. Technically good double contrast arthrograms can be performed if a horizontal beam technique is used, and if lateral and oblique films are large enough to include the entire knee and the suprapatellar

pouch. The synovial surfaces are coated by a thin film of positive contrast substance and shadowed by air (Figs. 6A, B), and excess positive contrast pools in the dependent portion of the knee. Any small air bubbles stay just above the fluid level of the positive contrast substance and do not interfere with the evaluation of the synovial surfaces.

The arthrographic appearance of the diffuse nodular lesions of the synovium (Fig. 5) is not specific for pigmented villonodular synovitis, but the diagnosis is strongly suggested if the appearance is combined with the aspiration of bloody or xanthochromic fluid.

Other synovial abnormalities that may have a similar appearance are synovial chondromatosis, rheumatoid arthritis (Fig. 7), tuberculosis, synovial hemangioma, and lipoma arborescens. The synovial abnormalities seen in hemophiliac arthritis are very similar to pigmented villonodular synovitis; however, they present no diagnostic problem if the patient is a known hemophiliac. Pigmented villonodular synovitis may occasionally produce only one synovial nodule (Figs. 6A, B).

RHEUMATOID ARTHRITIS

In rheumatoid arthritis, knee arthrography is performed primarily for the diagnosis of the giant popliteal cyst. It dissects into the calf, between the gastrocnemius and soleus muscles, and causes signs and symptoms that are often mistaken for thrombophlebitis (Figs. 3, 8). The arthrogram can also show the proliferative changes of the synovium (Figs. 7A, B) and opacification of lymphatic vessels (Fig. 8). The latter is a sign of inflammation but is not specific for rheumatoid arthritis.

Pannus formation and liberation of enzymes into the synovial fluid causes destruction of articular and meniscal cartilages. The degree of destruction can be evaluated by the arthrogram. There are few clinical indications for delineation of the destructive changes of the soft tissues within the knee. Occasionally arthrographic evaluation is requested when synovectomy or another surgical procedure is contemplated.

SYNOVIAL CHONDROMATOSIS

Synovial chondromatosis is caused by the formation of cartilage within the synovial villi. These microscopic cartilage bodies are extruded into the joint and grow, receiving their nourishment from synovial fluid. Multiple bodies are thus formed. Most of them are loose but some may be attached to the synovium. Usually, but not always, some of the cartilaginous bodies calcify or ossify and become visible on routine radiographs. If calcifications are not visible, plain films show only joint distention. Bone erosions are rarely seen in the knee. Chronic swelling of the knee and occasional locking caused by cartilaginous bodies caught between the articular surfaces are suggestive of synovial chondromatosis.

On arthrography, multiple filling defects, usually somewhat similar in size, are seen within the joint cavity (Fig. 9). In the absence of calcification these can be similar to the synovial nodules seen in pigmented villonodular synovitis. If synovial chondromatosis is suspected, the routine double-contrast arthrogram may present problems since air bubbles can closely simulate the appearance of the small chondromatous bodies (Fig. 10). A solid positive contrast arthrogram or an air arthrogram is therefore preferable. However, a double-contrast arthrogram can be performed by taking films of the entire knee with a horizontal X-ray beam in the lateral and oblique projections. This technique causes positive contrast to flow to the dependent portion of the knee and either leaves the chondromatous bodies covered by a thin film of positive contrast agent and shadowed by air or shows them as lucent filling defects in the dependent portion of the knee, which is filled by positive contrast agent (Fig. 11). Any air bubbles lie on the surface of the positive contrast fluid and do not interfere with the detection of intra-articular cartilaginous bodies.

The arthrogram is most useful for diagnosis of synovial chondromatosis when the cartilaginous bodies have not calcified or when only a few small calcifications can be seen on plain roentgenograms, and it is uncertain whether they lie within the knee or are capsular or extracapsular. If the calcification is surrounded by moderately radiolucent cartilage and is shadowed either by air or by positive contrast agent, a diagnosis of intra-articular location can be made.

CHONDROMATOUS AND OSTEOCHONDROMATOUS BODIES

Chondromatous and osteochondromatous bodies are common in the knee joint and are usually caused by a fragment of articular cartilage growing within the knee, nourished by synovial fluid. Only rarely are loose bodies the result of synovial chondromatosis. Most of these cartilaginous bodies are partially calcified and can be seen on routine examination of the knee. However, it is often uncertain whether ossifications are within the intrasynovial space of the knee joint, in the cruciate ligaments, within the menisci, in the capsule, or immediately peripheral to the capsule. An arthrogram with tomography helps pinpoint the location.

The arthrographic examination is technically difficult since a positive contrast arthrogram may obscure the loose bodies and the double contrast arthrogram may produce false positive findings if air bubbles are mistaken for cartilaginous bodies. Using air only, it is difficult to get all surfaces of the knee adequately covered, and an osteochondromatous body may not be completely surrounded even when it is intra-articular.

It is not uncommon to see one or more osteochondromatous bodies in popliteal cysts (Figs. 12, 13).

OSTEOCHONDRITIS DISSECANS

Osteochondritis dissecans is a disease of children and young adults. A fragment of articular cartilage—sometimes with attached subchondral bone—separates partially or completely from the femoral condyle (Figs. 14–16). It is thought to be caused by acute or chronic trauma. The anteromedial portion of the medial femoral condyle adjacent to the intercondylar notch is most commonly affected, but the lateral femoral condyle and patella are also subject.

Osteochondritis dissecans is usually visible by plain film examination and appears as a radiolucent defect in subchondral bone. A small osseous body may be seen adjacent to this defect or somewhat separated from it (Fig. 15A), occasionally lying within the knee joint as a loose body. Arthrography is helpful in determining whether the articular cartilage overlying the osseous defect is broken (Fig. 15B) or intact (Figs. 16A, B, C). If contrast material completely surrounds the osteochondral fragment, the articular surface is broken and the fragment is loose (Fig. 15B). If no contrast agent appears between the osseous fragment and its base, the articular cartilage is intact and spontaneous healing may occur, obviating the need for surgical intervention at this stage (Fig. 17).

Following the injection of contrast material, roentgenograms should be made with the involved side of the knee distracted. Tomograms are helpful in determining whether the osteochondromatous fragment is loose and whether cartilage is covering a subchondral defect seen on the plain films (Fig. 16C). Fractures of the articular cartilage can be diagnosed only on the arthrogram since they are not visible on the plain films.

Fragmentation at the posterior margin of the distal femoral epiphysis, seen more often laterally than medially in a child, is not osteochondritis dissecans, but a common variant of epiphyseal ossification (Fig. 18A). There is no need to perform an arthrogram in such cases but if it is done, the overlying articular cartilage is intact (Fig. 18B).

CHONDROMALACIA PATELLAE

Chondromalacia patellae is the most frequent cause of knee pain in teenagers and young adults. Pain in the knee is usually anteromedial, and increases when the patient climbs stairs or sits with the knees flexed. Other symptoms are instability, or giving way, and, occasionally, locking of the knee. Because these symptoms are similar to those of meniscal tear, particularly when there is a history of injury, the clinical differentiation between chondromalacia patellae and meniscus tear can be difficult.

Retropatellar pain produced by compression of the patella against the femoral condyles and a grating sensation when moving the patella are suggestive of chondromalacia but these findings do not exclude the possibility of a meniscal tear.

Examination Technique

Following the examination of the menisci, the knee is fully extended and placed in the lateral position. Spot films of the articular cartilage of the patella are taken in slight external rotation, making the lateral facet of the patellar cartilage tangential to the X-ray beam (Fig. 19A), and in slight internal rotation, making the medial facet tangential to the X-ray beam (Fig. 19B). A horizontal beam lateral view of the knee with the knee extended may also be helpful as the positive contrast-coated patellar cartilage can be seen through the air in the suprapatellar pouch. The patellar cartilage is also visible on the skyline view but is usually not seen completely since part of it is obscured by the femoral condyles (Fig. 19C).

Diagnostic Criteria

In the early stages of chondromalacia patellae there is softening and swelling of the articular cartilage, which is not demonstrated on arthrography. Later stages can be diagnosed by seeing positive contrast agent in fissures and erosions within the articular cartilage and by detecting the irregular, uneven surface of the cartilage coated by a thin layer of positive contrast agent and shadowed by air (Figs. 20, 21).

OSTEOARTHRITIS

Osteoarthritis primarily affects the hyaline articular cartilages, which become thinner and fragmented and may completely disappear in a portion of the knee joint (Figs. 22, 23). Characteristically in osteoarthritis, the thinning of the articular cartilages occurs unevenly in the three compartments of the knee, with either the medial or lateral femoral tibial articulation and the patellofemoral articulation primarily affected.

The diagnosis of moderately advanced to advanced osteoarthritis can be made by routine radiographs, particularly if the films are taken with the patient standing. Subtle early changes of the articular cartilages are not seen on plain films but can be demonstrated on the arthrogram (Fig. 23). With erosion and fragmentation of the articular cartilages, the adjacent meniscus can be affected. It may show changes ranging from minor degeneration such as blunting or fraying of the inner edge with slight opacification at the apex to major tears and complete disintegration of the meniscal cartilage (Fig. 23). It is usually not possible to determine whether a tear of the meniscal cartilage is secondary to the osteoarthritis or has preceded the osteoarthritic changes. The arthrographic examination can be important when corrective surgery such as tibial osteotomy is planned. If the meniscal cartilages are reasonably intact, the surgeon can perform the osteotomy without an arthrotomy.

MEDIAL COLLATERAL LIGAMENT TEARS

The medial collateral ligament is an important structure for stability of the knee. It is frequently ruptured by acute trauma, often in association with tears of the medial meniscus and/or the anterior cruciate ligament. Rapid diagnosis of an acute medial collateral ligament injury can be important in deciding whether or not to operate. Pain and muscle spasm after injury often prevent adequate physical examination of the ligament. Arthrography can diagnose the presence and severity of tears of the medial collateral ligament and provide information on the state of the menisci and cruciate ligaments. The arthrogram should be performed within 48 hours of the injury because later the capsule may become air- and watertight, preventing leakage of contrast agent even when the ligament is torn and the knee is unstable.

The medial collateral ligament has two major parts—a deep portion, which is closest to the joint capsule, and a superficial portion.

The deep portion of the medial collateral ligament is closely associated with the joint capsule, so if the ligament is torn, the capsule is also torn, causing contrast material to leak from the joint (Fig. 24). If only the deep portion of the medial collateral ligament is torn, leaked contrast material appears as a sharp linear streak as it lies against the intact portion of the superficial ligament (Fig. 25). If only the superficial portion of the ligament is torn, no contrast material leaks out of the joint and the diagnosis cannot be made by arthrography. If both the deep and superficial portions are torn, leaked contrast material has a feathery appearance as it infiltrates the extra-articular soft tissues (Figs. 24, 26). An increased width of the medial compartment of the knee joint when valgus stress is applied during the arthrogram is an indirect sign of a torn medial collateral ligament (Fig. 27). Tears of the medial collateral ligament are frequently associated with peripheral detachments or tears of the medial meniscus (Fig. 25).

The lateral collateral ligament is separated from the lateral joint capsule so that the ligament may be torn while the capsule remains intact. An abnormal increase in the width of the lateral joint space on varus stress is an indirect indication of lateral ligament tear. Capsular tears can occur at the suprapatellar bursa, caused by a tear of the adjacent quadriceps tendon (Fig. 28). The tendon tear is the clinically significant injury.

Rarely, a capsular tear can lead to a persistent extracapsular communicating cyst. The cyst is caused either by a herniation of the synovium or a synovial lining forming around a persistent leak of synovial fluid. The cyst may cause a painful swelling (Figs. 29A, B).

ADHESIVE CAPSULITIS

Contractures of the capsule and suprapatellar pouch may occur after trauma, surgery, or prolonged immobilization of the knee joint, and can cause symptoms of painful restricted motion. The condition is similar to the better known "frozen shoulder."

The arthrogram shows markedly reduced intra-articular volume caused by constriction of the capsule (Figs. 30–32), and the patient may complain of pain before the usual volume of contrast agent has been injected. Occasionally, particularly after knee surgery, intra-articular adhesions prevent complete filling of the knee joint cavity (Fig. 32).

PITFALLS

A distended, lax posterior capsular fold of the knee should not be mistaken for a popliteal cyst.

Synovial villous proliferation is not specific for pigmented villonodular synovitis, but can be seen in a variety of inflammatory diseases.

Air bubbles can be mistaken for loose cartilaginous bodies.

Leaks of contrast substance from the suprapatellar pouch, posterior capsule, or a popliteal cyst are usually caused by overdistention of the joint and should not be mistaken for a clinically significant tear.

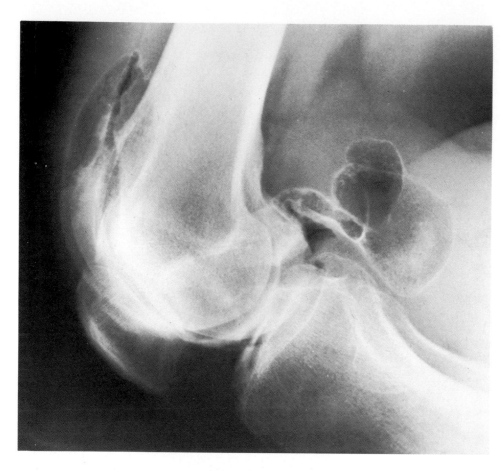

Figure 1
A popliteal cyst is an enlarged gastrocnemius, semimembranosus bursa that fills with air and positive contrast material through a narrow communication with the knee joint.

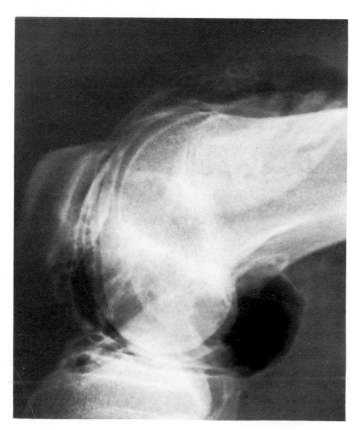

Figure 2
With the knee flexed, the capsule, distended by air and positive contrast material, bulges posteriorly. The bulge should not be confused with a popliteal cyst.

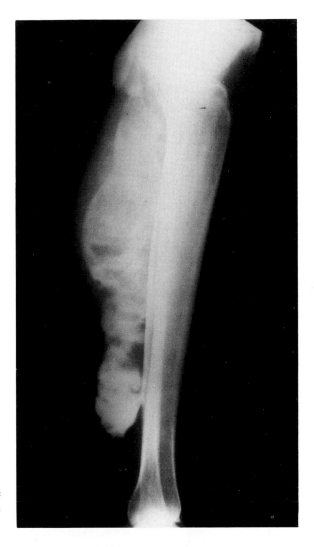

Figure 3
A giant popliteal cyst extends into the calf between the soleus and gastrocnemius muscles. It often causes pain, tenderness, and swelling which mimics thrombophlebitis.

A

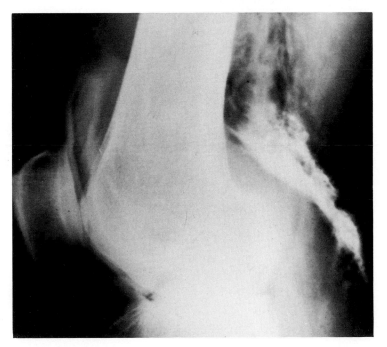

Figure 4
Extracapsular leakage of contrast agent from the knee joint can be caused by increased intra-articular pressure from the injection of contrast agents or from postinjection exercise.
A. Leakage usually occurs at the posterior capsular recess.

B

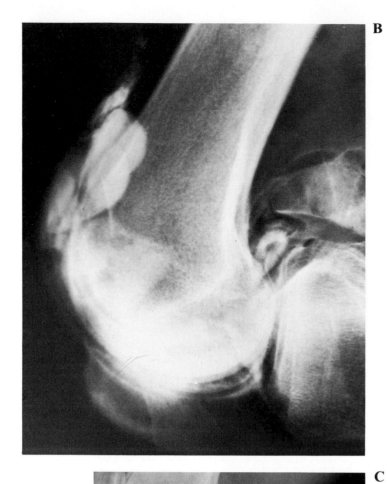

C

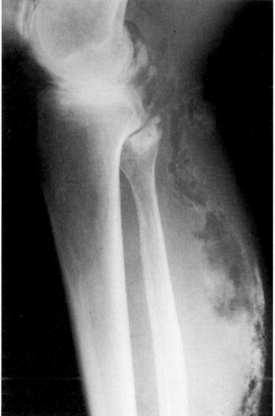

Figure 4
B. Contrast agents can also leak from the suprapatellar pouch, or (**C**) a popliteal cyst. These capsular ruptures are of no clinical significance.

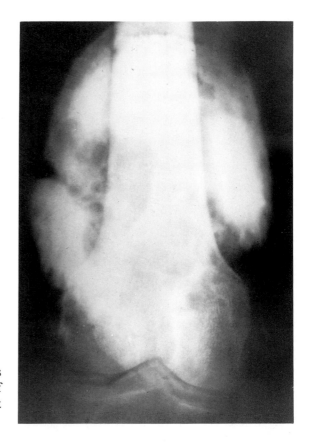

Figure 5
Pigmented villonodular synovitis in its diffuse form causes enlargement of the joint cavity and marked irregularity of the synovium. The large filling defects on a positive contrast arthrogram are synovial nodules.

A

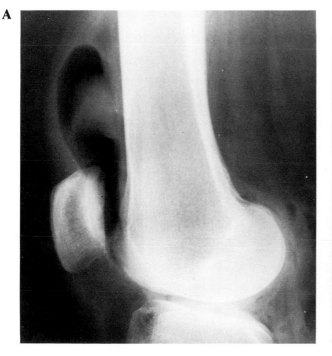

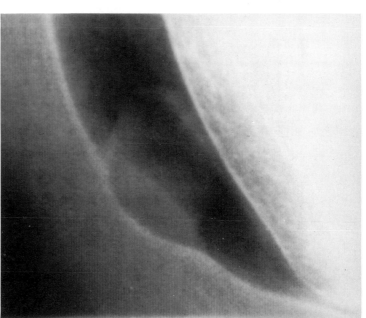

B

Figure 6
A,B. Pigmented villonodular synovitis appears as a single nodular mass on a double contrast study. Each patient had a palpable mass in the suprapatellar pouch which could not be seen on plain films.

A

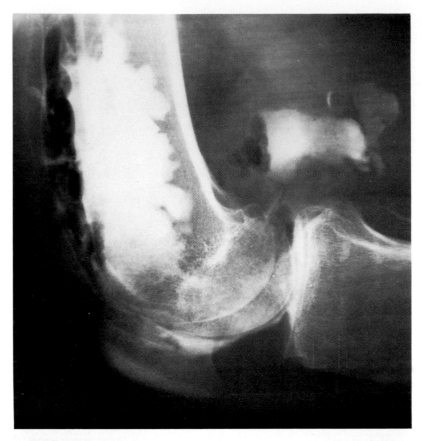

B

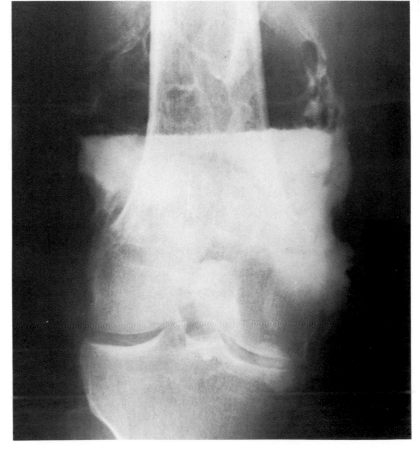

Figure 7

A,B. A double contrast arthrogram of a patient with rheumatoid arthritis shows an enlarged joint capsule. The shaggy irregular synovial surface caused by synovial proliferation can be seen in the dependent portion of the knee, which is filled with positive contrast, and in the superior portion where large synovial villi are covered by a thin layer of contrast agent and shadowed by air. A popliteal cyst is also present.

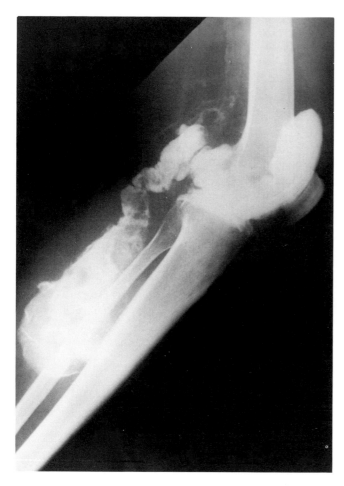

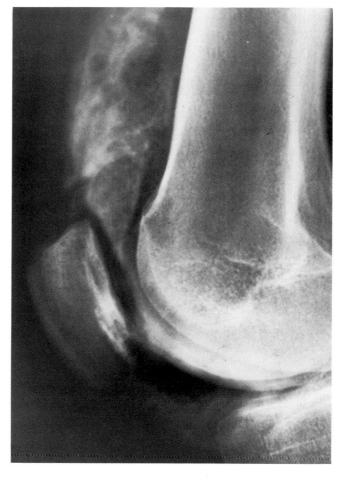

Figure 8
Rheumatoid arthritis of the knee produced a giant synovial cyst extending into the calf. Opacification of lymphatics (arrow) is seen, indicating inflammatory synovial disease.

Figure 9
Synovial chondromatosis causes multiple small radiolucent filling defects with irregularity of the synovial surface of the suprapatellar pouch as seen on a double contrast arthrogram. No calcifications were evident on plain radiographs.

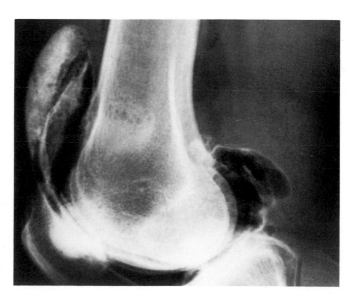

Figure10
Air bubbles in the suprapatellar pouch seen on a double contrast arthrogram can mimic the intra-articular radiolucent bodies of synovial chondromatosis. The synovial surfaces, unlike those in synovial chondromatosis, are smooth because the air bubbles are floating on the horizontal surface of the positive contrast agent.

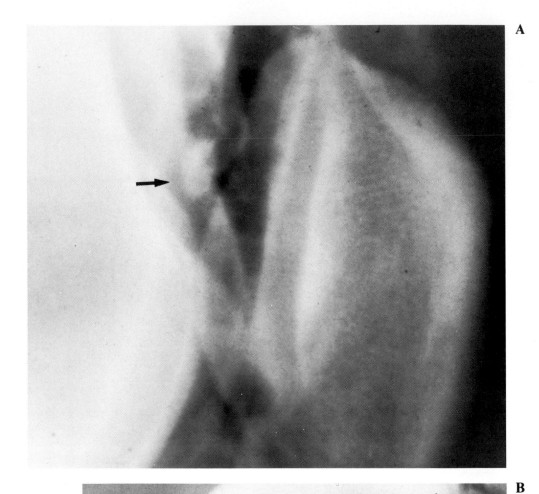

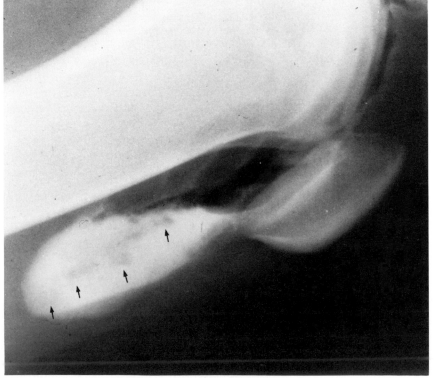

Figure 11
A. Only one small cartilaginous body coated by positive contrast and surrounded by air is seen between the patella and femoral condyles (arrow).
B. A film made with a horizontal X-ray beam and the patient prone shows the multiple filling defects (arrows) caused by loose bodies in the dependent portion of the suprapatellar pouch filled by positive contrast agent.

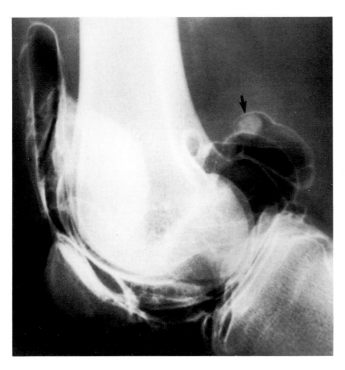

Figure 12
The lateral view of an arthrogram shows an osseous body lying within a popliteal cyst (arrow). On plain radiographs, a single small osseous body seen posterior to the knee could be mistaken for a fabella.

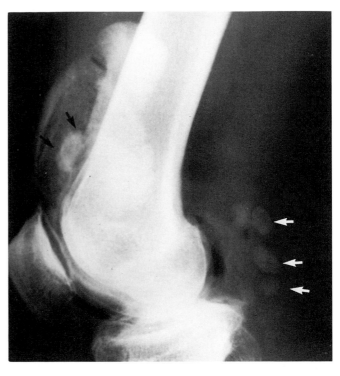

Figure 13
Multiple loose bodies (white arrows) lie in a popliteal cyst filled with air. An osteochondromatous body is seen in the suprapatellar pouch (black arrows).

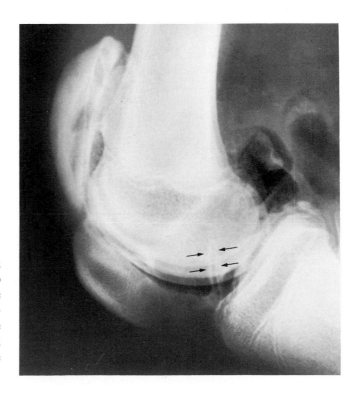

Figure 14
A linear radiolucent cartilaginous body (arrows), which was not seen on plain roentgenograms, lies anterior to the anterior cruciate ligament surrounded by positive contrast substance and shadowed by air. The arthrogram was performed for a suspected meniscus tear. The site of origin of this loose body could not be identified on the arthrogram, but at arthrotomy was found in the lateral femoral condyle.

A

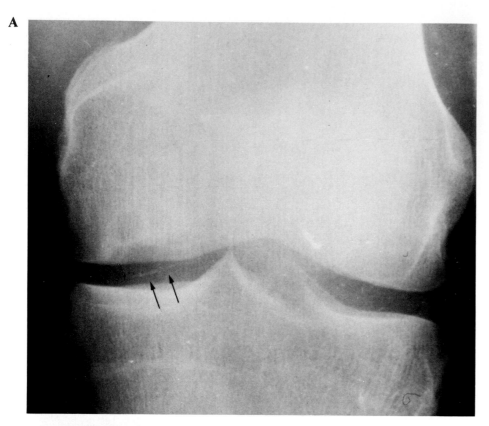

Figure 15
A. A plain radiograph of the knee shows a defect in the subchondral bone of the medial femoral condyle. A calcified body projects through the joint space on the medial aspect of the knee joint (arrows).
B. On the arthrogram, the large, predominantly cartilaginous body of osteochondritis dissecans is seen partially displaced from an osteocartilaginous defect in the medial femoral condyle. It is completely surrounded by contrast substance and therefore loose.

B

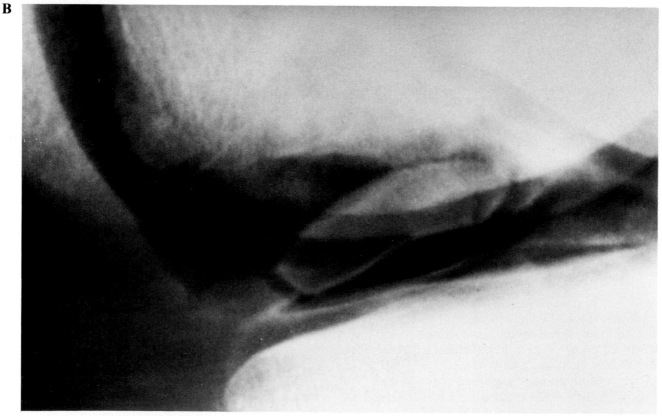

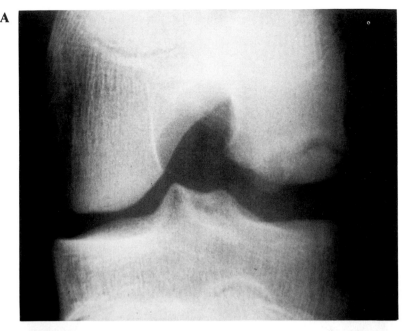

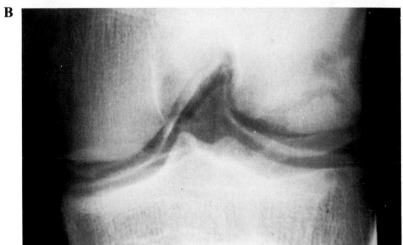

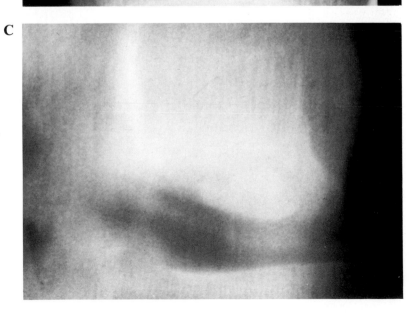

Figure 16
A. A large osseous body is seen at the osseous margin of the lateral femoral condyle.
B. A double contrast arthrogram shows that the articular surface over the osseous body is intact, and no contrast agent can be seen between it and its fossa. The osseous body is not loose.
C. A tomogram confirms the findings.

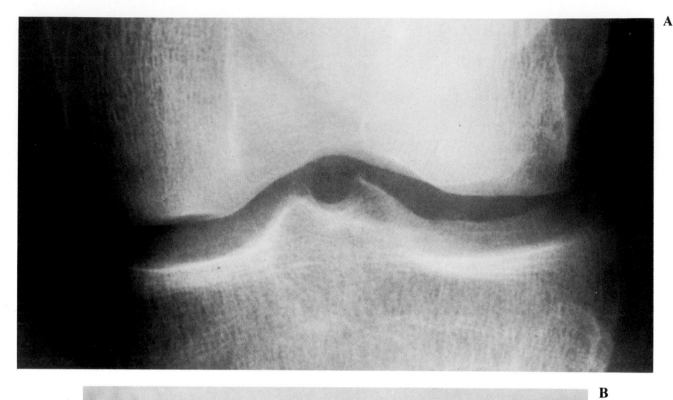

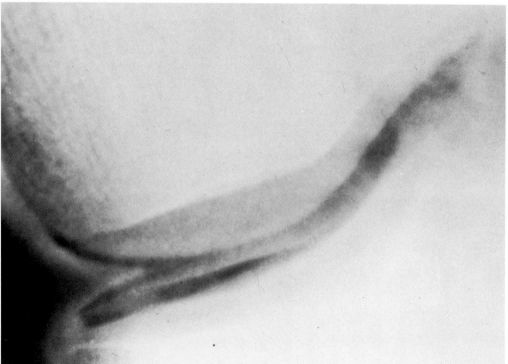

Figure 17
A. A shallow depression in the subchondral surface of the medial femoral condyle suggests a diagnosis of osteochondritis dissecans.
B. The arthrogram shows the overlying articular cartilage to be thick and intact.

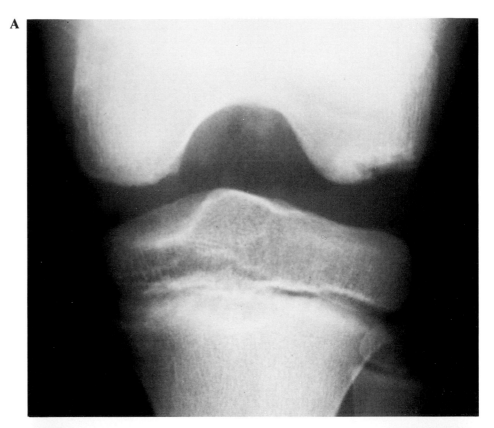

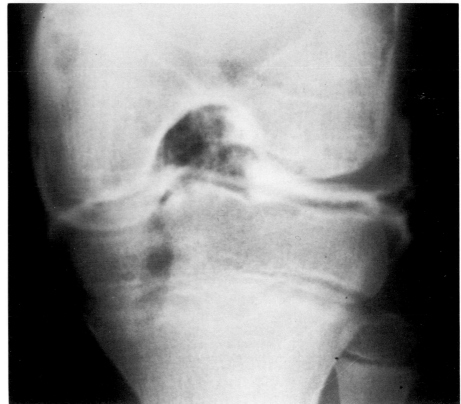

Figure 18
A. A plain roentgenogram shows a common ossification-center defect in the posterior portion of the lateral condyle of a child. This is a normal variant and not osteochondritis dissecans.
B. An arthrogram shows the intact articular cartilage over the defect.

A

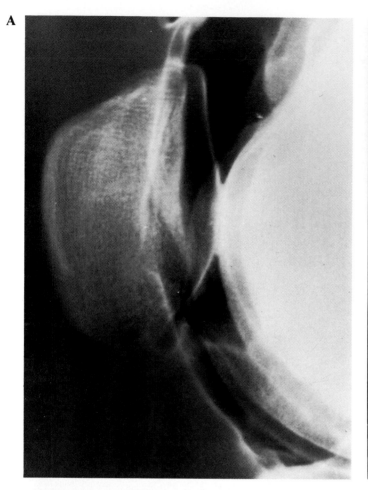

B

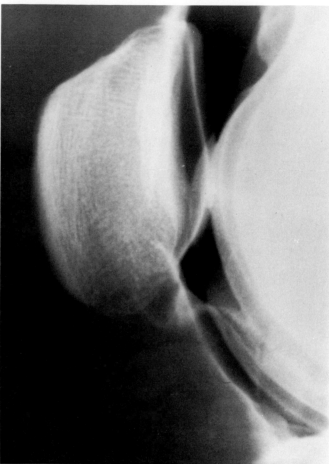

C

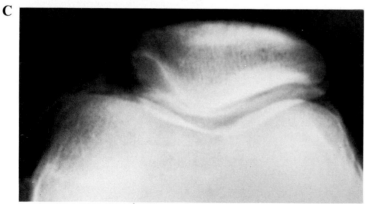

Figure 19
A. The normal articular cartilage of the lateral facet of the patella, seen on a slightly externally rotated lateral view of the knee, is thick and smooth.
B. The normal articular cartilage of the medial facet of the patella is seen on a slightly internally rotated lateral view.
C. The articular cartilages of the patella are visible on the tangential view of the patella, but are, as usual, partially overlapped by the articular cartilages of the femoral condyles.

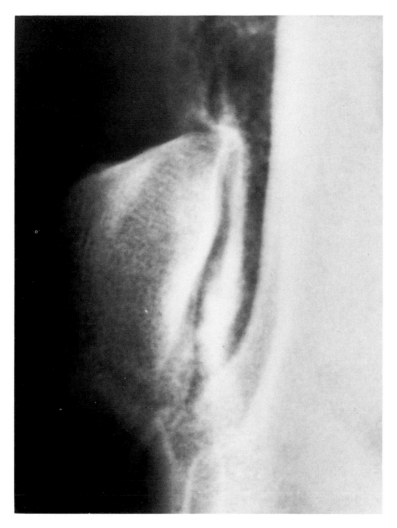

Figure 20
The irregularities and erosions on the surfaces of the articular cartilages of the patella apparent on the arthrogram are characteristic of an advanced stage of chondromalacia patellae.

A

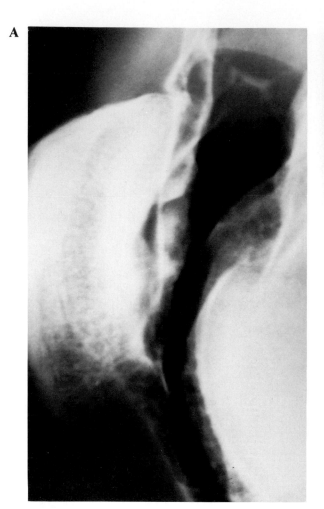

B

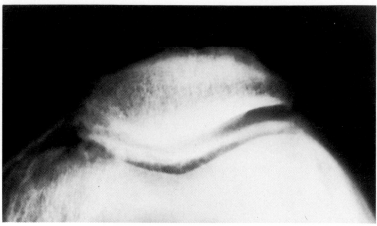

C

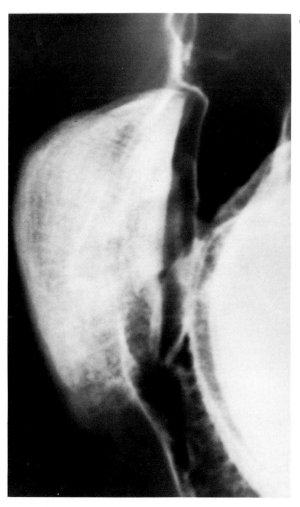

Figure 21
A. Marked irregularity of the surface of the articular cartilage of the medial facet of the patella is noted on a slightly internally rotated lateral view.
B. The tangential skyline view shows thinning and irregularity of the articular cartilage of the medial facet of the patella. The articular cartilage of the lateral facet is of normal thickness.
C. The lateral articular cartilage of the patella on a slightly externally rotated lateral view appears normal.

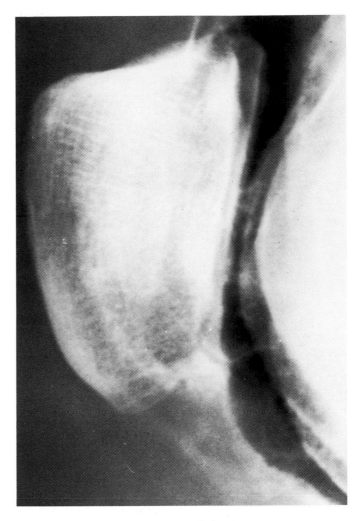

Figure 22
Thinning of the articular cartilage of the patella in an elderly patient is caused by patellofemoral osteoarthritis.

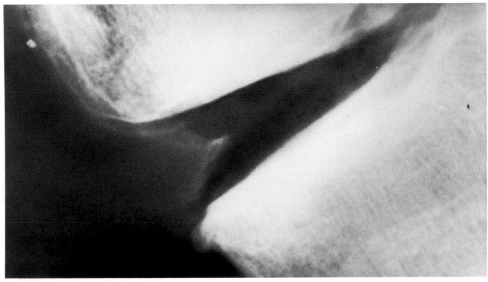

Figure 23
Osteoarthritis, causing thinning and complete erosion of the articular cartilages of the femoral and tibial condyles, is seen on a double contrast arthrogram. The meniscus is deformed and its apex is opacified, indicating degenerative tears.

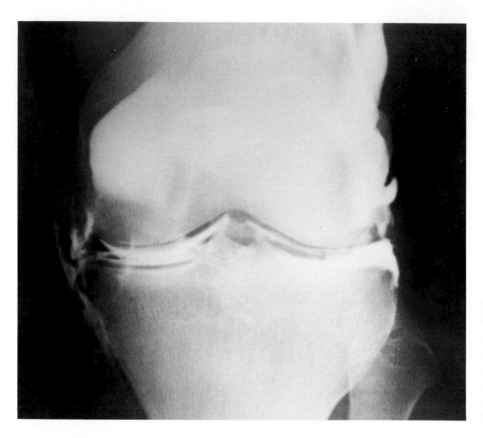

Figure 24
Twenty-four hours after an acute injury, an arthrogram shows positive contrast material leaking from the medial aspect of the knee joint, indicating a tear of the medial collateral ligament.

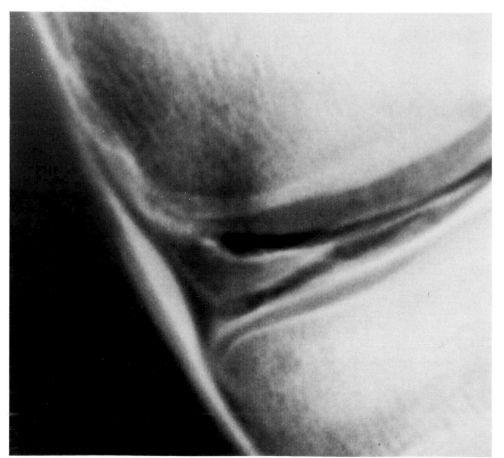

Figure 25
A peripheral vertical tear of the medial meniscus and a tear of the medial collateral ligament are demonstrated. The smooth peripheral margins of the contrast agent, which has leaked from the joint, indicates that the superficial portion of the medial collateral ligament is intact.

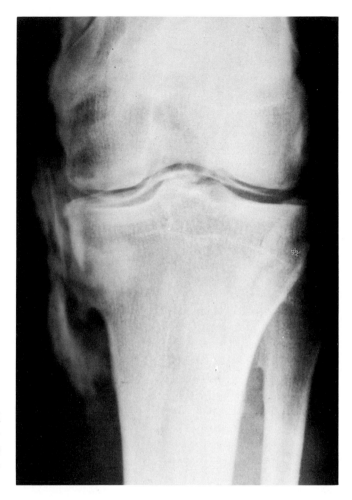

Figure 26
Leakage of contrast agent into the soft tissues on the medial aspect of the knee with a feathery pattern of the extra-articular contrast agent at the periphery indicates that both the deep and superficial portions of the medial collateral ligament have been torn.

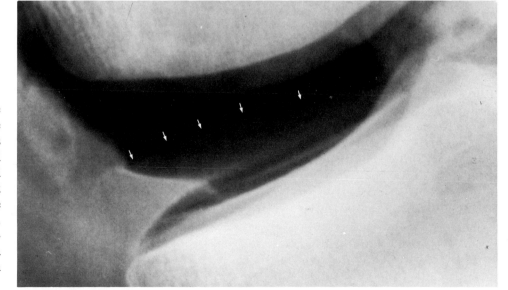

Figure 27
The abnormal increase in the width of the medial joint space of the knee with valgus stress indicates a tear or abnormal laxity of the medial collateral ligament. Leakage of contrast agent may not be seen if the tear is more than 3 days old. Because of the marked distraction of the articular surfaces, a portion of the meniscus is seen *en face* (arrows).

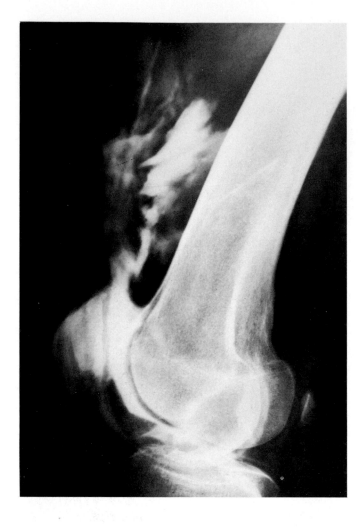

Figure 28
An arthrogram of a patient with an acute tear of the quadriceps tendon shows leakage of contrast agent into the region of the quadriceps tendon from a grossly distorted suprapatellar pouch.

A

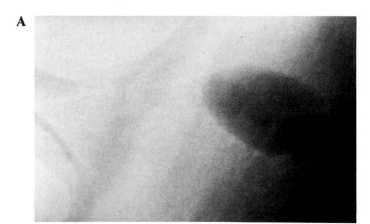

B

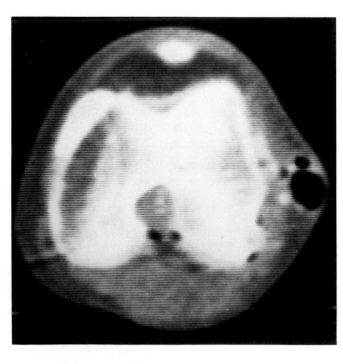

Figure 29
A. A communicating post-traumatic extra-articular synovial cyst on the lateral side of the knee fills with air injected into the knee joint.
B. A computed tomograph (CT) scan shows the air-filled cyst and its narrow communication with the knee joint. (Courtesy of Dr. J.C. Hirschy)

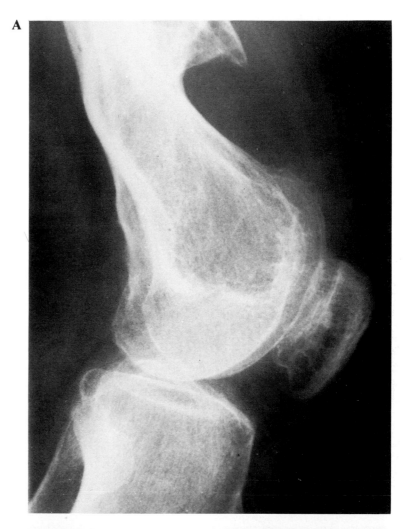

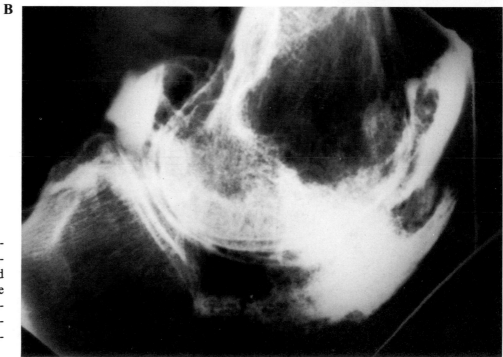

Figure 30
A,B. Adhesive capsulitis following injury and immobilization of the knee caused marked contracture of the capsule and diminution of intracapsular volume. The condition is analogous to the post-traumatic frozen shoulder.

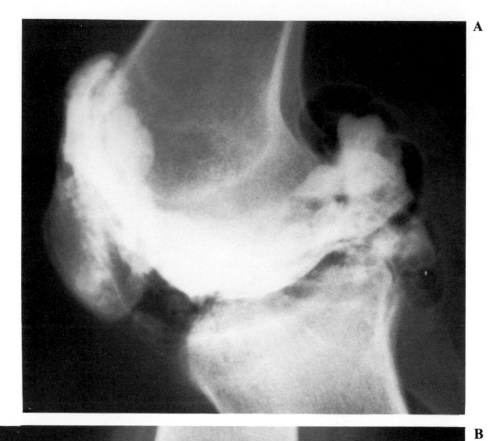

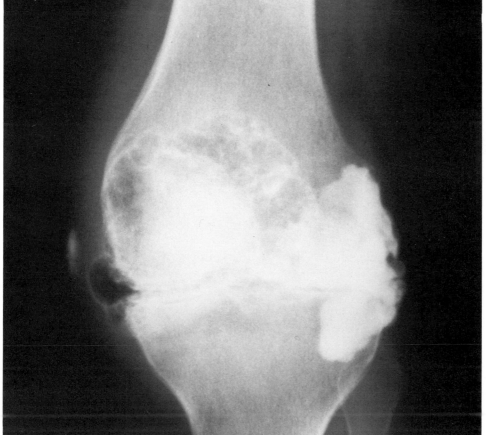

Figure 31
A,B. Adhesive capsulitis of the knee occurred following an injury that was treated by immobilization.

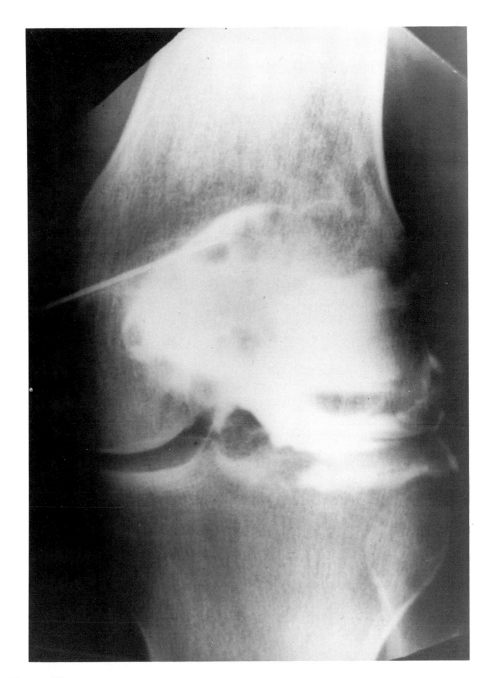

Figure 32
Postsurgical fibrosis within the knee joint prevents contrast filling of the medial compartment. The needle inserted from the medial side of the knee can be seen in the supracondylar region. The contrast medium is intra-articular since the lateral compartment is opacified.

7
Positive Contrast Shoulder Arthrography

Jeremy J. Kaye
Robert Schneider

Shoulder arthrography is useful in the diagnosis of complete and partial tears of the rotator cuff and of adhesive capsulitis, or the frozen shoulder, and in the evaluation of the degree of capsular deformity owing to previous shoulder dislocation.

TECHNIQUE

Preliminary anteroposterior roentgenograms are taken in internal and external rotation. An axillary projection and a bicipital groove view are also obtained. These are inspected prior to the arthrogram to detect or evaluate bony abnormalities.

The patient is then placed supine on a fluoroscopic table, preferably one with an overhead X-ray tube and undertable image intensifier to provide working space above the patient (Fig. 1). The shoulder is flat against the table and the arm, placed close to the body, is rotated so that the shoulder is in neutral position or in mild external rotation (Fig. 2). This position rotates the tendon of the long head of the biceps laterally and away from the projected needle path to avoid the possibility of injury to the biceps tendon by the needle. The articular surface of the glenoid faces slightly forward (Fig. 3) and should not be positioned so that it

is seen in tangent under the fluoroscope. When the articular surface of the glenoid is tilted slightly anteriorly and the shoulder is flat against the table, the needle tip can pass into the glenohumeral space without perforating the fibrocartilaginous glenoid labrum (Fig. 9).

Under image-intensified fluoroscopy, a lead "o" marker is placed over the glenohumeral joint space at about the junction of its middle and lower thirds (Figs. 4, 5). This point is then marked on the skin with an indelible felt-tipped pen. The patient should remain still because if the arm or shoulder is moved, the mark on the skin may no longer correspond to the glenohumeral joint space.

The standard arthrogram tray described in Chapter 1 is used with the addition of a 22-gauge, 3½-in. disposable spinal needle. Using aseptic technique, the shoulder is wiped with a solution of povidone-iodine and draped (Fig. 6). Using the 25-gauge, ⅝-in. needle, the skin beneath the mark is infiltrated with local anesthetic (1 percent lidocaine hydrochloride). The 22-gauge spinal needle is used for the joint puncture. The needle is inserted into the skin at the mark and directed downward absolutely vertically, toward the glenohumeral joint space (Fig. 7). The position of the needle should be checked frequently by fluoroscopy (Fig. 8). If the needle tip does not overlie the glenohumeral space it should be pulled back and redirected. If the patient experiences discomfort, additional local anesthetic can be injected through the spinal needle.

The normal glenohumeral joint space is relatively deep, so if the needle meets resistance after passing only a short distance, it is fairly certain that the needle is striking the humeral head and is not at its intended location. It is best to have the needle as close as possible to the medial border of the humeral head. If the needle is too close to the rim of the glenoid, it may strike that structure and pass downward medially over the anterior aspect of the scapula, which results in an extra-articular injection. The injection method employing the absolutely vertical needle position allows precise control of the medial-to-lateral course of the needle. Although its depth is not precisely known, this presents no problem.

When the needle meets resistance, it should be impinging on the articular surface of the glenoid. It should then be withdrawn a millimeter or two to free the tip, and a small amount of local anesthetic should be injected. If the needle is intra-articular, the anesthetic flows freely into the joint with little or no resistance to the plunger of the syringe. If the local anesthetic does not flow easily, either the needle tip is not in the joint cavity and needs to be advanced, or the needle tip is embedded in the articular cartilage of the glenoid and needs to be withdrawn a millimeter or two.

To definitively confirm the intra-articular location of the needle, a few drops of contrast material are injected. If the needle is intra-articular, the contrast material should flow away from the needle tip, outlining either the glenohumeral space or its recesses (Fig. 9). If the needle tip is extra-articular, the test injection of contrast material pools around the tip of the needle, infiltrating the soft tissues (Fig. 10). A small amount of extra-articular contrast material in this location does not interfere with the interpretation of an arthrogram because this is not where ruptures of the rotator cuff occur.

After the intra-articular position of the needle is confirmed, 10 to 12 cc of positive contrast agent are injected. If a large (20 cc) syringe is used, considerable pressure may be required to perform the injection through the 22-gauge needle. A 10 cc syringe is recommended for injection. Contrast material may also be injected through sterile connecting tubing, so that its flow into the joint can be observed fluoroscopically.

The shoulder of an average patient accommodates considerably more than the 12 cc of contrast material normally injected before the patient complains of discomfort caused by distention of the capsule. Patients with the diminished joint capacity of adhesive capsulitis (frozen shoulder) may feel pain after only 5 cc of contrast fluid have been injected. If the patient experiences significant pain during the injection, no further contrast material should be introduced.

After the injection of the contrast medium, the needle is removed. Roentgenograms in the anteroposterior projection in internal and external rotation are obtained as well as axillary and bicipital groove views (Figs. 16–19). These roentgenograms can be taken with the patient sitting, standing, or supine. The technician should work as fast as possible because the best roentgenograms are obtained soon after injection, before much of the contrast material is absorbed. While these first roentgenograms are being processed, the patient should exercise the shoulder.

If a complete rotator cuff tear is seen on the first set of roentgenograms (Figs. 25A, B), the examination is completed.

If no abnormality is seen, or if a partial rotator cuff tear is present on the initial set of radiographs (Figs. 32–34), a second postexercise set should be obtained, but with only the internal and external rotation views.

The patient may experience mild discomfort for 24 to 48 hours after the arthrogram and should be so advised.

In addition to the anterior approach with a directly vertical needle path, the arm can be externally rotated and the needle inserted until its tip hits the humeral head. The arm is then internally rotated, so that the needle should slide into the joint space. This method is not recommended, because internal rotation of the humerus usually causes the needle to slide over the glenoid into an extra-articular location, and there is danger that the needle may bend or break when the arm is moved. With a superior approach for needle placement, even a small amount of contrast material injected extra-articularly is in the region of the rotator cuff and can interfere with the interpretation of the arthrogram. An axillary approach for injection has a greater potential for damage to the axillary vessels and nerves. A posterior approach can be utilized, but fluoroscopic control is awkward. The anterior approach with a vertical needle path is simple, and has no drawbacks.

ANATOMY

A fibrous capsule surrounds the joint and is attached medially to the glenoid just beyond the glenoid labrum. Laterally, the capsule is attached to the anatomic neck of the humerus (Fig. 11). The capsule is generally thin, but is thickened anteriorly by the superior, middle, and inferior glenohumeral ligaments. These thickenings of the capsule cannot be appreciated on an arthrogram and play no part in its interpretation. The synovial membrane lines the inner surface of the joint capsule.

The axillary recess is an area of laxity of the inferior and medial portion of the joint capsule (Figs. 11, 17). This recess is obliterated when the arm is raised (Fig. 16). There is normally an opening in the joint capsule anteriorly, beneath the coracoid process, through which the shoulder joint communicates with the subscapularis bursa or recess (Fig. 12). The synovial membrane of the shoulder joint lines the subscapularis bursa, which is an integral part of the shoulder joint (Fig. 16). The synovial-lined capsule also forms the biceps tendon sheath which surrounds the tendon of the long head of the biceps as it exits from the joint in the bicipital groove (Figs. 11, 17). The subscapularis recess or bursa and the reflections of the synovial sheath around the long head of the biceps tendon are the two weakest areas of the joint, as they are in part covered only with a thin synovial membrane.

The glenoid labrum is a rim of dense fibrous tissue and fibrocartilage that completely surrounds the osseous glenoid and its covering of articular cartilage (Fig. 12). On a longitudinal section of the shoulder, it is a triangular structure with a broad base attached to the glenoid. Superiorly, the labrum is continuous with the origin of the tendon of the long head of the biceps.

The musculotendinous portions of the subscapularis, supraspinatus, infraspinatus, and teres minor muscles form the rotator cuff. Surrounding the humeral head, they have a conjoint tendon (Fig. 13). The subscapularis muscle arises from the anterior aspect of the scapula and its tendon inserts onto the lesser tuberosity. The supraspinatus muscle arises from the superior and posterior aspect of the scapula, and its tendon inserts onto the greater tuberosity. The infraspinatus muscle arises from the posterior inferior portion of the scapula, and its tendon inserts onto the greater tuberosity behind the supraspinatus tendon. The teres minor muscle arises from the posterior and inferior portion of the scapula and its tendon also inserts onto the greater tuberosity below and posterior to those of the supraspinatus and infraspinatus muscles. The tendinous portions of these muscles join together and with the joint capsule form a thick covering over the humeral head. The rotator cuff is slightly less than 1 cm in thickness and it separates the joint capsule and cavity from the subacromial–subdeltoid bursa. No normal communication exists between the shoulder joint and the subacromial–subdeltoid bursa (Fig. 14).

The subacromial bursa lies beneath the acromion process and above the rotator cuff. It is continuous with the subdeltoid bursa, which lies beneath the deltoid muscle and above the rotator cuff (Figs. 14, 25).

The subcoracoid bursa, which is not always present, lies anterior to the subscapularis muscle underneath the coracoid process. It is separated from the subscapularis bursa by the thickness of the supscapularis muscle belly. The subcoracoid bursa is not normally connected with the joint capsule but is sometimes connected with the subacromial–subdeltoid bursa.

The tendon of the long head of the biceps muscle arises from the superior rim of the glenoid process, passes intra-articularly over the humeral head, and leaves the joint through the bicipital groove, which lies between the greater and lesser tuberosities. In the groove, the tendon is surrounded by a synovial sheath (Fig. 15).

THE NORMAL ARTHROGRAM

On the anteroposterior radiograph made in internal rotation, the humeral head should be perfectly hemispherical in shape. The injected contrast material covers the articular surface of the humeral head, opacifying a very narrow space between the articular cartilage and the capsule superiolaterally. No contrast material is above the joint capsule, directly beneath the acromion process, or lateral to the joint capsule (Fig. 16). In internal rotation, the subscapularis bursa is well opacified. There is normally an indentation or notch between the subscapularis bursa and the axillary recess. The tendon of the long head of the biceps is rotated medially and is projected over the humeral head near the glenohumeral joint space. A portion of the glenoid labrum surrounding the posterior aspect of the glenoid is seen as a semicircular radiolucent filling defect projected through the humeral head and the contrast-filled joint capsule.

On the anteroposterior radiograph made in external rotation (Fig. 17), the injected contrast material covers the articular surface of the humeral head to the anatomic neck of the humerus where the capsule attaches. In external rotation, the subscapularis bursa is only partially opacified because the subscapularis muscle pushes against it, and some contrast material is squeezed out. In external rotation the tendon of the long head of the biceps muscle overlies the lateral aspect of the humeral head. When the biceps tendon projects over the lateral margin of the humeral head, the opacified synovial sheath must not be mistaken for filling of the subdeltoid bursa (Figs. 20, 21). The origin of the tendon of the long head of the biceps and the superior margin of the glenoid labrum cause a filling defect in the contrast-filled joint just above the superior margin of the glenoid. Contrast material above these structures should not be confused with a partial rotator cuff tear. The biceps tendon is seen as a lucent filling defect within its contrast-filled synovial sheath (Fig. 17).

On the radiographs taken in the axillary projection, a thin layer of contrast material can be seen in the glenohumeral joint space outlining the articular cartilages of the humeral head and the glenoid (Fig. 18). The subscapularis bursa or recess is seen anteriorly, near the base of the coracoid process. The joint capsule is somewhat lax posteriorly, forming the posterior recess. Contrast material can usually be seen in the biceps tendon sleeve located anteriorly, between the greater and lesser tuberosities. The axillary recess is obliterated, since the arm is in abduction. The glenoid labrum is seen as a radiolucent triangular filling defect at both the anterior and posterior margins of the glenoid.

Bicipital groove radiographs (Fig. 19) show the long head of the biceps tendon as an oval filling defect in the contrast-filled synovial sheath. The sheath and tendon are within the bicipital groove between the greater and lesser tuberosities.

LEAKAGE OF CONTRAST MEDIUM

Overdistention of the shoulder joint caused by the injection of too much contrast material or vigorous exercise by the patient can cause contrast material to leak from the subscapularis bursa (Figs. 20, 21) or from the distal end of the synovial sheath surrounding the long head of the biceps tendon (Figs. 22, 23). These are the two weakest areas in the capsule. Contrast material that has leaked from the joint presents a characteristic feathery appearance in the soft tissues. Leaks of contrast medium from the subscapularis bursa are of no clinical significance and do not interfere with the interpretation of the shoulder arthrogram. Leaks from the biceps tendon sleeve usually are of no clinical significance, except in the rare occasion when there is rupture of the biceps tendon, a condition that is readily apparent on clinical examination.

THE ABNORMAL ARTHROGRAM

Complete Rotator Cuff Tears

The term complete rotator cuff tear does not imply that the entire rotator cuff is torn, but only that the tear goes through the complete thickness of that musculotendinous structure (Fig. 24). When such a tear occurs, a communication is established between the glenohu-

meral joint space and the subacromial–subdeltoid bursa, and injected contrast material flows from the joint into the subacromial–subdeltoid bursa (Figs. 25A, B). The opacified subdeltoid bursa extends considerably further down the humeral shaft than the normal capsular insertion. Between the intracapsular contrast material and the bursal contrast material is the residual rotator cuff which may be difficult to evaluate on the positive contrast arthrogram.

When a complete rotator cuff tear is present, it is usually apparent on both the internal and external rotation views of an arthrogram. If not, the axillary view can clarify the diagnosis by showing contrast material in the subdeltoid bursa overlying the humeral shaft well below the normal area of the capsular insertion (Fig. 26). The axillary view is particularly helpful in identifying bursal opacification when chronic disease has caused contraction and deformity of the subacromial–subdeltoid bursa.

On the radiograph taken to show the bicipital groove, bursal filling can be seen anterior to the bicipital tendon sheath.

Neither the size nor the configuration of the opacified subacromial–subdeltoid bursa reflects the size of the tear through the rotator cuff. If only a very small amount of contrast material has passed into the subacromial–subdeltoid bursa on the initial postexercise radiographs, or if no contrast material is seen within the bursa prior to exercise and only on the postexercise roentgenograms, the tear is probably very small.

The precise location of the tear is not ordinarily identified by single contrast shoulder arthrography.

The internal rotation view of the arthrogram can occasionally yield some information about the thickness of the residual rotator cuff, which may interest the surgeon planning an operative repair (Fig. 25B).

When a complete rotator cuff tear is extensive and chronic and there is considerable degeneration of the residual cuff, the diagnosis can be made on routine roentgenograms by identifying narrowing of the space between the humeral head and the acromion and faceting of the undersurface of the acromion process (Figs. 27, 28). Opacification of the acromioclavicular joint (which lies immediately above the subacromial–subdeltoid bursa) can occasionally be seen (Figs. 28B–30). In these cases, a soft tissue mass representing the distended acromioclavicular joint may be palpable.

Partial Rotator Cuff Tears

A partial rotator cuff tear is a tear that does not extend through the full thickness of the musculotendinous rotator cuff (Fig. 31). Opacification of the subacromial–subdeltoid bursa is not seen with this type of tear (Figs. 32, 33). Partial tears which are within or at the superior surface of the rotator cuff are not demonstrable by shoulder arthrography. Only those partial tears that begin on or extend to the undersurface of the rotator cuff and are in contact with the injected contrast medium are visualized.

When a partial rotator cuff tear is present and the tear extends to the undersurface of the cuff, the shoulder arthrogram shows an ulcer-like collection of contrast material within the cuff, usually best seen on the external rotation views (Fig. 32). The contrast material tends to spread within the substance of the cuff, and thin linear streaks of contrast may be identified (Figs. 33, 34).

Many partial rotator cuff tears are seen only on radiographs taken after exercise. Also, what appears to be a partial rotator cuff tear on the pre-exercise films may, after exercise, prove to be a complete, full-thickness tear.

Adhesive Capsulitis (Frozen Shoulder)

An injury, surgery, or pain can cause a patient to limit the motion of the shoulder joint; when movement is curtailed, the joint capsule tends to contract. This contraction may further limit motion and increase shoulder pain. The preliminary films may show demineralization of the humeral head.

The patient who has an adhesive capsulitis or frozen shoulder may be very apprehensive about positioning the shoulder in external rotation for the injection procedure. Because of the contraction of the capsule it may be more difficult to place the tip of the needle into the joint. Additionally, injection of more than a small amount (5 to 6 cc) of contrast material into the joint causes the patient to complain of severe pain and a pronounced sensation of tightness. When the syringe containing the contrast medium is disconnected from the needle, there can be a brisk return flow of fluid from the shoulder joint.

In a shoulder with adhesive capsulitis (Figs. 35A, B), the capsular insertion tends to have a serrated appearance and a more vertical orientation than is noted in the normal shoulder arthrogram. In external rotation, the axillary recess is small and has a pinched-off appearance. In internal rotation, little or no contrast material is seen in the subscapularis bursa. The synovial extension around the long head of the biceps tendon usually fills with contrast material, but it may be tighter than usual. An axillary view shows a smaller than normal posterior recess.

Although it is not abnormal to have contrast mate-

rial leak from the region of the subscapularis recess or from the synovial reflection around the long head of the biceps tendon, leakage is more common in a patient with a frozen shoulder. Contrast material may even leak through the needle puncture site, which is never seen in a joint with a normal capacity.

Postdislocation Capsular Deformity

When the shoulder dislocates anteriorly, it strips the capsule from the anterior rim of the glenoid. After the dislocation has been reduced, the resultant deformity of the capsule can be seen on the arthrogram. On the internal rotation view, the normal notch separating the subscapularis bursa from the axillary recess is obliterated (Figs. 36A, B).

The shoulder arthrogram does not usually provide much information on the subluxing shoulder, but occasionally the external rotation view may show an enlarged axillary recess, and the internal rotation view may show partial obliteration of the notch between the subscapularis bursa and the axillary recess.

Bicipital Abnormalities

Most patients with a rupture of the long head of the biceps tendon do not undergo arthrography, since the diagnosis is obvious from the history and physical examination (Fig. 37A). When the tendon ruptures, both portions retract. If an arthrogram is performed, contrast material is seen within the bicipital tendon sheath, but the radiolucent filling defect of the tendon is absent (Fig. 37B). Leakage of contrast material from the shoulder joint through the bicipital tendon sheath does not in itself indicate a biceps tendon rupture.

If the biceps tendon dislocates from its groove, the external rotation view of the arthrogram shows the medially displaced, contrast-filled synovial sheath and the tendon within it (Fig. 38A). The bicipital groove view best shows the displacement of the tendon (Fig. 38B).

Loose Bodies

Loose bodies appear as filling defects in the opacified joint. They may be fracture fragments of cartilage, with or without subchondral bone, resulting from anterior dislocation. The loose bodies may lodge in any part of the joint and its extensions, such as the biceps tendon sleeve (Figs. 39A, B, C) or subscapularis bursa.

Synovial Abnormalities

When the shoulder joint is involved by rheumatoid arthritis or any of the other diseases producing a villous synovitis, the synovial surface is irregular and corrugated (Fig. 40). In inflammatory arthritis, lymph vessel and lymph node opacification are often seen (Figs. 40, 41). In chronic rheumatoid arthritis, complete rotator cuff tears are common (Fig. 40). Para-articular synovial cysts may opacify.

PITFALLS

There are only a few potential causes of error in the interpretation of shoulder arthrograms. In external ro-tation, the contrast material in the synovial sheath of the long head of the biceps tendon may extend beyond the lateral margin of the humeral head and may be mistaken for the opacified subdeltoid bursa (Figs. 20, 21). Near the origin of the long head of the biceps tendon, it is quite common to see a thin streak of contrast material above the radiolucent tendon. This must not be mistaken for a partial rotator cuff tear (Fig. 17).

Rarely, the subacromial–subdeltoid bursa is inadvertently injected while attempting to inject the glenohumeral joint. In this situation, the arthrographic appearance superficially mimics that of a complete rotator cuff tear, but no contrast material fills the glenohumeral joint space (Fig. 42).

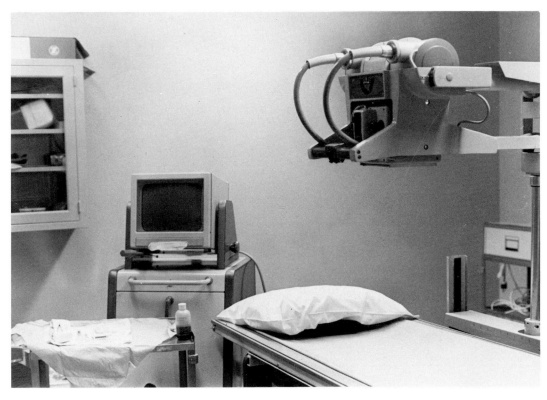

Figure 1
Fluoroscopic equipment with an overhead tube and under table image intensifier is preferred because it allows adequate space above the patient to keep needles and gloved hands sterile. The arthrogram tray, to which a 22-gauge disposable spinal needle has been added, is near the table.

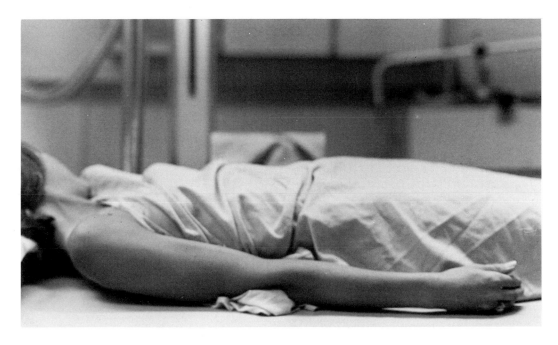

Figure 2
The patient lies supine with the arm close to the side and the thumb up. A pillow under the elbow keeps the patient comfortable.

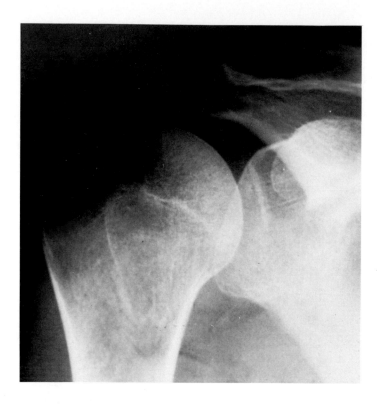

Figure 3
A roentgenogram of the shoulder, taken with the patient supine, shows the humeral head in moderate external rotation. The glenoid articular surface appears oval because it is tilted anteriorly.

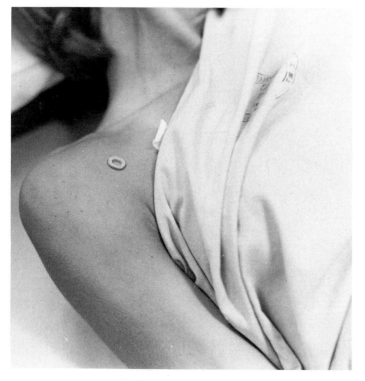

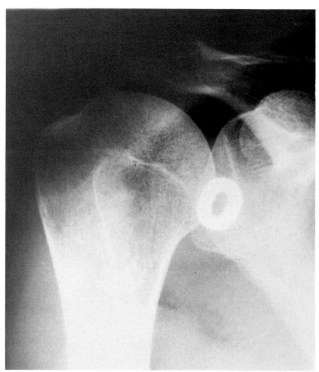

Figures 4 and 5
With fluoroscopic guidance, a lead marker is placed on the patient's skin overlapping the inner margin of the humeral head at the junction of the middle and lower thirds of the glenoid process. The spot is marked on the skin with indelible ink.

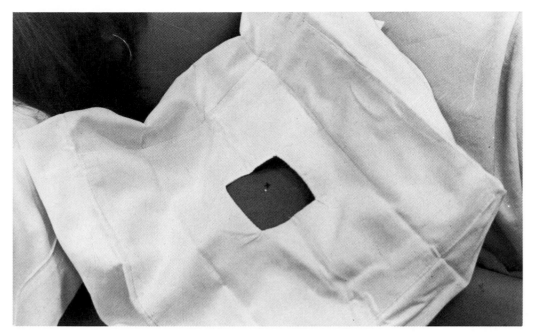

Figure 6
After an area at and around the mark made on the skin has been scrubbed with po-vidone-iodine solution, a drape sheet with a 2 × 2 in. hole is placed over the shoulder.

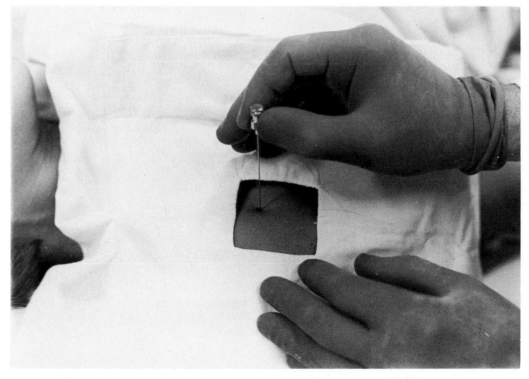

Figure 7
After subcutaneous local anesthesia with 1 percent lidocaine hydrochloride, the 22-gauge disposable spinal needle is inserted at the skin mark in a perfectly vertical di-rection. Local anesthesia is injected through this needle into the deeper tissues.

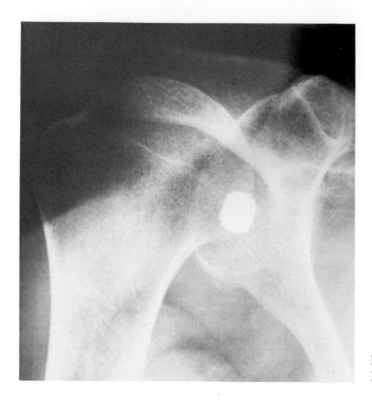

Figure 8
Progress of the needle is checked fluoroscopically.

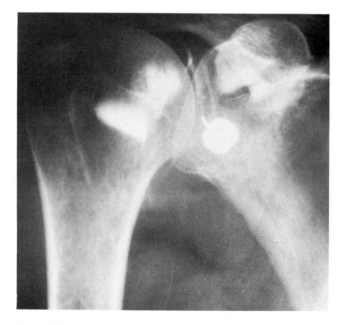

Figure 9
When fluoroscopic observation and reduced resistance to the injection of local anesthesia indicates that the needle has perforated the capsule and that its tip is within the joint, a small amount of positive contrast is injected. The contrast substance immediately leaves the needle tip and opacifies the subscapularis bursa, the glenohumeral space, or a portion of the joint behind the humeral head.

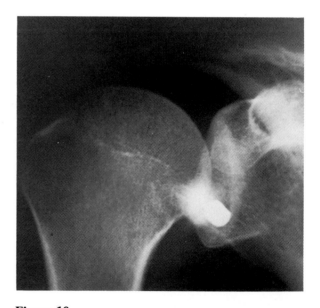

Figure 10
The cloud-like opacification at the tip of the needle after injection of a few drops of positive contrast agent indicates that the needle tip is in an extra-articular location. Extra-articular contrast substance in this location does not interfere with interpretation of the arthrogram. After the needle has been advanced a little further and its tip lies within the joint, the arthrogram can proceed.

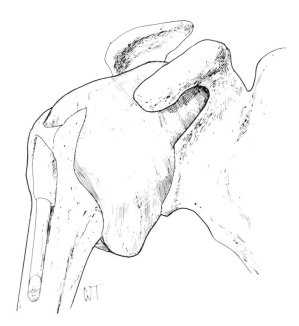

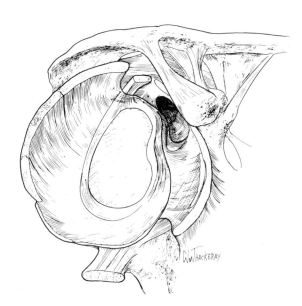

Figure 11

The shoulder joint capsule is shown extending from the glenoid to the anatomic neck of the humerus including the subscapularis bursa and the biceps tendon sheath. The redundant fold of capsule between the inferior margin of the glenoid and the humerus, called the axillary recess, is obliterated when the arm is fully abducted.

Figure 12

The glenoid fossa with the capsule partially resected is seen *en face.* A fibrocartilagenous glenoid rim deepens the glenoid fossa. The cut biceps tendon is visible superiorly. Anterior to the superior glenoid rim and inferior to the coracoid proccss is a hole through which the subscapularis bursa communicates with the shoulder joint.

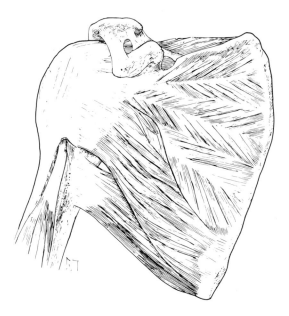

Figure 13

The musculo-tendinous rotator cuff is shown from the front (A) and the back (B). The rotator cuff is formed by the subscapularis, which inserts anteriorly at the lesser tuberosity, and by the supraspinatus, infraspinatus, and teres minor, which insert into the greater tuberosity from an anterosuperior to posteroinferior direction.

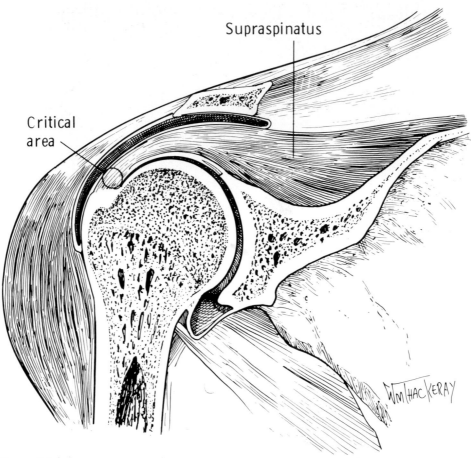

Figure 14
The space between the rotator cuff and the acromion process and deltoid muscle is occupied by the normally collapsed subacromial subdeltoid bursa. There is normally no communication between this bursa and the shoulder joint. Tears of the rotator cuff occur most frequently in the supraspinatus near its insertion.

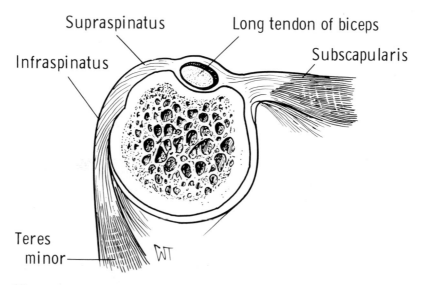

Figure 15
The tendon of the long head of the biceps muscle lies within its sheath in the bicipital groove between the greater and lesser tuberosities of the humerus.

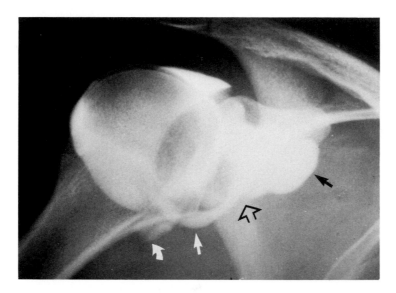

Figure 16
The humerus is internally rotated. Contrast agent envelops the humeral head and fills the subscapularis bursa (black arrow), which lies inferior to the coracoid process. The axillary recess (white arrow) appears small because the arm is partially abducted. The border between the subscapularis bursa and axillary recess is well defined (open black arrow). The opacified biceps tendon sleeve (curved white arrow) is rotated medially, and its distal end is seen medial to the upper shaft of the humerus. The glenoid labrum forms a sharply defined oval filling defect. There is no contrast agent beneath the acromion process.

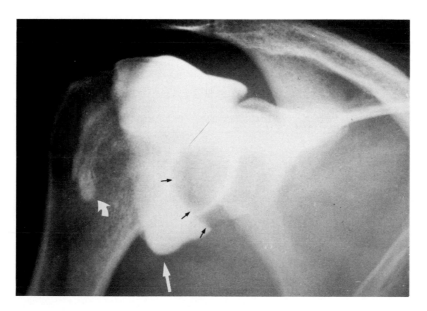

Figure 17
With the humerus in external rotation and with the arm at the side, the axillary recess is well filled with contrast substance (white arrow). The subscapularis bursa is only partially opacified because it is compressed by the subscapularis muscle. The opacified biceps tendon sleeve (curved white arrow) has rotated laterally and the longitudinal filling defect within the sleeve represents the biceps tendon. The intra-articular portion of the biceps tendon cannot be identified. The glenoid labrum forms an elliptical filling defect (black arrows).

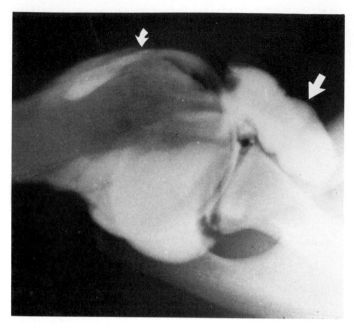

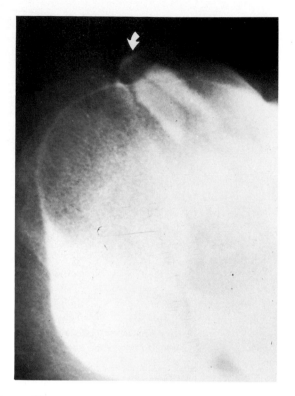

Figure 18

The axillary view shows the contrast-filled subscapularis bursa (white arrow), and the contrast-filled biceps tendon sleeve anteriorly (curved white arrow), and the opacified posterior capsular recess. No contrast agent crosses the humerus distal to the anatomic neck. The glenoid labrum can be identified at the margins of the glenoid tuberosity; however, its sharp edge is not clearly seen on a single positive contrast study.

Figure 19

The bicipital groove view shows the biceps tendon as a filling defect within its contrast-filled sleeve (arrow) and lying normally in the bicipital groove.

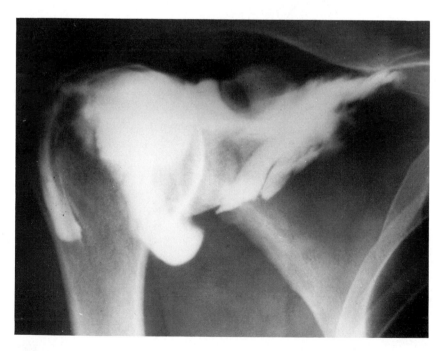

Figure 20

Leakage of positive contrast agent from the subscapularis bursa, particularly if occurring after the patient has exercised the shoulder, is not by itself a sign of shoulder joint pathology.

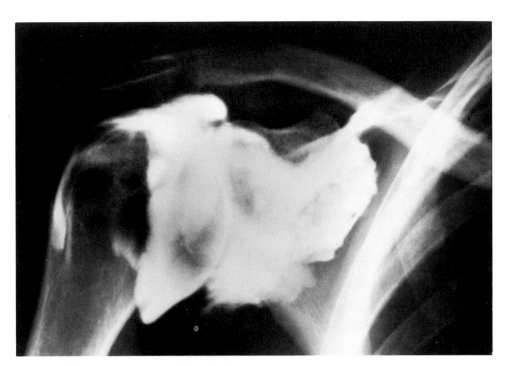

Figure 21
Positive contrast agent has leaked from the subscapularis bursa. This by itself is of no clinical significance, but the shoulder capsule appears tight and the edge of capsular insertion at the anatomic neck has a serrated appearance. The biceps tendon sleeve and axillary recess appear contracted, suggesting an adhesive capsulitis (frozen shoulder). The leak is caused by overdistension of a contracted capsule.

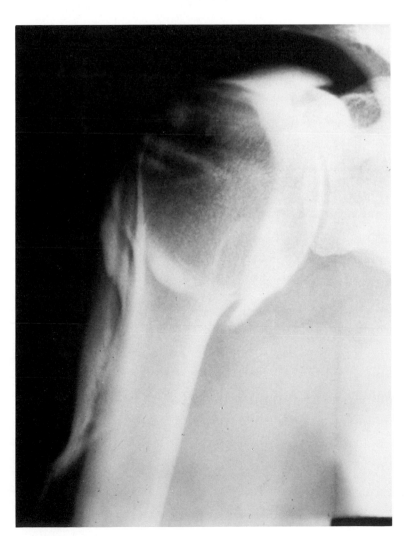

Figure 22
Leakage of contrast agent from the end of the biceps tendon sleeve similar to leakage from the subscapularis bursa is not a sign of specific shoulder joint disease. It occurs with overdistension of the joint capsule or with vigorous exercise which raises intracapsular pressure. The axillary recess appears pinched-off, and the lateral border of the contrast-filled capsule appears serrated and somewhat irregular, suggesting a diagnosis of frozen shoulder.

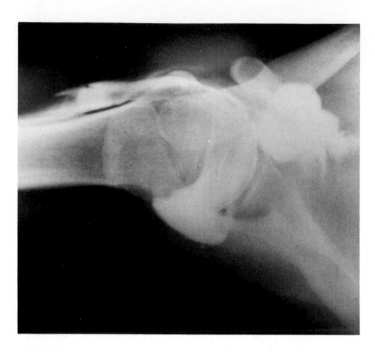

Figure 23
Leakage of contrast agent from the end of the biceps
tendon sleeve is seen on an axillary view.

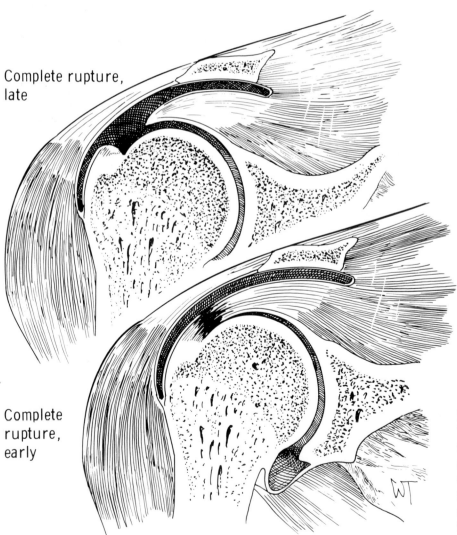

Complete rupture,
late

Complete
rupture,
early

Figure 24
The drawings of a coronal section through the shoulder joint
show how a complete rotator
cuff tear forms a communication between the shoulder joint
and the subacromial–subdeltoid bursa.

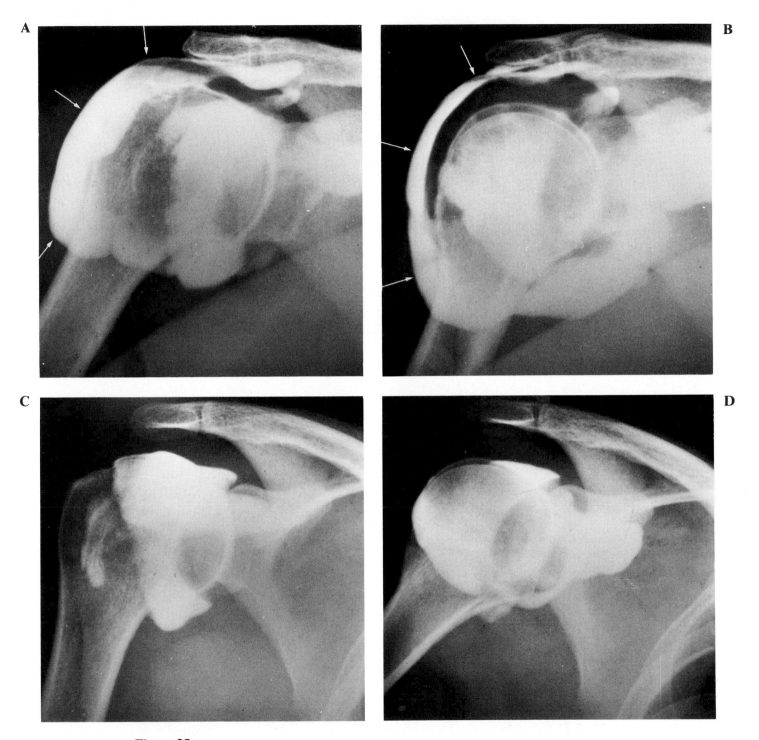

Figure 25
A. On the external rotation view, contrast agent is within the joint as well as within the subacromial–subdeltoid bursa (white arrows).
B. On the internal rotation view, the wide space between the humeral head and the undersurface of the subacromial–subdeltoid bursa indicates that the rotator cuff is not totally degenerated and that the tear is relatively small. The exact size of the tear cannot be evaluated from this positive contrast study.
C,D. The external and internal rotation views of a normal arthrogram show no contrast agent in the subacromial bursa.

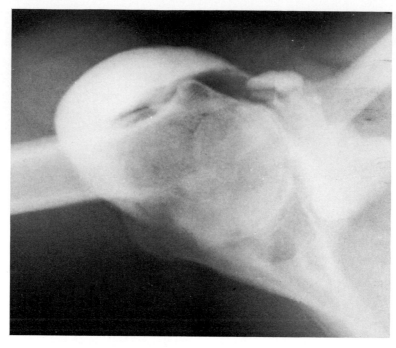

Figure 26
A complete rotator cuff tear is indicated on an axillary view by seeing contrast agent within the subdeltoid bursa. The positive contrast overlies the humeral shaft well below the anatomic neck of the humerus where the joint capsule inserts.

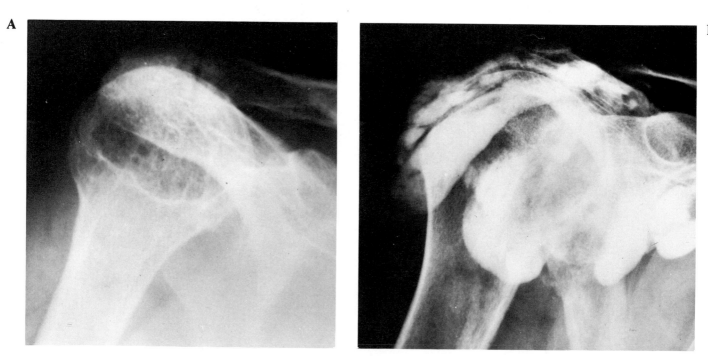

Figure 27
A. Upward displacement of the humeral head which articulates with the undersurface of the acromion is diagnostic of a large, chronic degenerative rotator cuff tear.
B. The arthrogram showing an opacified subacromial–subdeltoid bursa confirms the diagnosis of rotator cuff tear.

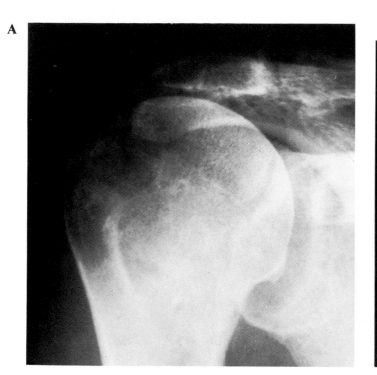
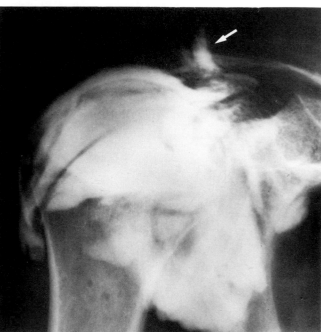

Figure 28
A,B. Upward displacement of the humerus and articulation with a faceted under-surface of the acromion indicates a large chronic rotator cuff tear. The arthrogram shows opacification of both the subacromial–subdeltoid bursa and the acromiocla-vicular joint (arrow).

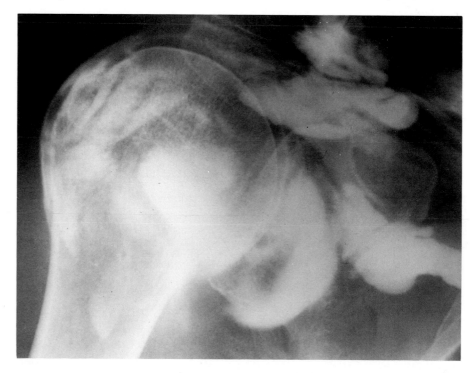

Figure 29
A rotator cuff tear with contrast agent extending from the shoulder joint into the subacromial bursa, and from there into the acromioclavicular joint, is demonstrated.

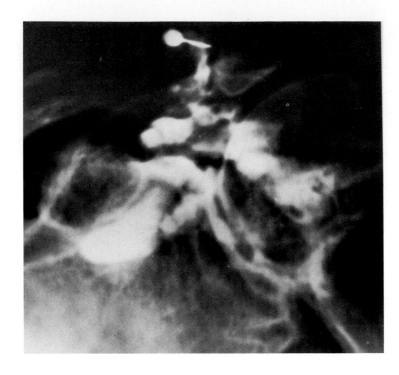

Figure 30
Contrast agent injected into an osteoarthritic acromioclavicular joint shows communication with the subacromial bursa and the shoulder joint, indicating a rotator cuff tear.

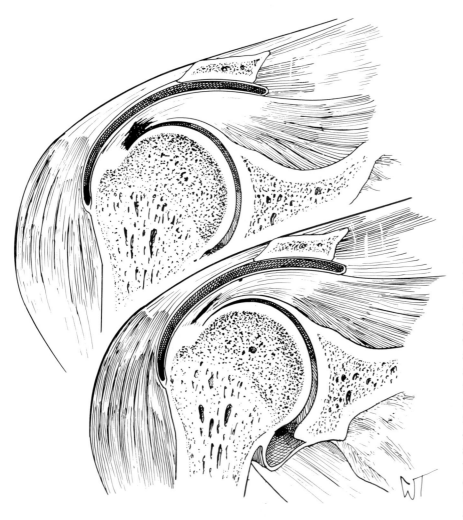

Figure 31
A partial rotator cuff tear on the undersurface of the rotator cuff is shown on drawings of a coronal section of the shoulder. Such tears are usually located in the region of the supraspinatus tendon insertion and extend into, but not through, the thickness of the rotator cuff. There is no communication between the shoulder joint and subacromial-subdeltoid bursa. Partial tears that do not extend to the undersurface of the cuff cannot be seen on a shoulder arthrogram.

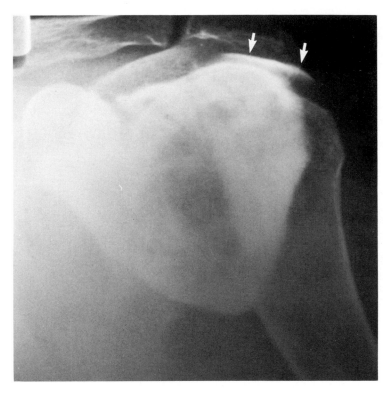

Figure 32
A partial rotator cuff tear shows positive contrast agent within the rotator cuff (arrows) but not in the subdeltoid bursa.

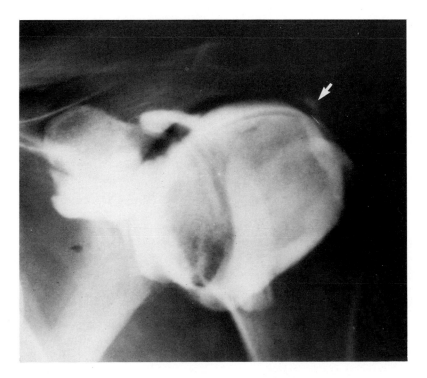

Figure 33
A very small partial rotator cuff tear is indicated by faint opacification within the rotator cuff in the region of the supraspinatus tendon (arrow).

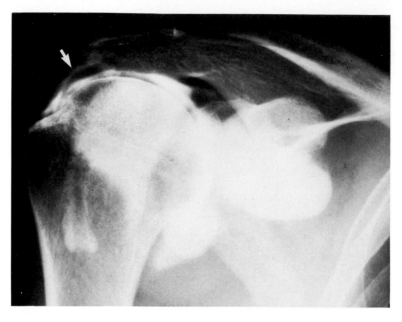

Figure 34
A partial rotator cuff tear is indicated by a crescentic streak of contrast agent within the rotator cuff (arrow). The bursa is not opacified.

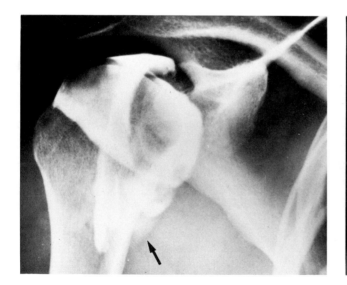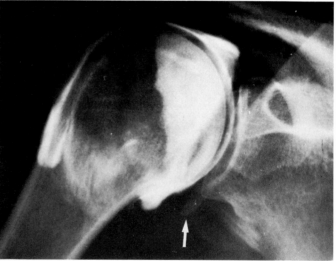

Figure 35
A,B. The capsule is very tight and the patient complained of pain after the injection of 5 cc of fluid. The capsular insertion at the neck of the humerus is serrated, the axillary recess is small, and the biceps tendon sleeve appears tight. Some leakage of positive contrast agent from the needle hole (arrows) has occurred at the inferior medial aspect of the joint. On the external rotation view (B), the opacified biceps tendon sleeve should not be mistaken for an opacified subdeltoid bursa.

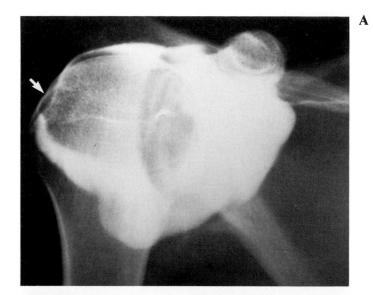

A

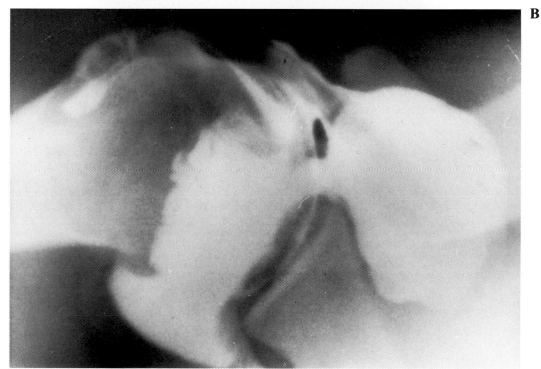

B

Figure 36
A. After an anterior subcoracoid dislocation of the humeral head, the anterior intra-capsular space is enlarged. The sharp distinction between the subscapularis bursa and axillary recess is lost and the axillary recess is much larger than normal. A Hill Sachs compression deformity on the lateral aspect of the internally rotated humeral head is accentuated by adjacent intra-articular positive contrast substance (arrow).
B. The enlarged axillary recess is seen particularly well on the axillary view.

A

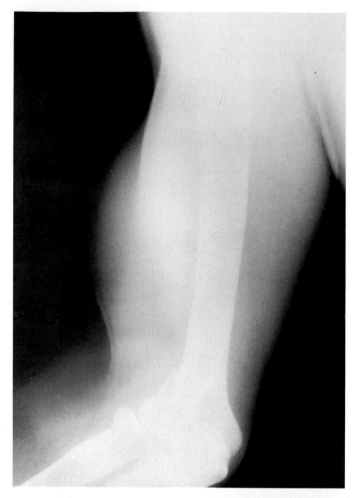

B

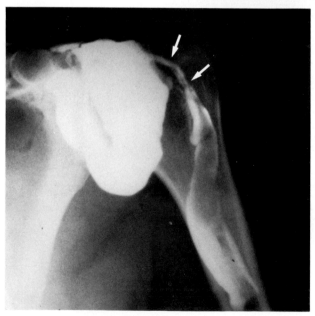

Figure 37
A. Rupture of the biceps tendon causing a bunching up of the biceps muscle above the antecubital fossa is evident on clinical examination and can be seen on a soft tissue roentgenogram.
B. An arthrogram shows the absence of the biceps tendon from its sleeve (arrows) and leakage of contrast agent from the distal end of the biceps tendon sleeve. Although leakage of contrast agent can occur after biceps tendon rupture, the finding of leakage by itself is rarely an indication that the biceps tendon is ruptured (see Figs. 22, 23).

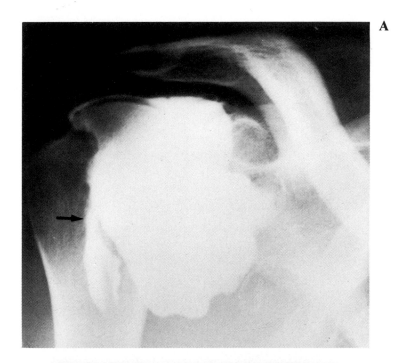

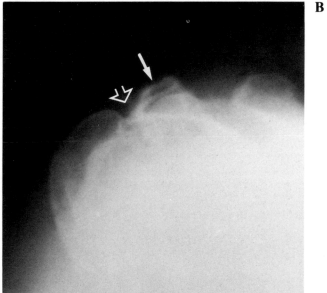

Figure 38
A. A dislocated biceps tendon (arrow) is seen on an external rotation view, far medial of its normal location.
B. The bicipital groove view shows the empty bicipital groove (open arrow) and the biceps tendon in its opacified sheath lying medially to the groove (arrow).

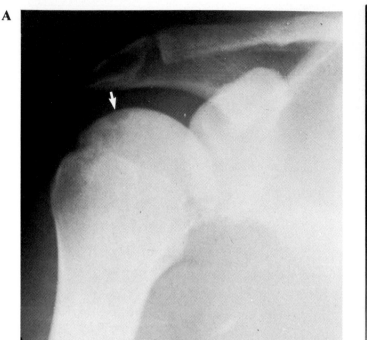

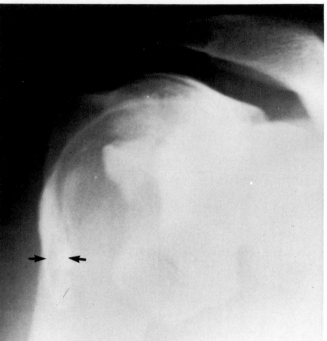

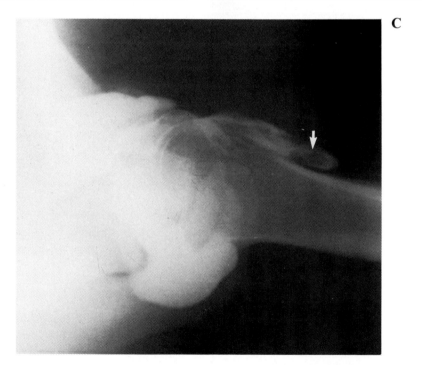

Figure 39

A. A routine roentgenogram of the shoulder with the humeral head in internal rotation shows a compression fracture on the posterolateral margin of the humeral head (arrow) caused by a previous anterior dislocation.

B. The arthrogram shows a cartilaginous body (arrows) appearing as a filling defect in the biceps tendon sleeve.

C. The axillary projection best shows the filling defect (arrow) in the biceps tendon sleeve.

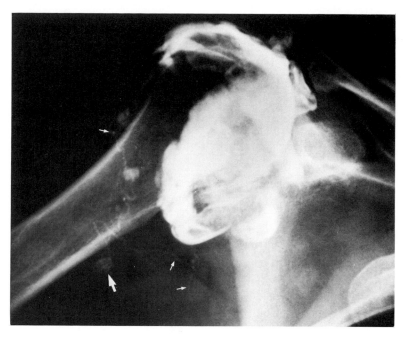

Figure 40
Inflammatory arthritis (rheumatoid arthritis) of the shoulder shows a rotator cuff tear causing filling of a contracted subacromial subdeltoid bursa. The synovial lining of the joint and bursa is irregular because of villous synovitis. Lymphatic vessels and nodes are opacified, indicating inflammatory joint disease (arrows).

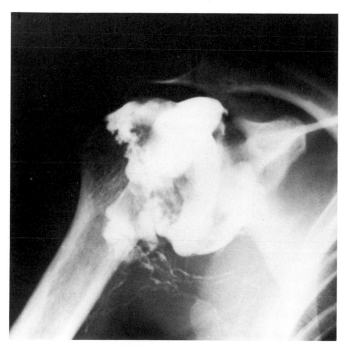

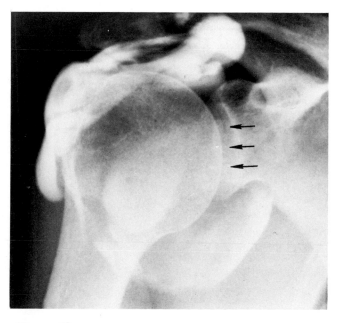

Figure 41
Rheumatoid arthritis of the shoulder shows villous synovitis and lymphatic opacification.

Figure 42
An inadvertent injection opacified the subacromial–subdeltoid bursa which was distended by an effusion. There is no contrast agent within the shoulder joint (arrows). A few days later, an intra-articular injection of positive contrast agent showed no bursal opacification, ruling out a rotator cuff tear.

8
Double Contrast Shoulder Arthrography

Amy Beth Goldman

The general indication for all shoulder arthrograms is persistent pain and/or weakness, in the presence of nondiagnostic plain film studies. Specific indications include injuries to the tendons of the rotator cuff and the long head of the biceps brachii, deformities or erosions of the articular cartilages, and abnormalities of the joint capsule.

For all these abnormalities, double contrast shoulder arthrograms may provide clinically pertinent information not available from positive contrast studies.

TECHNIQUE

Preliminary roentgenograms of the shoulder with internal and external rotation of the humerus as well as axillary and bicipital groove views are taken.

The injection is performed with the patient supine and the shoulder held in minimal external rotation (Fig. 1A). Placing the patient in a posterior oblique position to visualize the joint in tangent is not advisable because it rotates the fibrous labrum of the glenoid over the joint space, obstructing the needle path. Under fluoroscopic control, a lead marker is placed over the center of the glenohumeral joint and the point is marked on the skin (Figs. 1B, C). Following the ad-

ministration of local anesthesia, and using sterile technique, a 22-gauge, 3½-in. spinal needle is directed straight down into the joint space (Fig. 1D). If the needle is aimed too high, leakage of extra-articular contrast medium obscures the area of the rotator cuff. If the needle is aimed too low it is possible to miss the joint by passing through the axillary recess or to administer an axillary block with local anesthetic. When the needle is within the joint, a test injection demonstrates positive contrast material flowing away from the needle around the humeral head and across the humeral neck (Fig. 1E). If the needle is extra-articular, the contrast remains pooled around the tip. After successful positioning of the needle, 3 to 4 cc of 60 percent meglumine positive contrast agent are injected, followed by 10 cc of room air (Fig. 1F), and the needle is removed. Four routine roentgen studies are obtained: an internal and external rotation view with the patient standing, then an axillary view and bicipital groove view with the patient supine. The exposure setting for the standing views should be less than those used for the preinjection radiographs, so that the soft tissues coated by contrast and outlined by air are not overexposed. The axillary and external rotation views can be overpenetrated for optimum visualization of the articular cartilages. For the internal and external rotation

165

studies, the standing patient holds a 5-lb sandbag to produce distraction of the joint. The X-ray beam is angled 15° toward the feet to project the area of the rotator cuff away from the acromion process (Figs. 2A, B). The axillary view is filmed with the patient supine because the anterior glenoid labrum is outlined by a thin coating of positive contrast and air while most of the positive contrast material remains pooled in the posterior recess. If it is suspected that the patient has had a posterior dislocation, then a prone axillary view is added for better visualization of the dorsal aspect of the glenoid labrum. For the bicipital groove view, the patient may be either standing or supine.

If the initial films show a complete rotator cuff tear, the examination is terminated. If the initial studies appear normal, the patient is asked to exercise the shoulder and the films are repeated, since the second set may demonstrate a partial or complete cuff tear.

The amount of contrast material injected is critical. Excessive injections of air produce leakage via the subscapularis bursa (Fig. 3A) and/or the distal end of the sheath of the biceps tendon (Fig. 3B)—the normal weak points in the capsule. Excessive injection of positive contrast obscures the articular cartilages.

ANATOMY

Both the humeral head and glenoid are covered by hyaline cartilage. The glenoid has an additional fibrous labrum making it a more cup-shaped structure than it appears on routine roentgenograms (Fig. 4A).

The glenohumeral joint is surrounded and reinforced by three distinct soft tissue envelopes. Closest to the bone and cartilage is the synovial-lined joint capsule (Fig. 4B). It attaches to the humerus at the anatomic neck and to the osseous rim of the glenoid (Fig. 4B). The capsule has two normal outpouchings: the axillary recess, which extends between the scapula and the humerus, and the subscapularis bursa immediately below the coracoid process (Fig. 4B). Surrounding the synovial-lined capsule, and actually incorporated into it, is the second strong reinforcing sheath composed of the tendons of the rotator cuff: the subscapularis, the supraspinatus, the infraspinatus, and the teres minor (Fig. 4C). The tendons of these muscles occupy most of the space between the humeral head and the acromion process. Outside the rotator cuff is the third thin envelope composed of the subacromial bursa which, as its name suggests, is below the acromion process, the subdeltoid bursa, which is below the deltoid muscle, and, in some individuals, the subcoracoid bursa. The subacromial and subdeltoid bursae communicate with each other and are actually a single sac that covers the outer surface of the rotator cuff (Fig. 4D). They can communicate with the joint capsule only if there is a complete tear of the intervening rotator cuff.

The tendon of the long head of biceps brachii originates just proximal to the superior lip of the glenoid labrum (Fig. 4E). From its origin to the bicipital groove, it is an intra-articular structure, and for a short distance below the groove it is covered by a synovial-lined capsular reflection, the biceps tendon sheath, which communicates with the joint (Fig. 4E).

THE NORMAL ARTHROGRAM

Compared with the positive contrast arthrogram, the double contrast technique provides superior visualization of (1) the inferior surface of the rotator cuff, which is seen to best advantage on the radiographs taken with the patient standing; (2) the proximal portion of the tendon of the long head of the biceps, which is visualized on all four routine views; and (3) the anterior aspect of the glenoid labrum, outlined clearly on the external rotation and axillary views.

The internal and external rotation views (Figs. 5A, B) demonstrate the attachment of the contrast-filled capsule to the humeral neck, the axillary recess, which provides the necessary redundancy to elevate the arm, and the subscapularis bursa. Air rising to the top of the joint clearly outlines the contrast coated superior capsule which is part of the inferior surface of the rotator cuff. The entire proximal portion of the tendon of the long head of the biceps is visualized as a soft tissue density within the air-distended capsule and synovial-lined sheath (Fig. 5). On the internal rotation view, the biceps tendon is superimposed on the humeral head lateral to the glenoid (Fig. 5A). On the external rotation view (Fig. 5B), the biceps tendon parallels the superior surface of the humeral head and turns downward and laterally into the bicipital groove where it lies within its synovial sheath. The articular cartilages are seen to best advantage on an external rotation view with the patient in a 15° posterior oblique position to obtain a tangential view of the joint.

A normal supine axillary view (Fig. 5C) shows that the opacified capsule does not extend below the neck of the humerus. There is no contrast material superimposed on the proximal humeral shaft. The sharply pointed anterior glenoid labrum is demonstrated. Both the normal axillary and bicipital groove views (Figs. 5C, D) reveal the contrast-coated tendon of the long head of the biceps and its air-filled sheath resting between the greater and lesser tuberosities.

THE ABNORMAL ARTHROGRAM

Rotator Cuff Tears

The diagnosis of a rotator cuff tear is difficult to establish clinically. The classic textbook description of shoulder pain accompanied by an inability to elevate the arm and maintain abduction occurs in a minority of patients. In the majority, the intact tendons are sufficient to initiate and hold abduction. In most instances, when plain roentgenograms are negative for fracture and calcium deposits, a rotator cuff tear is suspected clinically because the patient is middle-aged, and complains of chronic pain and weakness. Most tears are the result of trauma and degenerative changes in the tendons of a middle-aged person. Both single and double contrast arthrograms provide an accurate means of confirming a diagnosis of tear.

A complete rotator cuff tear does not refer to rupture of all four tendons. Rather it indicates that the interruption extends through the entire width of one or more of the four muscles. The most common site of injury is at the insertion of the supraspinatus tendon on the greater tuberosity. A partial tear refers to an interruption that does not extend through the entire width of the cuff. Partial tears can occur on both the superior and inferior surfaces of the cuff, but only those on the inferior surface that tear the adjacent capsule can be diagnosed by shoulder arthrography.

The extension of injected contrast material into the subacromial and subdeltoid bursae is the arthrographic criterion for a complete rotator cuff tear (Figs. 6–10). On the internal and external rotation views, contrast is seen beneath the acromion process, lateral to the humeral head and below the greater tuberosity. On the axillary projection, an abnormal collection of contrast material within the subdeltoid bursa extends across the proximal end of the humeral shaft (Fig. 6C). Partial tears appear roentgenographically as abnormal collections of air and/or positive contrast material extending above the articular cartilage of the humeral head (Figs. 11, 12). These small interruptions in the inferior surface of the tendons are frequently only visualized on the postexercise study (Fig. 11).

Once the diagnosis of a rotator cuff tear is established, two decisions in clinical management remain: first, the choice of surgical candidates, and second, in operative cases, the choice of the optimum incision to achieve a tension-free repair. The indications for surgery include acute traumatic tears and chronic tears which even after a course of conservative therapy still produce pain and weakness. The principal contraindication to surgery is severe degeneration of the tendons, leaving the surgeon, as stated by McLaughlin, "only

rotten cloth to sew." The double contrast arthrogram has the advantage over the single contrast study of visualizing cuff fragments coated by contrast and shadowed by air. Thus the size of the tear and the quality of the remaining tissues can be visualized. A traumatic tear shows the torn tendons to be smooth, of normal width, and occupying almost the entire space between the humeral head and the acromion process (Fig. 6). If there are also degenerative changes, the arthrogram reveals irregularity of the surfaces of the torn tendons, air and/or contrast within the fragments, and thinning of the torn tendons (Figs. 7–10). On plain radiographs, a decrease in the distance between the humeral head and the acromion process, or a faceting of the undersurface of the acromion, is a sign of a large chronic rotator cuff tear. Should an arthrogram be performed, it will reveal a large rotator cuff tear with severe degenerative changes in the small remaining portions of the cuff. Patients with rheumatoid arthritis frequently have destruction of the rotator cuff involving all of the tendons (Fig. 10).

Evaluation of the width of the tear is important because a good surgical result requires complete resection of dead tissue and a tension-free suture line. Preoperative recognition of a wide tear may alter the surgical approach or indicate that a planned repair is not feasible.

Biceps Tendon Abnormalities

The double contrast arthrogram is superior to a positive contrast study for the evaluation of the long head of the biceps because the entire intra-articular portion of the tendon can be seen and there are fewer cases of failure to fill the sheath.

The double contrast technique shows the proximal portion of the tendon of the long head of the biceps coated by contrast material within the air-distended capsule and its synovial-lined sheath (Fig. 5). Complete rupture of the long head of the biceps is diagnosed arthrographically by failure to visualize the shadow of the tendon within the capsule or sheath, and/or by distortion or dilation of the sheath (Figs. 13, 14). The leakage of contrast from the distal end of the biceps tendon sheath by itself is not an indication of a biceps tendon tear (Fig. 3B). The synovial reflection is normally a weak point in the capsule and leakage is usually the result of increased intracapsular pressure caused by vigorous exercise, overdistension of the joint from injecting too much contrast agent, or diminution of the capacity of the capsule. Leakage is rarely associated with abnormalities of the tendon itself.

Incomplete tears and tenosynovitis of the tendon of

the long head of the biceps are conditions that produce chronic, nonspecific shoulder pain. Both entities are characterized arthrographically by an increase in the width of the tendon and irregularity or loss of the sharp margin of the sheath caused by edema (Fig. 15).

Medial dislocation of the biceps tendon results from a combination of trauma and anatomic variations in the bicipital groove. The displacement is usually a temporary but recurrent phenomenon related to the position of the arm. It results in chronic shoulder pain associated with a snapping sensation. The condition can be recognized if the tendon does not show its normal shift in its projection on internal and external rotation films. The opacified biceps tendon sheath has an irregular margin and is displaced medial to the bicipital groove (Fig. 16A). The diagnosis is most reliably made on the bicipital and axillary views because the displaced tendon can be seen outside of its normal osseous intertubercular groove (Figs. 14, 16). On the axillary view, the subluxed tendon projects anterior to the lesser tuberosity (Fig. 16B). On the bicipital groove view the dislocated biceps tendon is seen medial to the tuberosities (Figs. 14C, 16C).

Articular Cartilage Abnormalities

The articular cartilage abnormalities that result from shoulder dislocations are best seen on the double contrast arthrogram. Capsular deformities are seen equally well on a single contrast study (Fig. 17). On a single contrast arthrogram, the articular cartilages are partly obscured by the density of the positive contrast medium, while on double contrast studies, they are clearly outlined. The Bankart deformity, a compression or avulsion defect of the anterior inferior rim of the glenoid, is infrequently identified on plain films (Fig. 18A) because it rarely involves the subchondral bone. On double contrast arthrograms, the cartilage deformity can be visualized with the glenoid articular surface tangent to the X-ray beam on the 15° posterior oblique radiograph taken with the patient standing (Figs. 17, 18B). On the axillary view, taken with the patient supine, the blunted positive contrast-coated anterior labrum shadowed by air is seen (Fig. 18C). If the patient is referred for a suspected previous posterior dislocation—a rare occurrence—the axillary view should be performed with the patient prone to evaluate the posterior aspect of the labrum.

The Hill-Sachs compression defect is frequently seen on plain films. However, a small deformity limited to the articular cartilage is best detected by a double contrast arthrogram (Fig. 19B).

In addition to documenting irreversible capsular and cartilage changes the arthrogram can also detect coexisting rotator cuff tears that may produce persistent pain (Figs. 19A, B).

Loose Bodies

The localization of loose osteocartilaginous fragments can also be an indication for double contrast shoulder arthrography. The loose cartilaginous fragments which can result from Bankart fractures, osteonecrosis, and osteoarthritis tend to collect in the axillary recess (Fig. 20), the subscapularis bursa, and the biceps tendon sheath (Fig. 21).

Adhesive Capsulitis (Frozen Shoulder)

If adhesive capsulitis is present and a double contrast arthrogram is performed, the patient may not feel the characteristic discomfort experienced by a positive contrast injection. The probable reason is the immediate decompression of the capsule owing to leakage of air and contrast from the joint, usually from the subscapularis bursa or biceps tendon sheath. On double contrast arthrograms, the diagnostic criteria for adhesive capsulitis are contraction of the capsule with pinching of the axillary recess, reduced volume of the subscapularis bursa, and a saw-tooth deformity at the insertion of the capsule into the humerus (Fig. 22).

PITFALLS

On the external rotation view, the contrast-filled biceps tendon sleeve must not be mistaken for the contrast-filled subdeltoid bursa. The air-shadowed soft tissues—particularly those of the rotator cuff—can be too dark if the exposure settings used for the preliminary roentgenograms are not reduced. Injection of more than 10 cc of room air usually causes leakage from the joint. Contrast-coated air bubbles should not be mistaken for loose cartilaginous bodies. If the subdeltoid bursa is opacified, a careful check should be made to determine whether there is contrast agent in the shoulder joint since it is possible to inject the bursa directly. The opacification of the bursa after inadvertent injection is not indicative of a rotator cuff tear.

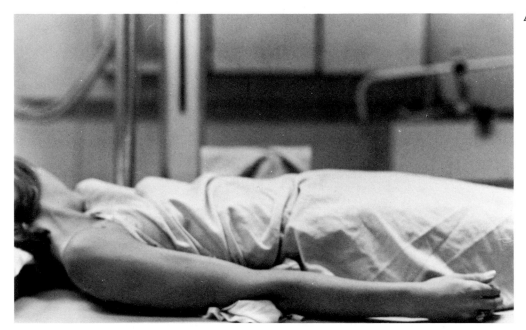

A

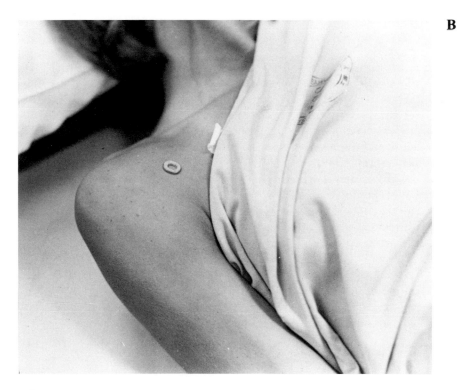

B

Figure 1

A–F. The technique of needle placement for double contrast arthrography is identical to that of the single contrast study, although the amount of contrast media injected differs.

A. The patient is placed supine on the table with the shoulder in minimal abduction and external rotation.

B, C. A lead marker is placed on the skin, and under fluoroscopic control is adjusted until it rests over the center of the glenohumeral joint. This point is then marked on the skin with indelible ink. (**C** on next page)

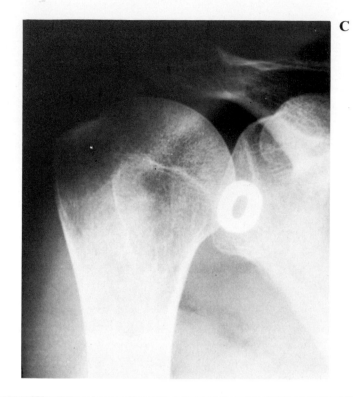

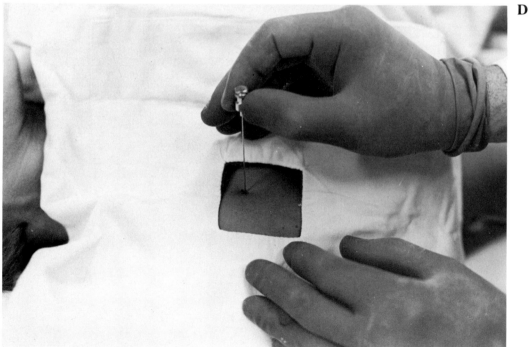

Figure 1
D. Following sterile preparation of the shoulder and administration of local anesthesia, a 22-gauge spinal needle is directed straight down into the joint space.

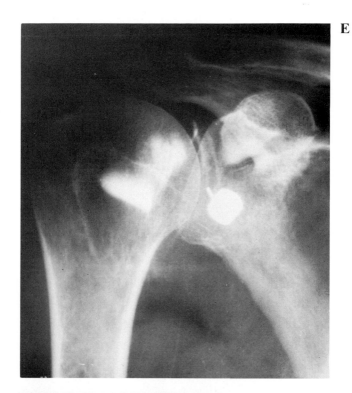

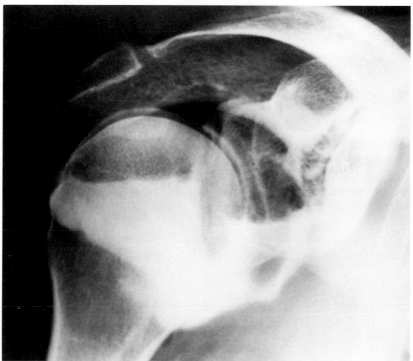

Figure 1
E. A test injection performed with a small amount of positive contrast agent shows contrast agent around the humeral head or across the humeral neck, or in some cases in the subscapularis bursa, indicating intra-articular needle placement.
F. After successful positioning of the needle, 4 cc of a meglumine positive contrast agent followed by 10 cc of room air are injected and the needle is removed.

A
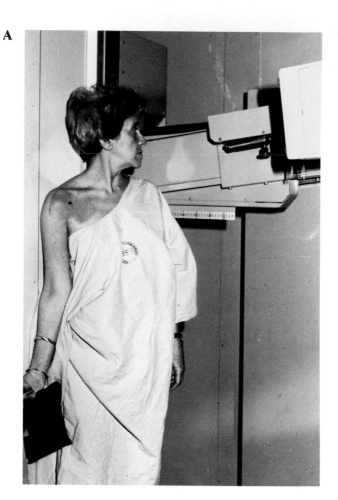

B
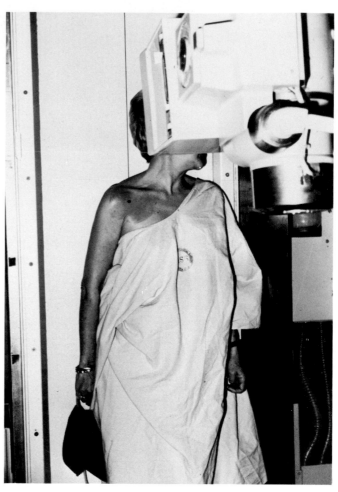

Figure 2

The routine arthrogram includes external and internal rotation views of the shoulder taken with the patient standing and holding a 5-lb sandbag to produce distraction on the joint.

A. The external rotation view is filmed with the shoulder in a slight posterior oblique projection to view the joint in tangent for optimum visualization of articular cartilage.

B. The internal rotation view is obtained with the shoulder flat against the table. Soft tissue technique enhances detail in the region of the rotator cuff.

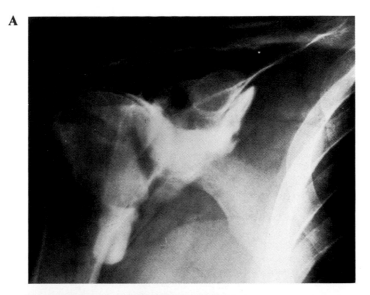

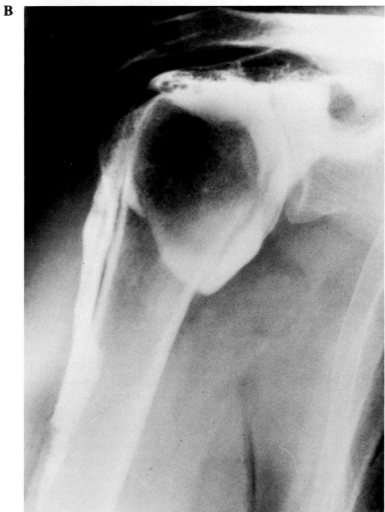

Figure 3
Leakage from the subscapularis bursa (A) or biceps tendon sheath (B) is related to
the capacity of the capsule, the amount of contrast injected, and the amount of
pressure generated by motion or exercise.

A

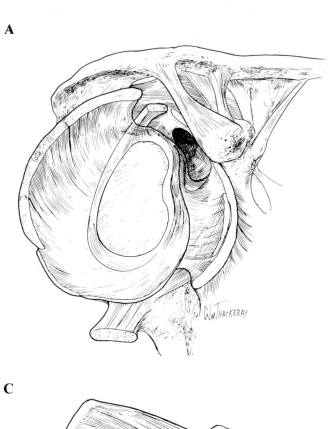

B

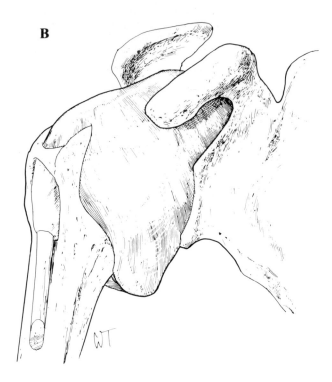

C

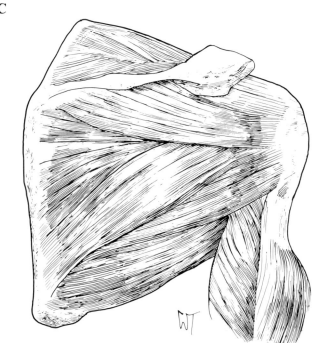

Figure 4

A. The glenoid articular surface has a fibrous labrum surrounding the articular cartilage.

B. The joint capsule inserts on the humeral neck, proximal to the greater tuberosity, and attaches to the osseous rim of the glenoid adjacent to the articular cartilage. The axillary recess is a capsular fold between the humerus and glenoid which becomes smaller as the arm is abducted. The subscapularis bursa communicates with the capsule and is located below the coracoid process.

C. The rotator cuff is a thick envelope surrounding the capsule and actually incorporated into it. The cuff is composed of the combined tendons of the subscapularis, supraspinatus, infraspinatus, and teres minor.

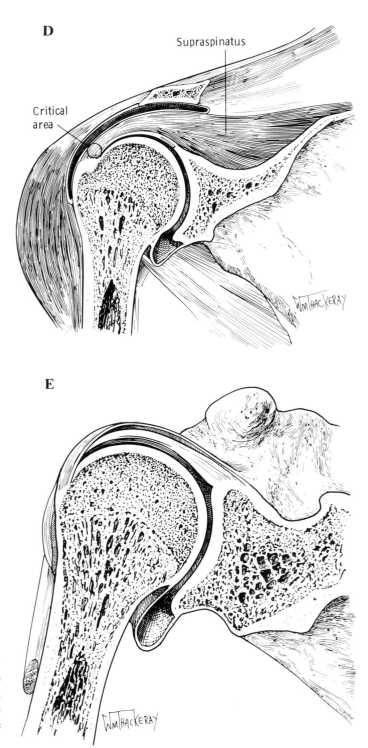

Figure 4
D. The subacromial–subdeltoid bursae communicate.
E. The tendon of the long head of the biceps originates from the superior glenoid labrum. Its proximal portion is intra-articular. A capsular reflection covers it in the bicipital groove and for a variable distance below the groove.

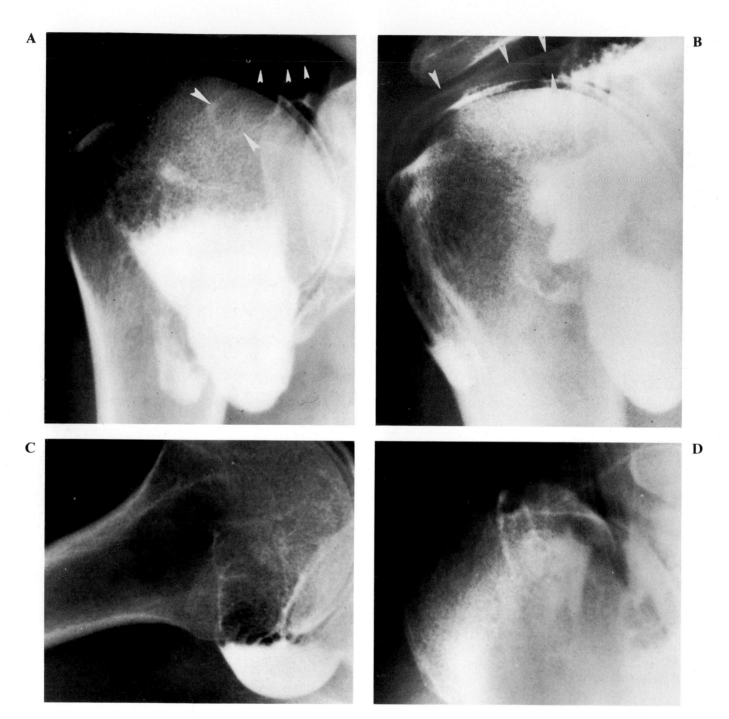

Figure 5

A. On the normal double contrast arthrogram, the standing internal and external rotation views demonstrate the capsular attachments to the humeral head and glenoid, the axillary recess hanging between the humerus and scapula. The undersurface of the rotator cuff is coated by positive contrast and outlined by air (small arrowheads).

B. The tendon of the long head of the biceps is seen as a soft tissue density within the capsule and within its synovial sheath (large arrowheads).

C. On the axillary view, the tendon and sheath are seen between the greater and lesser tuberosities. The axillary view also demonstrates the sharp triangular anterior glenoid labrum.

D. The bicipital groove view best shows the position of the biceps tendon.

A
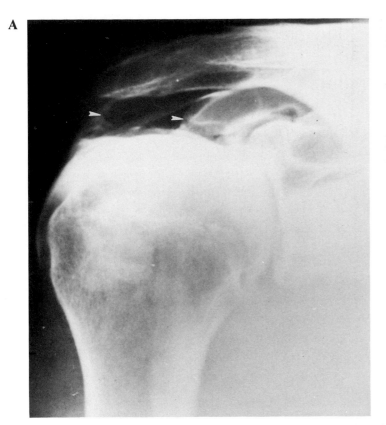

B
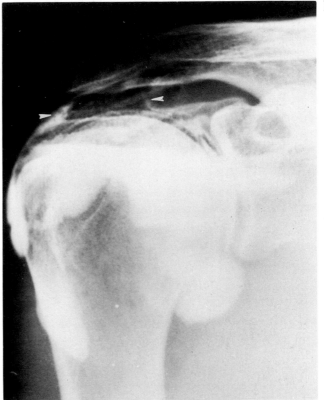

C
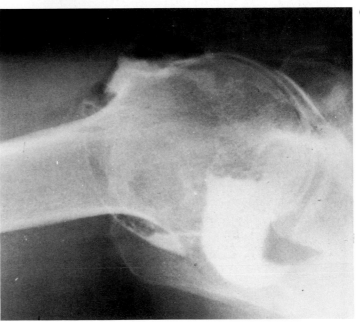

Figure 6
A, B. A complete rotator cuff tear is demonstrated on the standing internal and external rotation views. Abnormal collections of air and contrast are seen in the subacromial subdeltoid bursa below the acromion, lateral to the humeral head and below the greater tuberosity. The fragments of the torn cuff are smooth and of normal width (arrowheads). The tear is wide, extending over two-thirds of the humeral head.
C. The axillary view reveals air and contrast material within the subdeltoid bursa projected across the proximal humeral shaft.

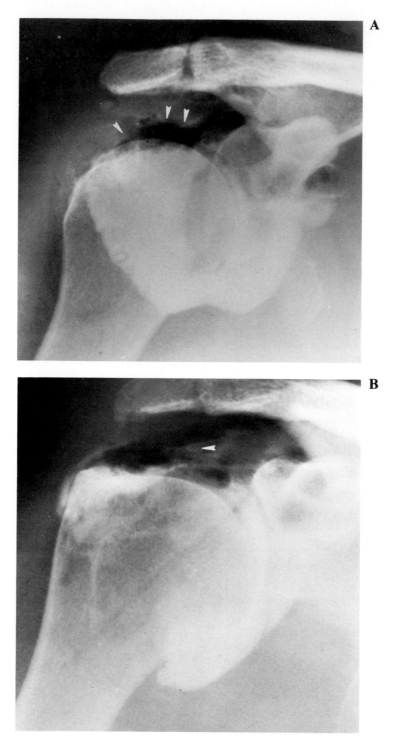

Figure 7
A, B. A complete rotator cuff tear with air and contrast in the subacromial–subdeltoid bursas. The torn cuff (arrowheads) has irregularities along its surface but still occupies most of the space between the articular cartilage of the humeral head and the acromion. Such findings indicate mild degenerative changes. The tear is not wide.

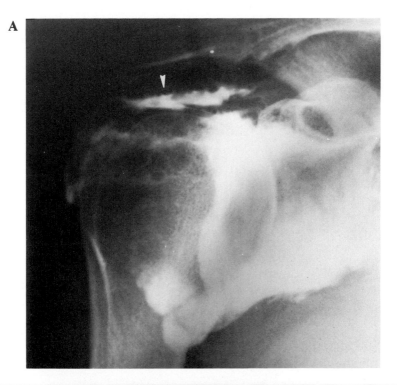

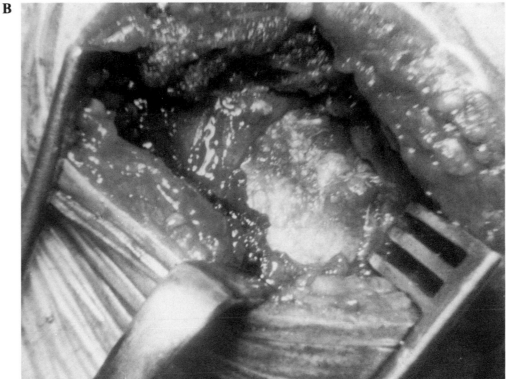

Figure 8
A. A complete rotator cuff tear with air and contrast in the subacromial subdeltoid bursa below the acromion, lateral to the humeral head and below the greater tuberosity. The arthrogram demonstrates moderate degenerative changes in the torn cuff with surface irregularities and loss of width (arrowhead).
B. At surgery the arthrographic findings were confirmed. The humoral head is visible through the tear in the rotator cuff.

A 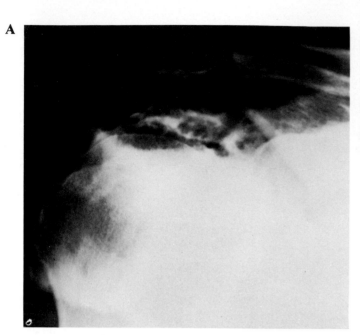 B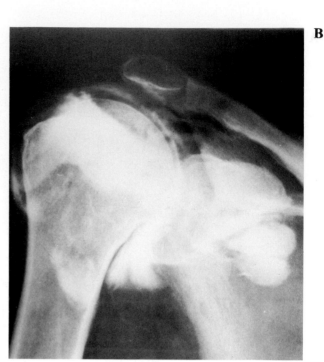

Figure 9
A, B. A complete rotator cuff tear is seen with severe degenerative changes in the tendons. The air and positive contrast outline irregular small tissue fragments containing contrast within their substance.

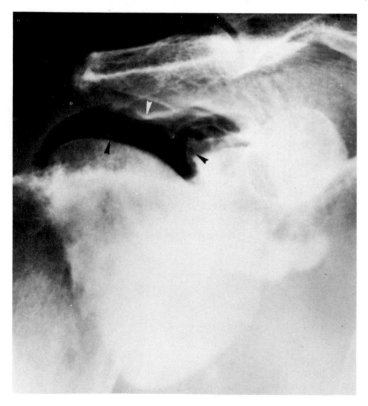

Figure 10
Rheumatoid arthritis has almost completely destroyed the rotator cuff, leaving only a small nubbin (white arrowhead). The articular cartilages on both sides of the joint have also been destroyed (black arrowheads).

A

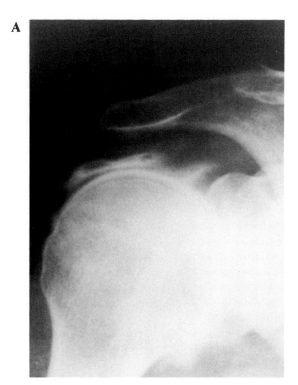

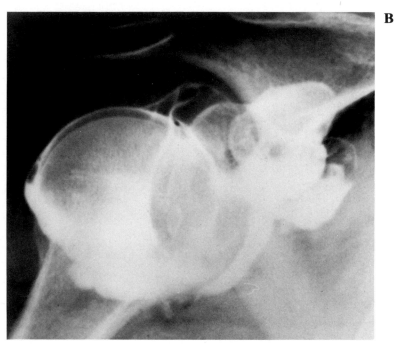

B

Figure 11
A. A partial rotator cuff tear is seen on a postexercise study. An abnormal collection of air and contrast is seen above the articular cartilage of the humeral head. Since it does not reach the acromion or extend below the insertion of the cuff on the tuberosities, the tear is partial.
B. The preexercise internal rotation view is negative.

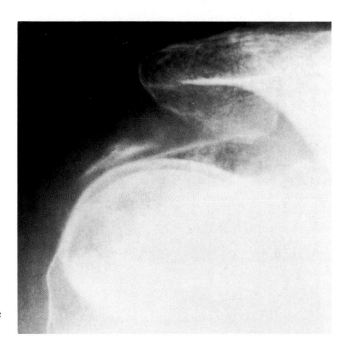

Figure 12
A partial rotator cuff tear is filled with both air and positive contrast.

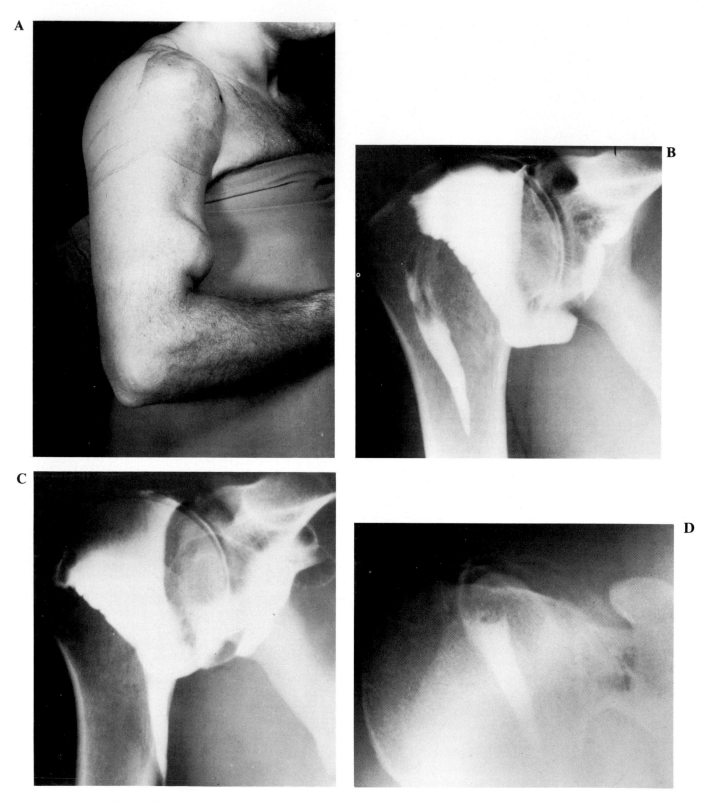

Figure 13
A. A complete tear of the tendon of the long head of the biceps can usually be diagnosed clinically by an abnormal protuberance of the biceps muscle on the anterior aspect of the arm.
B, C, D. The arthrogram demonstrates air and contrast within the sheath, but the soft tissue shadow of the tendon is absent.

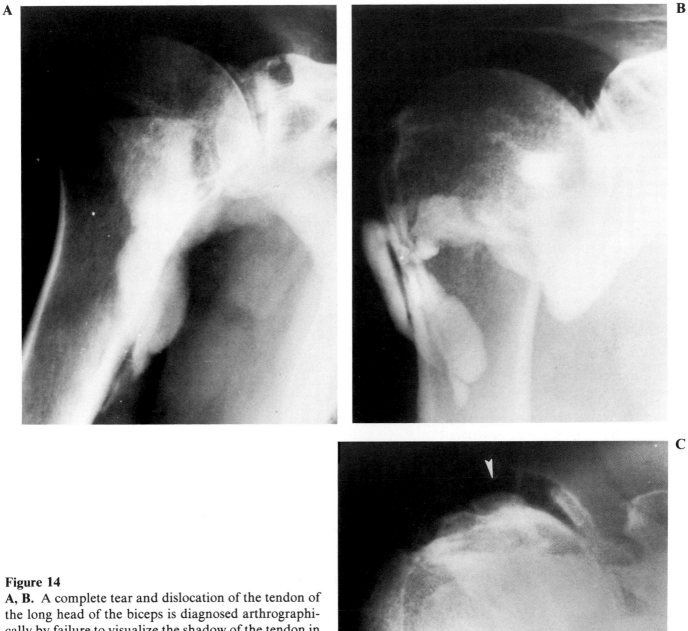

Figure 14
A, B. A complete tear and dislocation of the tendon of the long head of the biceps is diagnosed arthrographically by failure to visualize the shadow of the tendon in the sheath and by distortion and dilation of the sheath. **C.** The bicipital groove view shows displacement of the sheath from its normal osseous intertubercular groove (arrowhead).

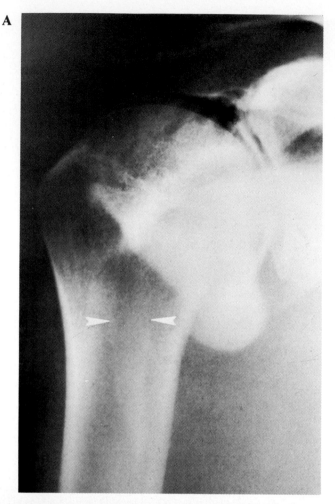

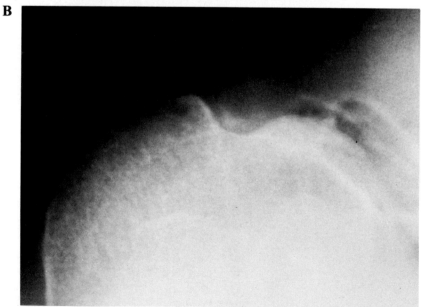

Figure 15
A, B. An incomplete tear of the tendon of the long head of the biceps is diagnosed arthrographically by an increase in the width of the tendon and loss of the sharp margin of the sheath (arrowheads).

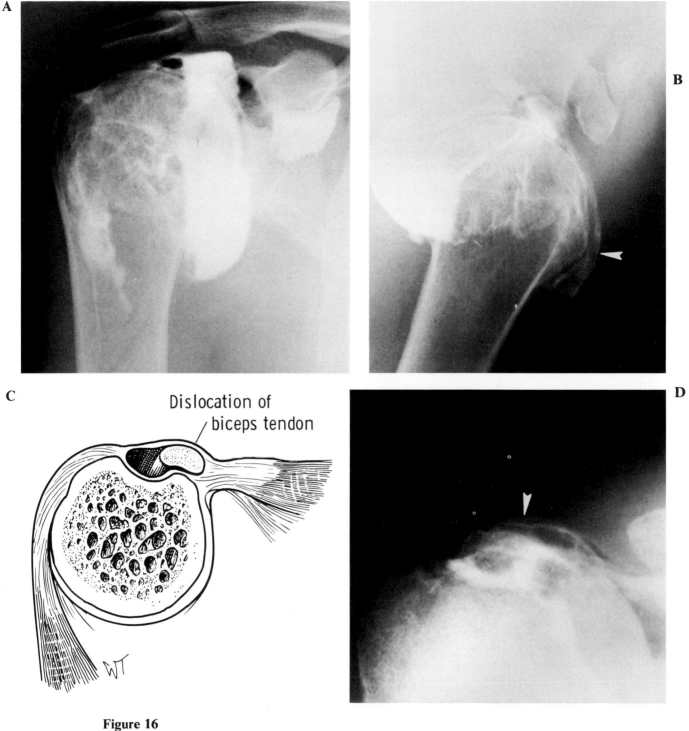

Figure 16
A. Medial dislocation of the tendon of the long head of the biceps can be suspected on the external rotation view since the sheath appears medial to the tuberosities and there are minor irregularities in its outline. However, the diagnosis of dislocation is definitively established on the axillary view (**B**) and bicipital groove views (**C, D**), with both the tendon and sheath (arrowheads) medial to the osseous intertubercular groove.

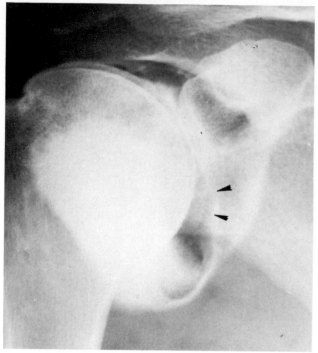

Figure 17

Following the reduction of an anterior dislocation, the double contrast arthrogram demonstrates capsular laxity with loss of the normal indentation between the subscapularis bursa and axillary recess. The absence of the inferior aspect of the articular cartilage of the glenoid (arrowheads) indicates a Bankart deformity.

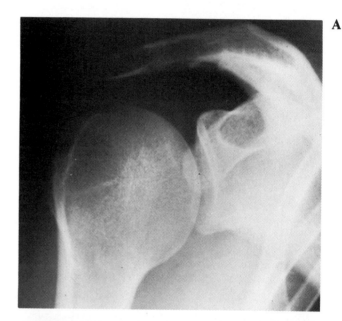

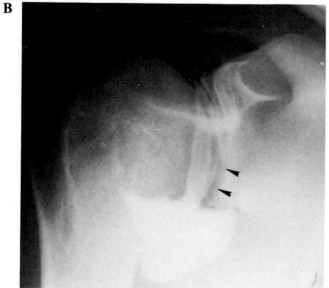

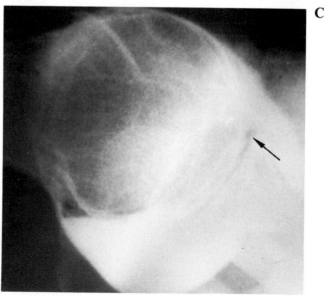

Figure 18

A. Following the reduction of an anterior dislocation, plain films appeared normal.
B. A 15° posterior oblique external rotation view and a supine axillary view (**C**) demonstrate a Bankart deformity (arrowheads and arrow) with both blunting and avulsion of the inferior glenoid labrum.

A 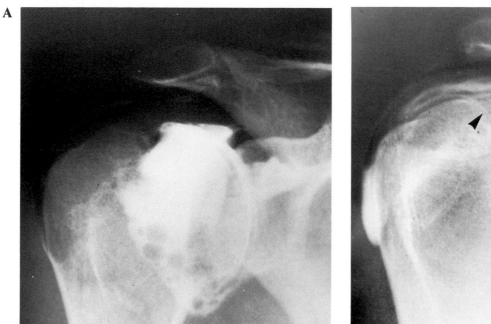 B

Figure 19
A, B. Following the reduction of an anterior dislocation, the double contrast arthrogram demonstrates an unusually positioned Hill-Sachs deformity (arrowheads) and a rotator cuff tear.

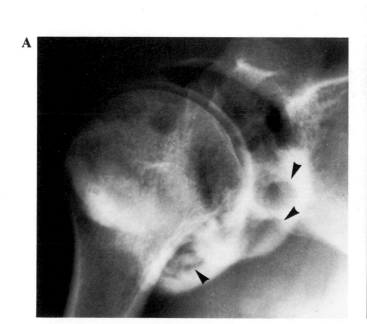 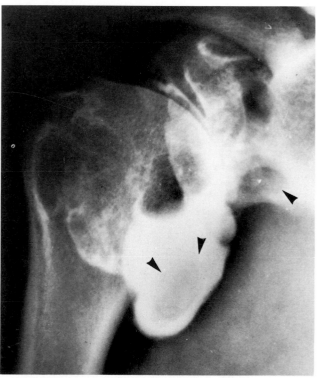

Figure 20
A, B. On both internal and external rotation views loose cartilaginous bodies (arrowheads) are seen in the axillary recess.

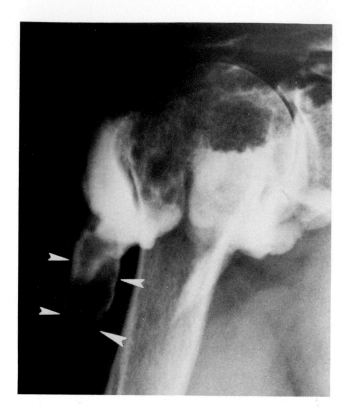

Figure 21
Lucent osteocartilaginous fragments (arrowheads) are lodged within the biceps tendon sheath. This patient also has a complete tear of the rotator cuff.

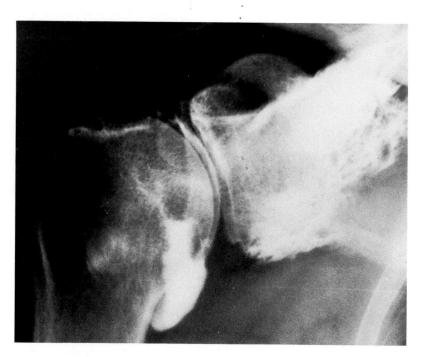

Figure 22
Arthrographic criteria for a diagnosis of adhesive capsulitis are: reduced capacity of the capsule, irregularities of the capsular insertion, a small axillary recess, and leakage of contrast prior to exercise.

9

The Adult Hip

Bernard Ghelman
Robert H. Freiberger

In adults, hip arthrography is performed for several reasons. When infection of the hip joint is suspected and if, after needle insertion, no fluid is aspirated, the injection of a few drops of positive contrast agent verifies the position of the needle tip. The complete arthrogram following the aspiration may also show periarticular abscess or sinus formation. When calcifications or ossifications are seen near the hip on plain films, the arthrogram can determine their intra- or extra-articular location. An arthrogram can also detect intra-articular cartilaginous bodies or synovial masses not visible on plain films. The arthrographic evaluation of cartilaginous joint surfaces and joint congruity, which is very important in the infant and child, is less important in the adult, since the articular cartilages are thin and conform to the shape of the subchondral bone. A major application of hip joint arthrography is to evaluate painful hip prostheses by detecting loosening and verifying infection.

EQUIPMENT

Although hip joint arthrography can be performed with all types of fluoroscopic equipment, the most convenient is an image-amplified fluoroscope with an overhead tube and an under-table image amplifier (Fig. 1). This setup permits adequate working space above the hip joint with less chance of contaminating needles and gloved hands than under a conventional fluoroscopic tower. The standard arthrogram tray is used with the addition of a 22-gauge or a 20-gauge, 3½-in. disposable spinal needle, saline solution without preservatives, and containers for aerobic and anaerobic cultures.

INJECTION PROCEDURE

The patient lies supine on the fluoroscopic table with the hip in neutral position. A small pillow placed under the knee makes the patient more comfortable, flexes the hip joint slightly, and relaxes and hip joint capsule. Placing the leg in traction (Fig. 2) increases the width of the space between the femoral head and the acetabulum for better opacification. Traction also provides good immobilization of the lower extremity, which is particularly important if subtraction studies are to be made. With fluoroscopic guidance, a metallic marker is placed over the midpoint of the femoral neck slightly to the medial side, and the point is marked on the skin with indelible ink (Fig. 1). When a pendulous abdomen overlaps the hip joint, the patient is asked to retract the abdominal wall by hand. Alternatively, adhesive strapping may be used to hold the abdomen above the working area.

When the hip is in neutral position, the point marked on the skin is lateral to the femoral artery, but if the hip rotates externally, the femoral vessels and nerves move laterally and may underlie the marked point. Therefore, external rotation of the femur should be prevented.

After antiseptic skin preparation and draping, the 22-gauge, 3½-in. spinal needle is inserted using 1 percent lidocaine hydrochloride local anesthesia. The needle insertion can be performed successfully in a number of ways. With the hip in neutral position it is possible to insert the needle vertically; however, a more lateral and inferior point of needle insertion, slanting the needle upwards and medially, appears to be preferable as the femoral vessels and nerves are definitely avoided (Fig. 3A). With this approach, the tip of the needle slides more easily and completely beneath the capsule than with vertical needle insertion. A more lateral needle placement (Fig. 3C) may be preferred when a metallic prosthesis prevents fluoroscopic visualization of a vertically placed needle.

As the needle is being inserted, the position of the needle tip is checked by intermittent fluoroscopy to ascertain that puncture of the capsule is achieved below the head–neck junction of the femur near the point selected by preliminary fluoroscopy (Fig. 3B). When the needle tip hits the bony femoral neck, aspiration may produce synovial fluid which should be smeared as well as cultured aerobically and anaerobically. After aspiration, up to 15 cc of positive contrast agent is injected into the hip joint and the needle is withdrawn. Should the patient complain of pain related to the distention of the hip joint, the injection is stopped. If contrast agent can escape from the hip joint through a sinus tract or communicating abscess, more than 15 cc of contrast agent may be injected.

If no synovial fluid is aspirated after the needle strikes the femoral neck, it is impossible to determine whether intra-articular placement of the needle tip has been achieved. For confirmation of placement, the injection and aspiration of saline solution can be tried. If the needle tip is intra-articular, there should be little resistance to the injection of about 10 cc of saline. Absolute verification of intra-articular needle position is obtained by injecting a few drops of positive contrast agent. With intra-articular placement, contrast agent will immediately flow from the needle tip and opacify one of the capsular recesses (Fig. 3B). If, however, the contrast agent hangs like a cloud at the tip of the needle, intra-articular needle position has not been

achieved and the needle must be repositioned. It is often helpful to flex the hip slightly and to bounce the needle tip against the cortex of the femoral neck to achieve an intra-articular position.

A few drops of contrast agent injected intra-articularly to verify the position of the needle do not interfere with culture of injected and reaspirated saline solution. A large quantity of intra-articular positive contrast agent should not be injected for verification of needle placement since the iodinated organic compound is slightly bacteriocidal.

After fluid for culture has been aspirated, contrast material is injected. If desired, the contrast fluid can be injected through sterile plastic tubing attached to the needle so that fluoroscopic observation is possible. Following the injection, the needle is removed. In general, two sets of roentgenograms with the hip in neutral, external, and internal rotation are made. The first set is taken immediately after injection with only minimal movement of the hip joint to distribute contrast agent. A second set is made following exercise. Other views and tomograms may be made if needed. The technique for subtraction studies for suspected loose prostheses begins on page 193.

HIP ANATOMY FOR ARTHROGRAPHY

The hip is a ball-and-socket joint with the femoral head fitting into the acetabulum. The articular surface of the femoral head comprises approximately two-thirds of a sphere, facing upward medially and forward. It is covered on its articular surface by hyaline cartilage except for a small central area where the ligamentum teres attaches. The acetabulum is less completely covered by articular cartilage than the femoral head. Its central area contains fat covered by synovial membrane. The hyaline articular cartilage is horseshoe-shaped and is referred to as the lunate surface. Cartilage extends beyond the osseous margins of the acetabulum, forming the labrum or limbus, (Figs. 4, 5) which is proportionately larger in infants and children than it is in the adult. The hip joint capsule attaches to the pelvis slightly peripherally to the labrum or limbus (Fig. 4). The femoral attachment of the capsule, a strong, thick structure, is at the level of the intertrochanteric line in front of the femur and slightly above the intertrochanteric crest in back of the femur. The joint cavity occasionally communicates with the iliopsoas bursa through a capsular defect that lies between the vertical band of the iliofemoral ligament and the pubofemoral ligament. These, as well as other reinforcing ligaments, are extra-articular and not seen on the arthrogram. The intra-articular ligamentum teres extends from the fovea capitis to the acetabular notch at the inferior aspect of the acetabulum. The notch is bridged by the transverse ligament.

The femoral vein, artery, and nerve, in medial to lateral order, lie anteriorly and slightly medial to the axis of the femoral neck when the femur is in neutral position and the femoral head is within the acetabulum. Rotation of the femur or abnormalities in the position of the femoral head alter the position of the vesssels with respect to the femur.

THE NORMAL ARTHROGRAM

A narrow space between the labrum or limbus and the capsular attachment fills with contrast material forming the limbus thorn (Figs. 4A, B). A very thin film of contrast agent outlines the space between the articular cartilages of a normal femoral head and the acetabulum. Sometimes the femur has to be put in traction or the patient has to exercise the hip in order to fill a normally congruous joint space with contrast agent. The capsule with its synovial lining roughly follows the contour of the femoral neck and constricts in the center of the neck, forming the orbicular zone. Most of the contrast agent collects at the base of the neck of the femur.

The transverse ligament bridging the acetabular notch inferiorly can often be identified as a small semi-circular impression in the contrast-filled capsule at the base of the acetabulum. The ligamentum teres cannot be seen in the normal hip, but does become visible when the femoral head is displaced laterally (Chapter 10, Fig. 11). Communications between the hip joint and the iliopsoas bursa are not normally seen by arthrography, but can become apparent when the abnormal conditions that produce chronic synovial effusions cause the communication to enlarge (Fig. 12).

The os acetabuli, a normal variant representing an unfused ossification center within the superior portion of the acetabular labrum, can usually be seen on conventional roentgenograms, but an arthrogram can prove that the ossicle lies within the cartilaginous labrum and not in the hip joint (Figs. 5A, B).

THE ABNORMAL ARTHROGRAM

Loose Bodies

The arthrogram verifies the intra-articular location of osseous or calcific bodies seen on plain films and is the only means of showing cartilaginous intra-articular loose bodies. A combination of arthrography and tomography helps in identifying the filling defects made by cartilaginous bodies in the opacified joint capsule. Although calcified or ossified bodies can be detected on routine radiography, their intra-articular or extra-articular location is often uncertain; the arthrogram establishes the position without doubt (Fig. 6). The most common cause of intra-articular loose bodies is degenerative arthritis when fragments of articular cartilage become loosened. Since these fragments are nourished by synovial fluid, they may grow until they are much larger than the original defect in the cartilage.

Rarely, an osseous body may arise from subchondral areas of incomplete ossification of the femoral head secondary to Legg Calve Perthes disease or other causes of osteonecrosis. The arthrogram establishes whether the osseous body is separated from the femoral head, and whether the overlying articular cartilage remains intact (Chapter 10, Figs. 19, 20). If the osseous body is separated from the femoral head, it can cause pain, interfere with motion of the hip joint, and perhaps call for surgical intervention. If it is not separated, surgical removal is not indicated.

Osteochondritis dissecans, a condition of children or young adults that is common in the knee joint, is rare in the hip joint. If present, the arthrogram combined with tomography can best establish whether the osseous body is separate or remains covered by intact articular cartilage.

The arthrogram is also useful in diagnosing and localizing intra-articular fragments of the femoral head or acetabulum due to prior posterior dislocation. These fragments, which may only be cartilaginous, are usually sheared from the articular surface of the femoral head as it displaces over the posterior acetabular rim. On plain radiographs (Fig. 7A), the presence of fragments is inferred by a slight lateral displacement of the femoral head, but otherwise they may not be visible. The arthrogram is able to outline these fragments (Figs. 7B, C).

A relatively uncommon cause of loose bodies within the hip joint is synovial chondromatosis (Fig. 8). In this condition, metaplasia within the synovium causes microscopic pieces of cartilage to be extruded into the joint. These cartilage fragments grow, and by the time the patient's hip is symptomatic there are usually numerous cartilaginous bodies in the joint, from the size of a pinhead to the size of a pea or larger. When these bodies calcify, diagnosis on plain roentgenograms is usually not difficult since the calcifications conform to the shape of the joint. However, when no or very few calcifications are present, diagnosis from routine radiographs becomes impossible, but the arthrogram is highly diagnostic.

Villous and Villonodular Synovitis

Pigmented villonodular synovitis is a condition in which radiolucent nodular filling defects may be seen on an arthrogram. These nodular masses do not calcify but may cause pressure erosions of the intra-articular surfaces of the femoral head, neck, and acetabulum (Fig. 9A). Although the synovial masses are visible by arthrography (Fig. 9B) and arthrotomography, it may not be possible to absolutely differentiate them from noncalcified synovial chondromatous masses.

Villous synovitis occurs in inflammatory joint diseases like infection and rheumatoid arthritis, and also with intra-articular osteoid osteomas. On the arthrogram the synovial surfaces have a finely to coarsely corrugated appearance. Opacification of lymphatics occurs occasionally in inflammatory joint disease but is not diagnostic of joint infection (Fig. 10).

Joint Deformity and Incongruity

When the shape of the femoral head and/or acetabulum is altered by disease, the arthrogram demonstrates the incongruity of the joint surfaces (Fig. 11). The normally spherical shape of the femoral head becomes flattened or oval. Pooling of contrast agent between the separated incongruous joint surfaces may be seen with the hip in the neutral position or with the femur abducted or rotated. The most common cause of hip joint deformity in the adult is degenerative osteoarthritis, and it is frequently accompanied by superolateral displacement of the femoral head with the joint space narrowing superiorly and widening medially (Figs. 12B, C). Less commonly, superomedial or medial displacement with respective joint space narrowing is present. Because the thin articular cartilage conforms to the shape of subchondral bone, arthrography is usually not necessary for evaluation of joint incongruity in the adult.

An evaluation of the state of the articular cartilages, particularly those of the acetabulum, may occasionally be of value if surgical intervention other than total hip replacement is contemplated. A varus osteotomy or the insertion of a femoral head prosthesis is only performed if the articular cartilage of the acetabulum is in a reasonably good condition—which the arthrogram can determine (Fig. 11).

The Opacified Iliopsoas Bursa

The iliopsoas bursa is normally not opacified by arthrography. Conditions causing chronic synovitis such as pigmented villonodular synovitis, rheumatoid arthritis, or degenerative arthritis—diseases associated with chronic synovial effusions—can enlarge the communication between the joint and bursa and so enlarge the bursa that it may be clinically detected as a pelvic or abdominal mass (Fig. 12A). The pathomechanics of distention of the iliopsoas bursa appear to be similar to the formation of a popliteal cyst at the knee joint. A patient with a painful palpable and visible groin mass, initially thought to be an incarcerated femoral hernia (Fig. 12A), was seen in an emergency room. The severe osteoarthritis of the hip documented on a roentgenogram of the pelvis (Fig. 12B) suggested the possibility of a distended iliopsoas bursa (Figs. 12C, D). The arthrogram confirmed the diagnosis of a distended iliopsoas bursa.

ARTHROGRAPHY OF HIP PROSTHESES

Two serious complications arising from the insertion of hip prostheses are infection and loosening. The former can be confirmed by aspiration, smear, and culture; the latter can often be confirmed by arthrography.

Injection Technique

A technical problem in performing arthrograms on patients with hip prostheses is that the needle is obscured by the metallic femoral component and it is difficult to confirm the intra-articular placement of the needle tip. Feeling the tip scrape against the metallic component is not a guarantee of intra-articular placement.

In order to facilitate intra-articular needle placement, a more lateral than usual point of insertion can be chosen. Occasionally, a point completely lateral to the hip, with the needle horizontal and parallel to the table top (Figs. 3C, 19), is selected in order to fluoroscopically visualize the entire length of the needle and the needle tip as it touches the lateral aspect of the metallic femoral component. A small amount of contrast agent is injected and, if intra-articular, it almost always outlines the base of the acetabular component of the prosthesis, which is seen fluoroscopically as a dense, straight line of contrast agent perpendicular to the neck of the prosthesis and close to the head–neck junction (Fig. 15B). If a cloud-like collection of contrast agent forms around the tip of the needle, the tip is extra-articular. A normal intracapsular space does not exist because the pseudocapsule that forms postoperatively is usually tight and irregular.

In a patient with a total hip prosthesis, placing the needle tip just beneath the polyethylene cup most often results in intra-articular location of the needle tip. If the femoral head has been replaced by an Austin–Moore or a Thompson prosthesis, insertion of the needle tip at the inferior margin of the metallic head appears most advantageous. Cup arthroplasties are the most difficult of all prostheses for aspiration and arthrography because the capsule is very tight and extends irregularly beneath the cup and femoral neck. Placing the needle tip beneath the edge of the cup is best for achieving an intra-articular location (Fig. 13).

After operative procedures on the hip, extracapsular ectopic bone formation can seriously interfere with the placement of the needle into the deformed and contracted capsule. Ectopic bone formation usually occurs superolaterally in the region of the greater trochanter (Figs. 17, 20). There are no specific guidelines for needle insertion except that the area of ossification must be avoided; occasionally an approach medial to the femoral vessels is successful.

NONCEMENTED PROSTHESES

The Austin–Moore prosthesis is never cemented into the femur and the Thompson prosthesis is usually not either. Normally, there is a tight fit between the stem of the prosthesis and the femoral shaft, with only a very thin layer of contrast agent seen between them. A wide zone of bone absorption around the stem and a layer of contrast agent more than a fraction of a millimeter wide, are signs of loosening (Figs. 14A, B).

CEMENTED PROSTHESES

Several years ago, when acrylic cement was first used to fasten the components of total hip prostheses to bone, the cement was radiolucent and therefore not visible on the roentgenogram (Figs. 15, 16A). No contrast agent was seen in the bone–cement interface of a normal solidly cemented prostheses (Fig. 15B).

By arthrography, a loose prosthesis could be detected easily because injected contrast agent was seen in the interface between the radiolucent cement and bone (Fig. 16B). To make the cement visible on plain roentgenograms, barium sulfate was added to it, imparting a radiographic density that is slightly greater than that of bone (Figs. 17–19). Although this development has been useful in permitting visualization of the cement and the cement–bone interface, it has made evaluation of arthrograms performed for loosening more difficult and sometimes impossible. A thin layer of opaque contrast agent usually cannot be seen in the interface between opaque cement and opaque bone.

Subtraction Technique

When the cement holding a prosthesis is radiopaque, a technique in which a preinjection roentgenogram is subtracted from a postinjection roentgenogram is helpful in visualizing the injected contrast agent. Theoretically, only the difference between the pre- and postinjection film, the injected contrast agent, should be visible on the subtraction study. In practice, however, a faint image of the subtracted parts remains and the technique is helpful in demonstrating radiopaque contrast filling of the interface between radiopaque cement and radiopaque bone (Figs. 18–20).

The patient is supine on the fluoroscopic table. The leg is in neutral position and a small pillow may be placed under the knee. A traction device is applied to the leg with as much weight as the patient can tolerate (Fig. 3). Sandbags placed medially and laterally to the leg in traction help prevent movement.

After the needle has been inserted and its intra-articular location verified, and after fluid has been aspirated for smear and cultures, the first roentgenogram is taken and a positive copy of it is made. Approximately 10 cc of radiopaque contrast agent is then injected and a second roentgenogram is made with patient, X-ray tube, and film in exactly the same position as it was for the first roentgenogram. It is sometimes possible to take a third roentgenogram before the patient moves. The extended time interval between injection and filming may permit more contrast agent to flow into the cement–bone interface. A print is made with the positive copy of the pre-injection radiograph superimposed on the post-injection radiograph. Even if there is slight motion of the femur between the initial film and subsequent ones, adequate subtraction studies of the components can usually be obtained by making two studies: The first superimposes the pelvis and acetabular component and the second matches the femur and femoral component.

Diagnostic Criteria for
Loose Prostheses

The diagnostic criterion for loosening of a cemented prosthesis is seeing contrast agent throughout the bone–cement interface (Figs. 16–20). The filling of 1 cm or less of the bone–cement interface at the super-olateral aspect of the acetabular component or its inferomedial aspect is common but is not an indication of complete loosening. Similarly, opacification less than 1 cm long at the cement–bone interface on top of the femoral component does not indicate total loosening.

Unfortunately, an arthrogram showing no contrast agent in the bone–cement interface, and therefore negative for loosening, cannot completely rule out the possibility of a loose prosthesis. The bone–cement interface can be filled with granulation tissue or its edges may be sealed by granulation tissue, preventing the entrance of contrast agent.

POSTOPERATIVE ABNORMALITIES

Leakage of contrast agent from the postoperatively deformed pseudocapsule of the hip joint is not unusual. Contrast agent can extend to fill a bursal cavity in the region of the greater trochanter (Fig. 21) and can also extend into the space between the separated osteotomy fragments of the greater trochanter (Fig. 22). Determination of whether these extra-articular communicating spaces are abscesses or sinus tracts caused by infection, or whether they are bursal cavities, is made by culture of aspirated fluid. When the culture is positive, the extra-articular contrast collections are abscesses (Figs. 23–26); when the culture is negative, they represent communicating bursae that are usually of no clinical significance.

The opacification of lymphatic channels (Figs. 21, 26) is a sign of inflammatory disease that may be infectious in origin. Lymphatic opacification, however, is not a specific sign of infection, and the diagnosis of infection can only be made reliably by aspiration and culture for aerobic as well as anaerobic organisms.

ARTHROGRAPHY AFTER PROSTHESIS REMOVAL

Following the removal of an infected total hip prosthesis and subsequent antibiotic treatment, an aspiration of the hip followed by an arthrogram can determine the activity of the infection. This is of particular importance when insertion of a new prosthesis is contemplated. Needle placement for aspiration is exceedingly difficult because of the severely deformed and contracted capsular space. Proof that the needle tip was in the intracapsular space is particularly important when no purulent fluid can be obtained or when the cultures of aspirated saline solution are negative. The injection of contrast agent following aspiration demonstrates that the needle tip is intra-articular and that aspiration was carried out from the intracapsular space (Figs. 27, 28).

PITFALLS

Do not assume that the needle tip striking the femoral neck or a metallic prosthesis means that the tip is intra-articular. The position of the needle tip must be confirmed by the injection of positive contrast agent.

Only saline solution without preservatives should be injected to avoid interference with culture of aspirated fluid.

Communications of the hip joint with extra-articular bursae, such as a trochanteric bursa, or a bursal sac formed in a pseudarthrosis of an osteotomized greater trochanter are not unusual in the postoperative hip and should not be interpreted as abscesses unless cultures are positive for infection.

Inadvertently injected air that forms one or more bubbles in the positive contrast-filled capsule must not be mistaken for loose bodies.

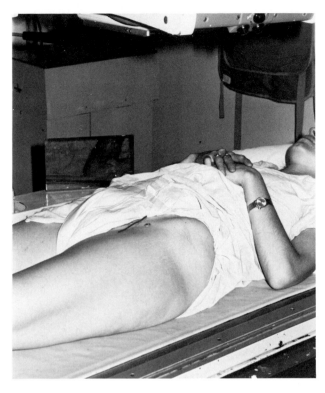

Figure 1
X-ray equipment with an overhead tube and under-table image amplifier is best for arthrography of the hip since it provides ample work space above the patient, and sterility is easily maintained during the injection procedure. A linear marker has been placed over the patient's femoral artery. Lateral to the artery, the lead marker over the center of the femoral neck indicates the intended site of capsule puncture.

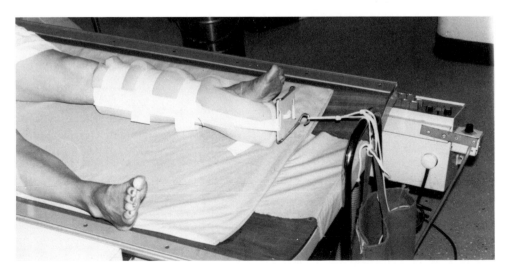

Figure 2
When the examination is done for the loosening of a total hip prosthesis, leg traction is used to increase the gap between the loose cement and bone. Traction also helps immobilize the extremity.

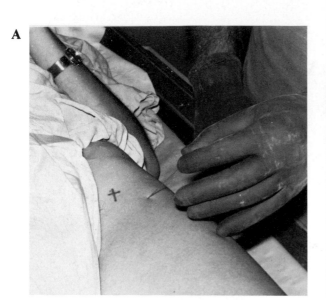

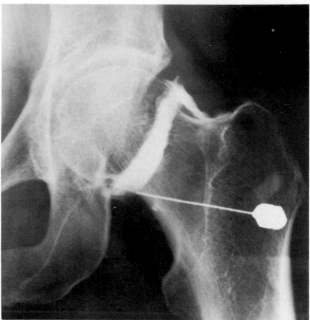

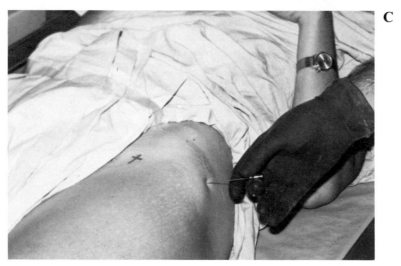

Figure 3

A, B. After antiseptic skin preparation and draping of the patient, a 22-gauge short-bevel spinal needle is aimed at the intended puncture site of the hip joint capsule. Most commonly, the skin is punctured slightly inferolaterally to the mark made on the skin and the needle is slanted upward and medially. Because a metallic femoral prosthesis hides a vertically placed needle on fluoroscopy, a more lateral approach (**C**) for those cases is preferable since it permits the needle tip to be seen fluoroscopically. Needle placement can vary from a practically vertical direction to a lateral approach. (The drape has been removed for the photograph.) The position of the needle can be seen on many of the following hip arthrograms.

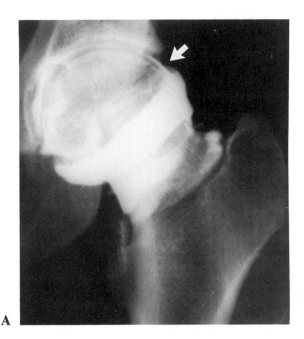
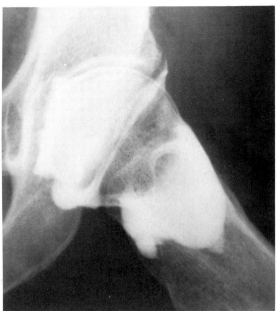

A

B

Figure 4

A, B. The normal hip arthrogram of an adult shows a thin, even layer of contrast agent between the articular surfaces of the femoral head and acetabulum on both anteroposterior and lateral projections, indicating congruity of joint surfaces. The limbus, a cartilaginous extension of the roof the acetabulum (arrow), is relatively smaller than in childhood. Contrast agent accumulates just below the femoral head and at the femoral insertion of the capsule. Less contrast agent is seen in the midportion of the femoral neck at the zona orbicularis.

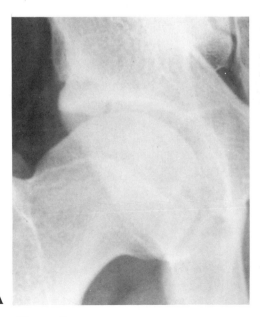
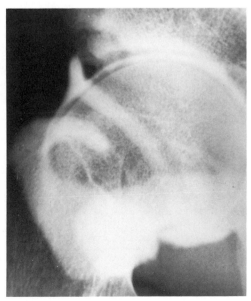

A

B

Figure 5

A. The patient had a clicking sensation when moving the hip, and the osseous body at the superior margin of the acetabulum was thought to be a loose osseous body.
B. The arthrogram clearly shows that the osseous body lies within the cartilaginous limbus, as no contrast agent is seen between the osseous body—an os acetabuli—and the roof of the acetabulum.

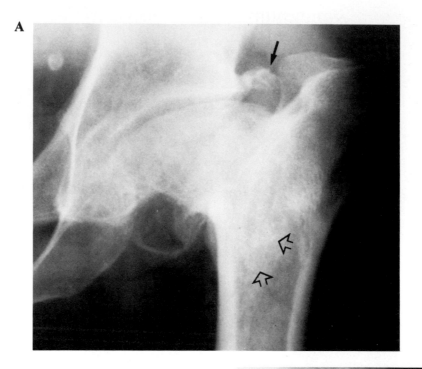

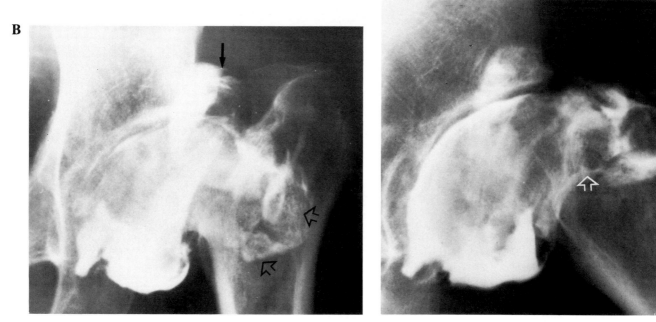

Figure 6
A. An osseous body at the lateral margin of the acetabulum (arrow) is seen on a plain roentgenogram of a hip joint deformed by a childhood fracture followed by avascular necrosis. A faint calcific density overlying the subtrochanteric area of the femur (open arrows) was not recognized as a loose body.
B, C. An arthrogram shows that the osteochondromatous body (arrow) is surrounded by contrast substance and is therefore intra-articular. Several other osteochondromatous bodies (open arrows) are seen within the hip capsule, and one of them corresponds to the faint calcification seen on the plain roentgenogram.

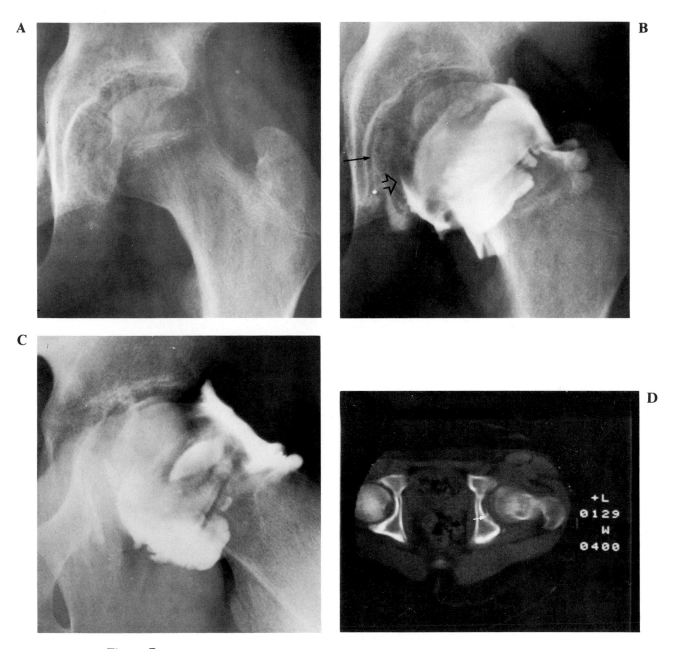

Figure 7
A. Following a hip injury, the patient had severe pain and limped. The femoral head is displaced laterally in the acetabulum. It seemed likely that a fragment of bone or cartilage was displacing the femoral head, but no fragment could be seen.
B, C. The arthrogram showed a layer of contrast agent on the articular cartilage of the acetabulum (arrow) and another on the articular cartilage of the femoral head (open arrow). This indicated that some object was lying between the two cartilages, since normally only a single line of contrast agent is seen.
D. The computed tomographic scan shows a small osseous and cartilaginous body (arrow) wedged between the femoral head and acetabulum. A defect in the articular surface of the femoral head could also be seen.

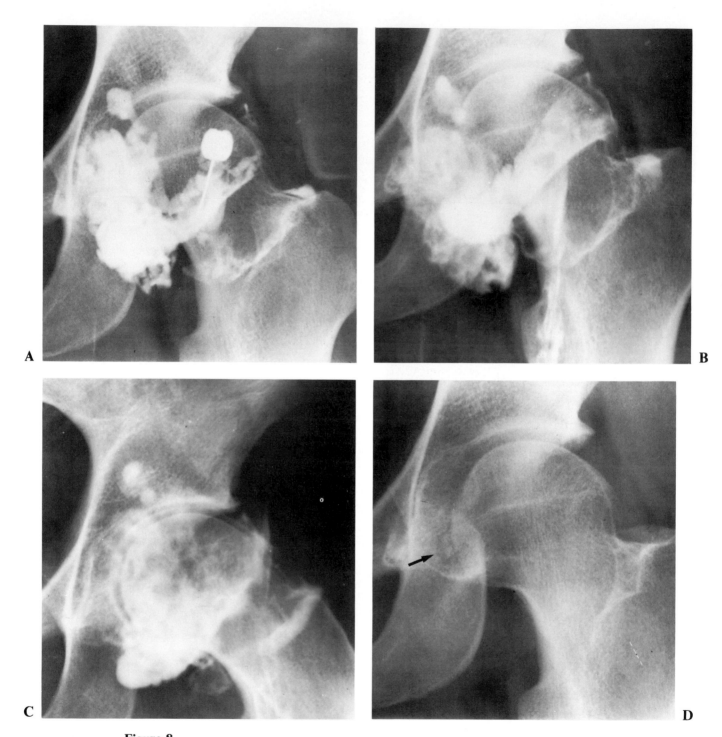

Figure 8
A-C. Synovial chondromatosis causes multiple radiolucent filling defects in the opacified hip joint.
D. A review of the preliminary plain radiographs of the hip shows a very faint calcific density (arrow) between the inferomedial segment of the femoral head and the acetabulum. This may be a partially calcified chondromatous body, but the diagnosis cannot be made without the arthrogram.

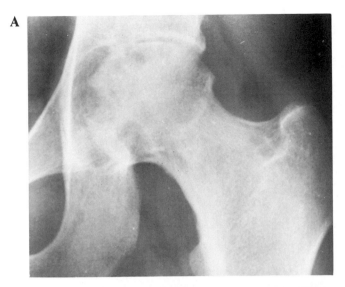

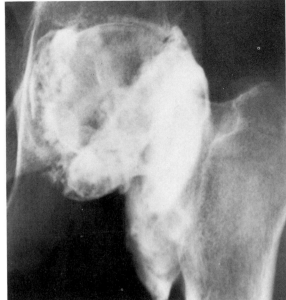

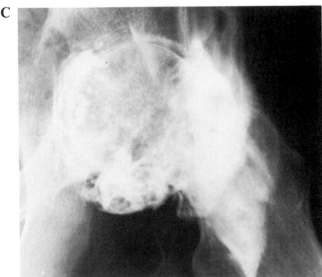

Figure 9
A. Pigmented villonodular synovitis causes erosions of the intra-articular bony surfaces of the hip joint.
B, C. The nodular synovial masses of pigmented villonodular synovitis are evident on the single positive contrast arthrogram.

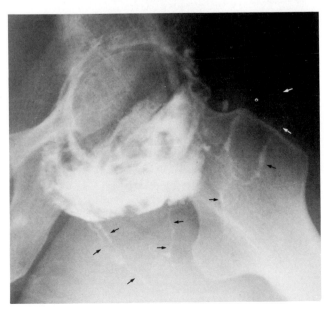

Figure 10
Irregular synovial surfaces and opacification of the lymphatics (arrows) indicate inflammatory disease.

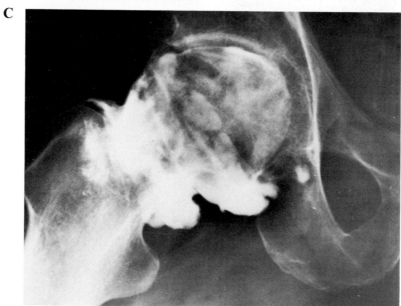

Figure 11
A–C. The reduced thickness and irregularity of the articular cartilage of the femoral
head is shown in a patient with osteonecrosis and moderate collapse of the superior
articular surface of the femoral head. The articular cartilage of the acetabulum is of
normal thickness but the surface is irregular. These findings prompted a decision to
perform a total hip joint replacement rather than a femoral head replacement.

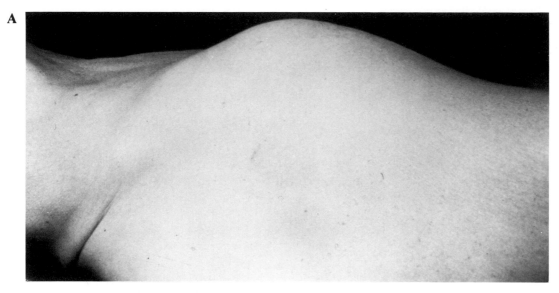

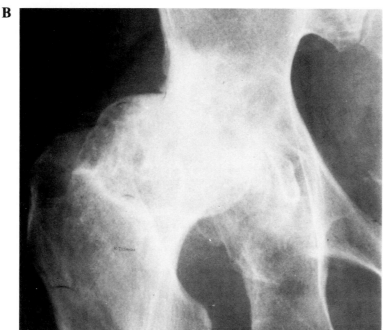

Figure 12
A. An elderly woman presented at the emergency room with a painful groin swelling that was initially clinically diagnosed as an incarcerated hernia.
B. The roentgenogram showing severe osteoarthritis of the hip suggested the diagnosis of a distended iliopsoas bursa and led to the performance of an arthrogram.

C

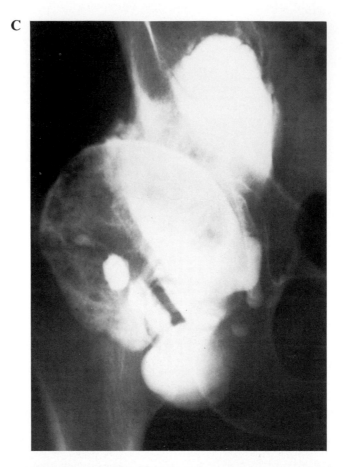

D

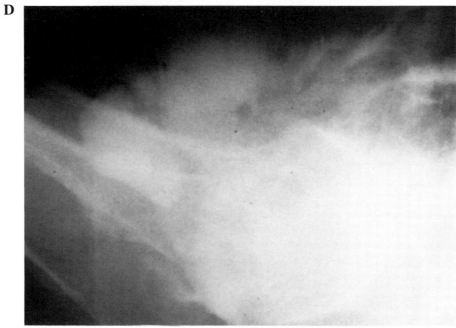

Figure 12
C. An abnormally enlarged iliopsoas bursa, opacified by radiopaque contrast substance, is seen on an anteroposterior view and (**D**) a lateral view.

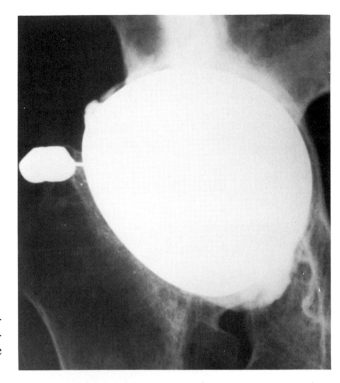

Figure 13

An aspiration was requested on a painful hip joint containing a cup arthroplasty. The best area for needle tip placement is at the inferior margin of the metallic cup. The arthrogram verifies intra-articular needle position.

A

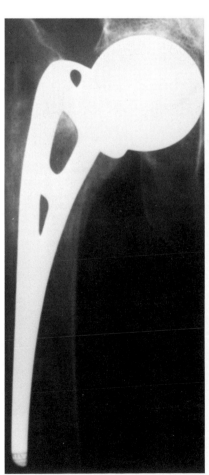

B

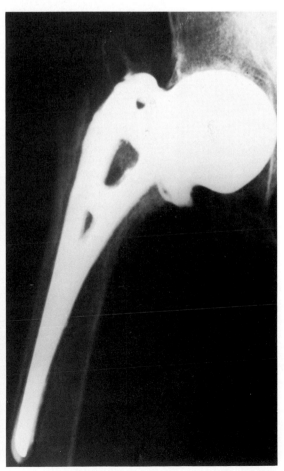

Figure 14

A. A routine roentgenogram of a painful Austin–Moore prosthesis shows more than the usual amount of bone resorption around the stem of the prosthesis.

B. An arthrogram performed after intra-articular injection of saline with aspiration for culture shows contrast agent surrounding the entire stem of the prosthesis. A thin layer of contrast agent is usually seen around the upper part of the stem of an Austin–Moore prosthesis which is not cemented into the femur, but in this case there is more positive contrast than normal, indicating that the stem is abnormally loose. The culture did not indicate an infection. This prosthesis was replaced by a total hip prosthesis.

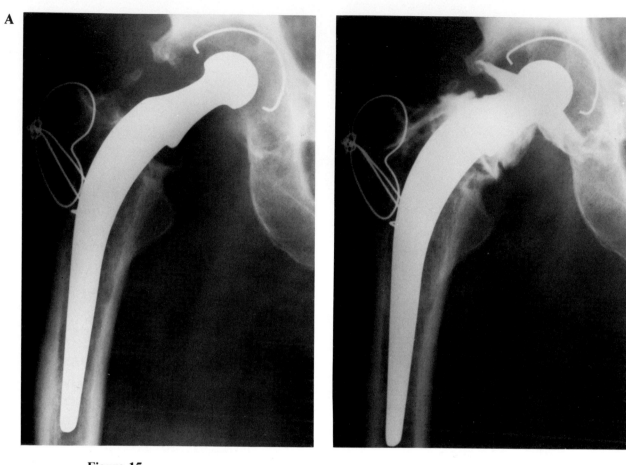

Figure 15
A. A Charnley–Müller prosthesis is fixed with radiolucent cement. The bone–cement interface is not visible.
B. An arthrogram was performed for aspiration and culture and for diagnosis of possible loosening. As no contrast agent can be seen in the bone–cement interface, a diagnosis of loosening cannot be made. The usual postoperative contracture of the pseudocapsule at the replaced hip joint is apparent.

A
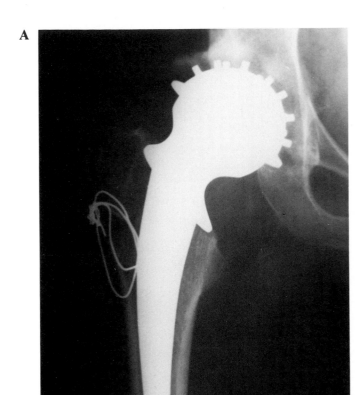

B
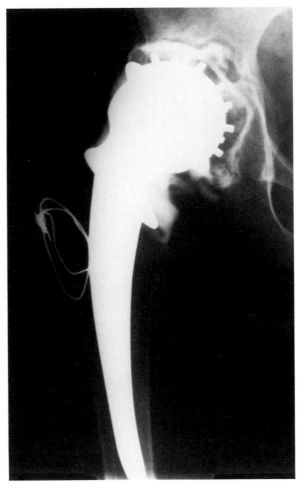

Figure 16
A. A McKee–Farrar prosthesis embedded in radiolucent cement was causing the patient pain.
B. An arthrogram performed after aspiration of fluid for culture shows positive contrast in the bone–cement interface of the acetabular component, indicating loosening. The culture was negative for infection.

A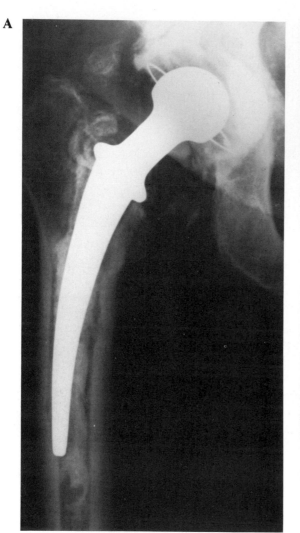

B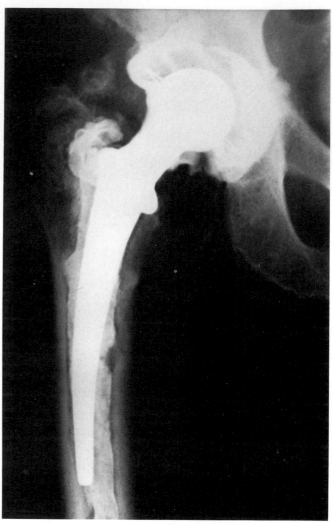

Figure 17

A. A total hip prosthesis is embedded in radiopaque cement. The bone–cement interface of the femoral component is abnormally wide and irregular, suggesting loosening. The bone–cement interface of the acetabular component is also somewhat prominent.

B. An arthrogram performed after aspiration for culture shows contrast agent in the femoral bone–cement interface, indicating loosening. No positive contrast agent can be identified in the acetabular bone–cement interface, but it would be difficult to see it between radiopaque bone and cement. A subtraction study might have provided further information.

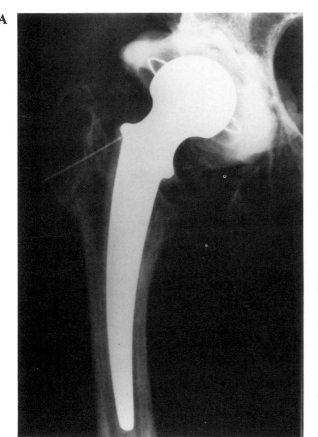

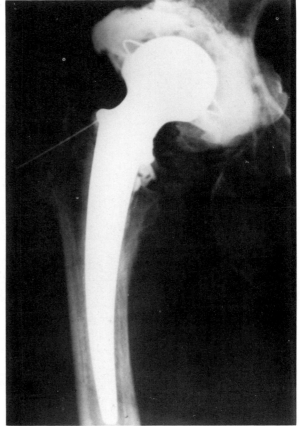

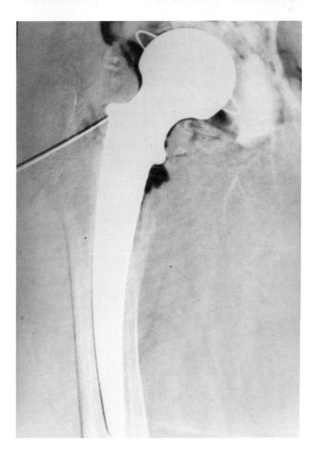

Figure 18

A. A Charnley–Müller prosthesis is embedded with radiopaque cement. The acetabular bone–cement interface is slightly prominent. The needle has been introduced by an anterolateral, somewhat inferior approach, and the tip of the needle is obscured by the neck of the prosthesis.

B. A thin layer of positive contrast agent can be seen at the neck of the prosthesis and where the cement protrudes into the pelvis (arrow). The contrast coating of the acetabular bone–cement interface cannot be seen well enough to determine loosening.

C. Subtracting the preinjection film from the postinjection film shows the positive contrast substance, now appearing black, completely surrounding the cement of the acetabular component. The acetabular component is loose. Despite immobilization, the patient moved the leg slightly and registration of the femur is not perfect. The misalignment is apparent at the needle and at the stem of the prosthesis where black shadowing can be seen on one side and a corresponding symmetrical white shadowing on the other. There is no evidence of loosening of the femoral component.

A

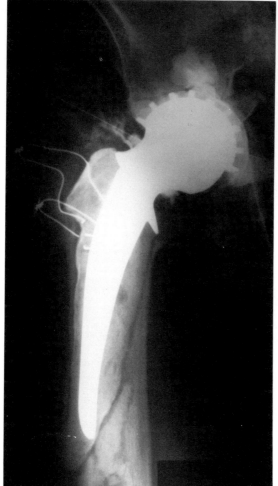

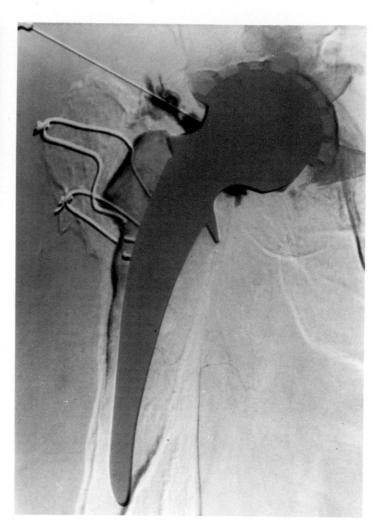

B

Figure 19
A. Following injection of positive contrast agent into a hip joint replaced by a McKee–Farrar prosthesis embedded with opaque cement, some positive contrast agent is seen medially at the acetabular bone–cement interface and at the bone–cement interface of the femoral component.
B. The subtraction study clearly shows loosening of both the acetabular and femoral components by demonstrating positive contrast medium at the bone–cement interfaces. The needle has been inserted from a superolateral direction.

A
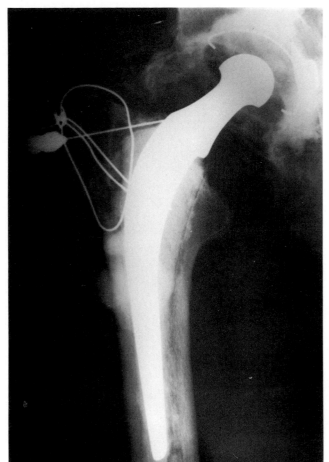

B
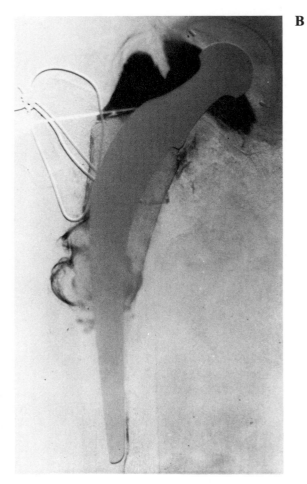

Figure 20
A. The loosening of either component of a Charnley prosthesis embedded with radiopaque cement is not conclusively demonstrated on the preinjection film.
B. The subtraction film clearly shows the radiopaque contrast agent in the bone–cement interface of the femur but not at the acetabular bone–cement interface. The
femoral component is loose.

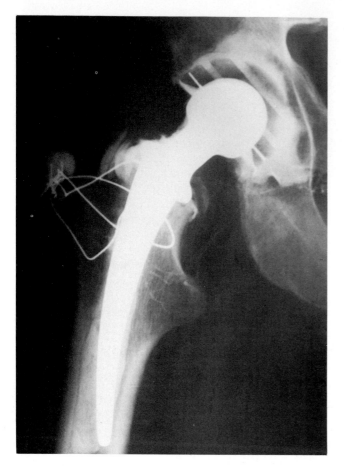

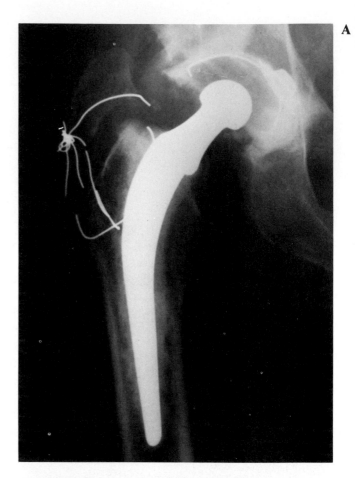

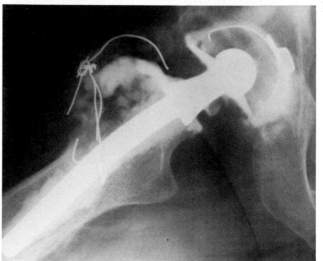

Figure 21
A small collection of contrast agent is seen on the outer margin of the osteotomized greater trochanter where the wires are twisted shut. If culture of aspirated fluid is negative, this collection, which is not unusual, is a small communicating bursa rather than an abscess.

Figure 22
A. The osteotomy fragments of the greater trochanter have separated and the wires that held them are broken.
B. The arthrogram shows a communication between the post-operative pseudocapsule and the separated trochanteric osteotomy fragments. Culture of aspirated fluid was negative, and there was no evidence of loosening of the prosthesis.

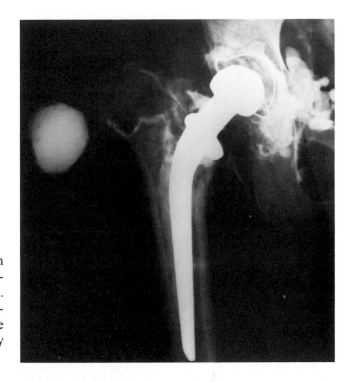

Figure 23

A positive culture was obtained from fluid aspirated from the hip joint prior to the arthrogram. The opacified soft tissue collections of contrast agent are therefore abscesses. Contrast agent in the acetabular bone–cement interface indicates loosening. Positive contrast agent is not seen in the femoral bone–cement interface, but a subtraction study might have shown it.

A

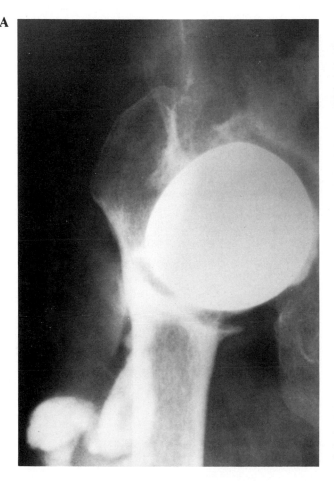

B

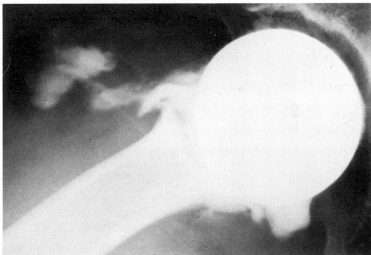

Figure 24

A, B. Aspiration and culture of fluid from a hip joint with a cup arthroplasty confirmed a clinical diagnosis of infection. The arthrogram opacifies a sinus tract and an abscess.

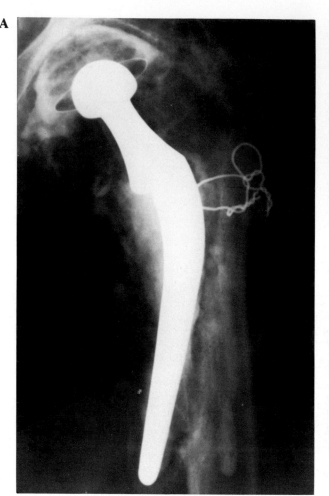
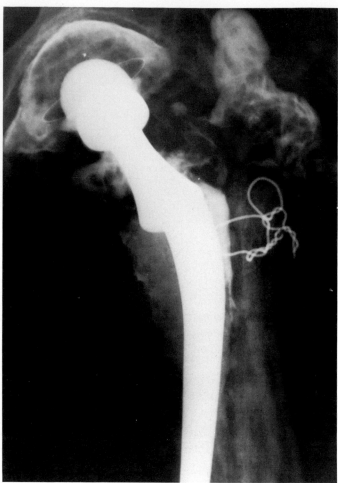

Figure 25

A, B. The bone–cement interface of the acetabular component is abnormally wide. The stem of the femoral component perforates the femoral shaft on its medial aspect. The bone–cement interfaces are abnormally wide and irregular, indicating loosening. Aspiration of the hip joint followed by an arthrogram was performed with the leg in traction. Joint fluid was sent to the laboratory and a positive culture was obtained. The arthrogram shows positive contrast agent in the acetabular as well as the femoral bone–cement interfaces, confirming the diagnosis of loosening. A soft tissue abscess located superolaterally is opacified with contrast medium. The diagnosis of infection and abscess is based upon obtaining a positive culture.

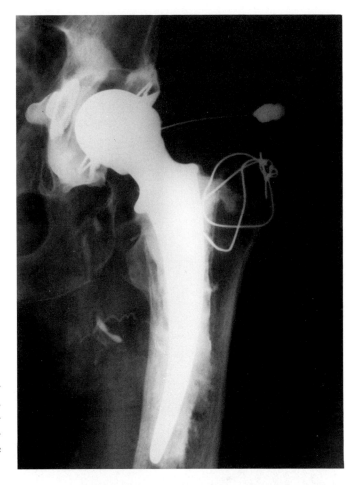

Figure 26
An arthrogram of a painful prosthesis faintly shows positive contrast agent in the femoral bone–cement interface, indicating loosening of the femoral component. Opacification of lymphatics suggests synovial inflammatory disease, but in this case infection was ruled out by negative cultures.

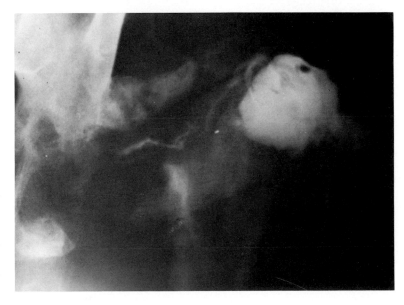

Figure 27
An infected total hip prosthesis has been removed and the patient had been treated with antibiotics. An arthrogram performed after aspiration of fluid for culture shows a distorted, constricted capsular space communicating with an irregular contrast-filled space near the greater trochanter. Culture of fluid indicated an infection.

A 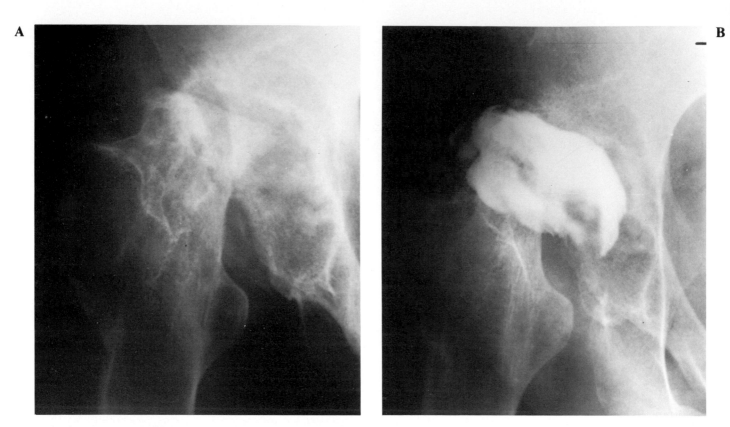 B

Figure 28
A. The nail stabilizing an infected subcapital fracture of the hip was removed and the patient was treated with a prolonged course of antibiotics.
B. Prior to insertion of a total hip prosthesis, a hip aspiration and arthrogram were performed to determine the state of the infection. Culture of aspirated fluid was negative for infection. The arthrogram provides proof that the needle had been placed intra-articularly and shows a distorted capsule with no evidence of abscess or sinus tract formation.

10
Hip Arthrography in Infants and Children

Amy Beth Goldman

A routine roentgenogram of an infant's or a child's hip joint is considerably less informative than that of an adult because the femoral head and acetabulum are incompletely ossified. Contrast arthrography is useful for evaluating the cartilaginous portions of the femoral capital epiphysis and the acetabulum, and for visualizing the joint space and synovial-lined capsule not visible on routine radiographs.

An important indication for contrast arthrography is a suspected septic hip. Fluoroscopy facilitates arthrocentesis of the hip and the arthrogram documents the intra-articular position of the aspiration needle, which is important when trying to obtain fluid for a culture. In the diagnosis of a neonatal infection, significant damage can occur if treatment is delayed. The arthrogram can also document damage of the unossified femoral capital epiphysis and show abscess and sinus formation.

A second indication for hip arthrography in infants and children is to evaluate the degree of displacement of the femoral head, the efficacy of closed reduction, and the degree of incongruity of the articular surfaces of congenital hip dislocation or subluxation. The severity of other congenital growth disturbances, such as proximal focal femoral deficiency and multiple epiphyseal dysplasia, can also be assessed more accurately by arthrography than by other means.

A third indication for contrast studies of a child's hip joint is to evaluate acquired hip deformities like those from aseptic necrosis or previous infection.

EQUIPMENT

Although any fluoroscopic equipment can be used for a hip arthrogram, the most convenient is one with an overhead X-ray tube and an under-table image amplifier (Fig. 1). Such equipment permits adequate working space above the hip joint with less chance of contaminating needles or gloved hands by touching the fluoroscopic tower. To perform hip arthrography in infants and children, the standard arthrogram tray with a 22-gauge, 1½-in. needle added is sufficient.

Injection Technique

The child is placed supine on the fluoroscopic table. Small infants may be placed transversely with the lower extremities toward the examiner (Figs. 2A, B). The hip is in neutral rotation and a small pillow can be placed under the knee to provide flexion of the hip joint and relax the capsule. Under fluoroscopic control, a lead marker is placed over the medial aspect of the femoral neck or, in older children, over the center of the femoral neck, to determine the location of skin puncture. The selected site is then marked on the skin with indelible ink (Fig. 2B). It is advisable to palpate the femoral artery and mark it on the skin as well in order to avoid its inadvertent puncture. Under sterile technique, a 22-gauge, 1½-in. needle is passed downward into the joint and aimed toward the medial aspect of the femoral neck (Fig. 3). If the femur is in a fixed, abducted position the needle can be inserted by a medial approach (Fig. 4). The position of the needle is checked fluoroscopically. If the infant is given appropriate sedation prior to the examination, it is not necessary to administer local anesthesia. In infants under 3 months, neither sedation nor anesthesia is required. General anesthesia is not used unless the arthrogram is performed in the operating room either immediately before or during an operative procedure, or unless it is needed by the surgeon for manipulation of the hip, or for application of plaster.

When the tip of the needle hits the femoral neck, aspiration of synovial fluid is attempted. If no fluid is obtained but cultures for suspected infection are desired, a few cubic centimeters of sterile saline without preservative are injected and reaspirated. Since contrast material is slightly bacteriostatic, large amounts should not be injected until the aspiration for culture is completed. Only 2 to 4 cc of a meglumine positive contrast agent diluted to 50 percent strength with sterile saline or water should be used for the arthrogram of an infant, because if there is too much contrast material or if it is too dense, the cartilaginous structures, the joint space, and the capsular recesses may be obscured (Fig. 5).

If the needle is intra-articular, the first drops of contrast material flow away from the needle tip and around the femoral head or across the femoral neck (Fig. 6). If, however, the injected contrast pools around the needle tip, it indicates that the needle is not within the joint and should be repositioned.

Following the injection procedure, the needle is removed and roentgenograms are obtained with the hip in neutral and frog-leg positions and usually with internal rotation of the femur. Additional projections may be obtained to determine the position of best fit of the femoral head in the acetabulum, or the best coverage of the femoral head by the acetabulum.

ANATOMY AND THE NORMAL ARTHROGRAM

The important features of the normal hip arthrogram (Fig. 7) are (1) a triangular limbus with a sharp point, (2) a thin limbus thorn with its tip not extending more than 2 to 3 mm above a horizontal line crossing

through the triradiate cartilage, (3) a spherical femoral head, (4) coverage of over half of the femoral capital epiphysis by the acetabulum, (5) a tight fit between the femoral capital epiphysis and the medial portion of the acetabulum in all positions of the femur, and (6) no visualization of the ligamentum teres.

Following the injection of positive contrast agent, the articular surface of the acetabulum is outlined by a thin, smooth line of contrast material. Its superior lateral aspect, called the limbus, is triangular in shape. It is relatively larger in children than in adults. Since the joint capsule inserts above the tip of the limbus, both its medial and lateral sides are covered by contrast material. The opacified space between the lateral margin of the limbus and the joint capsule is called the limbus thorn. It is a thin line with a sharp point and on anteroposterior projection, its superior tip should not extend more than 2 to 3 mm above a line drawn through the triradiate cartilages.

The femoral head is a perfect hemisphere, with its height (radius) equal to half its width (diameter), and most of its articular surface should be covered by the acetabulum. The ossified nucleus, if present, is in the center of the cartilaginous femoral head.

The synovial-lined capsule is also clearly outlined on the arthrogram. Contrast material pools at the insertion of the synovial membrane at the base of the femoral neck. In the center of the femoral neck, there is a relatively radiolucent zone referred to as the zona orbicularis. It is produced by the pressure of the orbicular ligament (a localized thickening of the capsular fibers), which leaves little room for the contrast medium. At the medial inferior aspect of the contrast-filled capsule is a small, rounded filling defect produced by the ligamentum transversum, which is a continuation of the cartilaginous labrum across the acetabular notch. It is flanked by two contrast-filled synovial pouches. The more proximal pouch is actually two superimposed folds of synovium creating ventral and dorsal recesses. The ligamentum teres, which originates from the medial side of the ligamentum transversum, runs between these folds of the proximal pouch and is not visible on a normal hip arthrogram. The joint space is narrow and uniform in width, and there should be no pooling of contrast material between the femoral head and the acetabulum.

THE ABNORMAL ARTHROGRAM

Neonatal Septic Hip

The primary role of contrast arthrography in neonatal septic arthritis of the hip is to confirm the intra-articular position of the needle tip. If joint fluid cannot be aspirated, sterile saline without bacteriocidal agents should be injected and reaspirated, followed by injection of positive contrast for the arthrogram. Aspirated fluid is sent for culture, and smears should be made for immediate examination. If bacteria are seen on the smear, treatment can be started at once. The neonatal septic hip is a medical emergency and studies should be performed immediately on the basis of clinical suspicion. The clinical diagnosis of joint infection in a neonate is difficult because systemic symptoms and signs may be entirely absent. A generalized sepsis can mask involvement of an individual joint. In the neonate, a hip held in fixed abduction, flexion, and external rotation or soft tissue swelling of the thigh suggests the diagnosis of hip joint infection. The infection usually reaches the joint by the hematogenous route, but direct innoculation can also occur from attempted femoral venopuncture.

Routine roentgenograms may be normal early in the course of joint infection. Pathologic dislocation secondary to pus distending the capsule and displacing the femoral head (Fig. 8A) and roentgenographically visible metaphyseal osteomyelitis occur only when the disease is already well advanced.

Hip aspiration aided by arthrography is the most reliable means of establishing an early diagnosis of neonatal septic hip and of evaluating the extent and type of cartilage destruction. Arthrocentesis of the hip joint may be difficult in septic joints, and several attempts at needle placement may be necessary before a successful aspiration is performed. Large quantities of contrast should not be injected until after aspiration because contrast material is moderately bacteriocidal. Once contrast is injected, superimposition of communicating soft tissue abscesses may complicate the interpretation of the arthrogram (Figs. 5, 8B). In addition to confirming the position of the needle, the arthrogram can demonstrate early cartilage destruction, capsular deformities which determine the severity of joint damage present before treatment. Occasionally, pathologic epiphyseal fractures can be detected (Figs. 9A, B). Early diagnosis and appropriate treatment can prevent the later, irreversible changes such as epiphyseal growth disturbances of the proximal femur and destruction of the acetabulum and/or femoral head.

Congenital Hip Dislocation

The diagnosis of congenital hip dislocation should be established in the first few days of life on the basis of the clinical examination with the Ortolani and/or Barlow maneuvers. The arthrogram is not used for diagnosis of congenital hip dislocation in the neonate.

Later, it can provide information concerning the severity of the dysplasia, the degree of incongruity of the joint, and the efficacy of therapy in infants or children in whom the diagnosis was not made and successful treatment not instituted in the neonatal period.

The contrast arthrogram is useful in differentiating between subluxation and complete dislocation. This distinction, which is unimportant in the neonate, becomes critical in older infants when treatment has not been instituted or successfully completed. In cases of subluxation (Figs. 10A–C), less than half of the femoral head is covered by the acetabulum and the limbus thorn is abnormally elevated by the laterally placed femoral head. In cases of dislocation (Fig. 11), the femoral head is displaced superiorly and laterally and is completely uncovered by the acetabulum. The elastic limbus is displaced downward to lie between the femoral head and the acetabulum. The capsule of the dislocated hip has a characteristic hourglass shape because it is pinched by the limbus, the iliopsoas, and constricted capsule. The ligamentum teres is readily seen.

The contrast study can also identify the cause of a failed reduction. The reduction can be obstructed by the interposition of the limbus between the femoral head and the acetabulum (Fig. 12) or by a thickened ligamentum teres that may occupy the acetabular cavity (Figs. 11, 12). On the arthrogram, an abnormal ligamentum teres appears as a ribbon-like radiolucent shadow on the acetabular side of the joint. An infolded limbus appears arthrographically as a lucent filling defect projecting between the femoral head and the articular surface of the acetabulum.

The contrast study is also useful in demonstrating femoroacetabular incongruity, flattening of the articular surface of the cartilaginous femoral head, pooling of contrast material in the medial aspect of the joint space, and inadequate coverage of the femoral head (Figs. 10, 13). This information helps identify candidates for iliac or femoral osteotomies or to plan conservative management.

Proximal Focal Femoral Deficiency

Proximal focal femoral deficiency is a congenital deformity of the proximal femur. It is characterized by the absence of, or abnormal modeling of the subtrochanteric region of the femur and shortening of the femoral shaft. Severe cases have an associated absence of the femoral neck and/or the femoral head. The acetabulum may be dysplastic or may appear completely absent. Contrast arthrography permits an early assessment of the deformity by confirming the presence or absence of a cartilaginous femoral head (Figs. 14A, B).

This information is important in determining prognosis and aids in planning surgical treatment.

In mild cases of proximal focal femoral deficiency where the cartilaginous femoral head appears to be normal, only a subtrochanteric osteotomy may be needed. With marked femoral shortening, a below-the-knee amputation and prosthesis may be required. In the severest deformities where the femoral head is absent, staged surgery can be planned to use the knee as a "hip joint," and to use a prosthesis designed for above-the-knee amputees. As in all dysplasias, ossification of the femoral head is frequently delayed, and without a contrast study to determine the presence of a cartilaginous femoral head, planning and instituting appropriate therapy may be delayed.

Legg Calve Perthes Disease

The early diagnosis of Legg Calve Perthes disease is established by plain film or radionuclide findings. In later stages, arthrography is a useful means of evaluating characteristics of the disease, including the degree of secondary cartilage abnormalities, the presence of incongruity, the efficacy of therapy, and the status of persistent unfused subchondral bone fragments.

During the early stages of this disease, the arthrogram is always normal because the abnormalities are only in the ossific nucleus. It is in the later stages of fragmentation and repair that the cartilaginous structures become involved (Fig. 15) and the arthrogram is useful in predicting the course of the disease. If the cartilaginous femoral head and acetabulum maintain their normal shape during the stages of fragmentation and repair of the ossification center, a well functioning hip joint can be expected. The arthrographic criteria that indicate a poor prognosis include:

1. An abnormal shape of the cartilaginous femoral capital epiphysis, with a decrease in the ratio of the height to half the width (Figs. 16–18)
2. Persistent enlargement of the unossified capital epiphysis
3. Irregularity of the contour of the cartilaginous femoral head (Figs. 17, 18)
4. Compression of the limbus and/or narrowing of the superior lateral aspect of the joint space (Figs. 17, 18)
5. Joint incongruity evidenced by pooling of contrast material medially between the femoral head and acetabulum (Figs. 15–18)
6. Inadequate coverage of the femoral capital epiphysis by the acetabulum.

Information obtained by arthrography may help in selecting candidates for iliac or intertrochanteric osteotomies.

An unusual finding is a persistent ununited fragment of the femoral head, sometimes erroneously referred to as osteochondritis dissecans, complicating a late, healed stage of Legg Calve Perthes disease. If the overlying articular cartilage of the femoral head is intact, the ununited bony fragment is not the cause of the patient's symptoms and does not need to be surgically removed (Fig. 19). If, however, the arthrogram shows contrast agent extending between the osseous body and the femoral head, indicating that the fragment is loose (Fig. 20), surgery may be required for relief of symptoms.

PITFALLS

Technical errors leading to incorrect interpretation of hip arthrograms in infants and children include the injection of too much positive contrast agent, and failure to dilute the contrast agent. In both instances, the cartilaginous portions of the femoral head and acetabulum are partially obscured, preventing adequate evaluation of cartilage surfaces and joint incongruity. Inadvertently injected air bubbles can be mistaken for loose cartilaginous bodies. In later stages of septic infections of the hip, intra-articular and capsular fibrosis may make intra-articular needle placement difficult. Persistence in attempting joint puncture in several different areas of the hip joint is often necessary before the injection of contrast agent indicates that an intra-articular location of the needle tip has been achieved. In infected hip joints, the opacification of communicating abscesses and sinus tracts may obscure the hip joint on one or more views, so multiple views in varying positions are necessary to detect destructive changes of the articular cartilages.

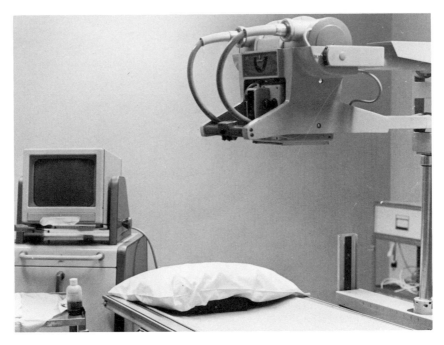

Figure 1
A fluoroscopic table with an overhead X-ray tube and an under-table image amplifier provides adequate working space above the patient and makes it easy to keep gloved hands and injection equipment sterile.

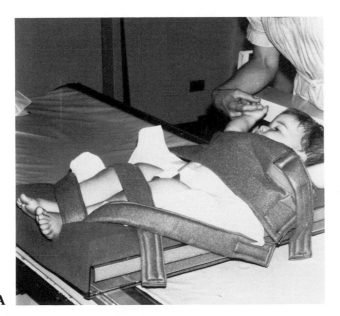
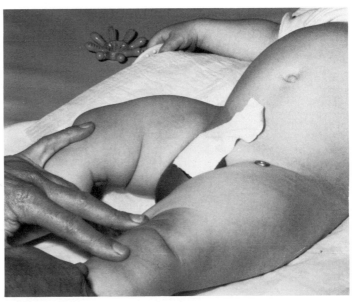

A   B

Figure 2
A. The infant is placed supine on the fluoroscopic table with the hip in neutral position. Small infants can be placed transversely on the table so that the examiner does not need to reach across the infant.
B. A lead marker is placed on the skin and moved under fluoroscopic controls to overlie the medial aspect of the femoral neck. The selected point for skin puncture is marked with indelible ink.

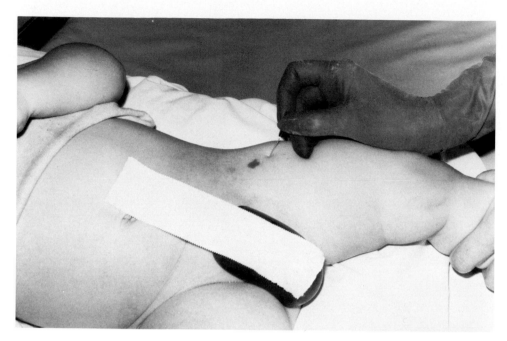

Figure 3
A 22-gauge, 1½-in. needle is directed toward the femoral neck to puncture the capsule immediately beneath the point marked on the skin. The sterile drape has been removed for photography. Alternatively, the needle may be slanted slightly upward and medially. The femur is held in neutral rotation.

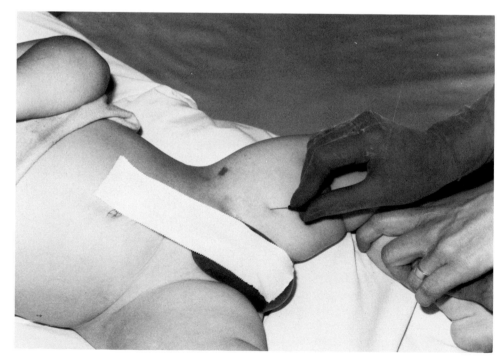

Figure 4
When the femur is fixed in abduction and external rotation, as might occur immediately after immobilization in this position for treatment of CDH or with an acute hip infection, the needle can be inserted from the medial aspect of the hip joint. The sterile drape has been removed for photography.

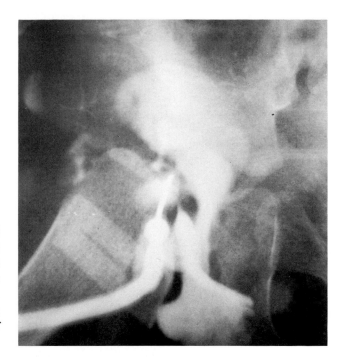

Figure 5

The injection of contrast agent through the medially inserted needle was made after aspiration of the hip joint. Plastic tubing attached between the syringe and needle permits fluoroscopic observation during injection. The periarticular collection of contrast agent is a communicating abcess. Smears and cultures indicated infection. The opacity of the contrast agent, undiluted in this case, obscures the details of the cartilaginous femoral head and acetabulum.

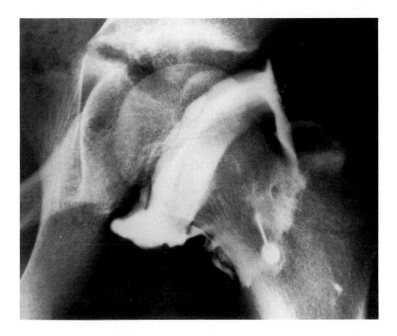

Figure 6

A roentgenogram made with the needle in place, immediately after the intra-articular injection of a moderate amount of contrast agent into the hip, shows no opacification of the joint space. This is a common finding in a normal congruous hip joint. Following the injection of contrast agent, the joint space can be opacified by traction on the leg or by having the patient exercise the hip.

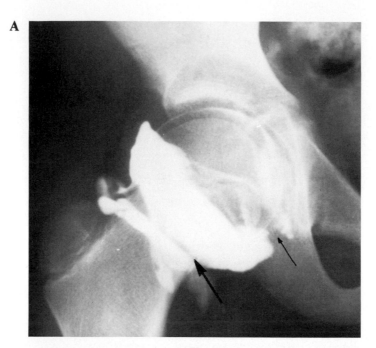

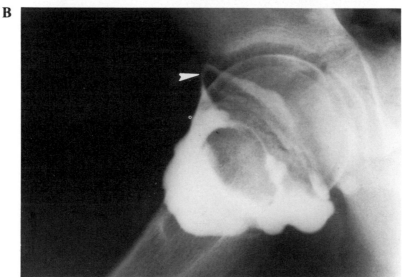

Figure 7

A, B. A thin layer of contrast agent is seen between the articular cartilages of the acetabulum and femoral head. Distraction of the joint surfaces or exercise may be necessary to opacify the joint space adequately. The triangular cartilaginous limbus at the superolateral margin of the acetabulum is outlined by contrast medium on its medial and lateral surface. The limbus thorn is the contrast-filled space between the lateral surface of the limbus and the capsule (white arrowhead). A normal limbus thorn is thin, and on the AP view its tip is less than 3 mm above a horizontal line drawn through the triradiate cartilage. The femoral head is hemispherical, and most of its articular surface is covered by the acetabulum. The zona orbicularis is an area of relative radiolucency crossing the middle of the femoral neck (large arrow). The ligamentum transversarium produces a notch at the interomedial aspect of the contrast filled capsule (small arrow).

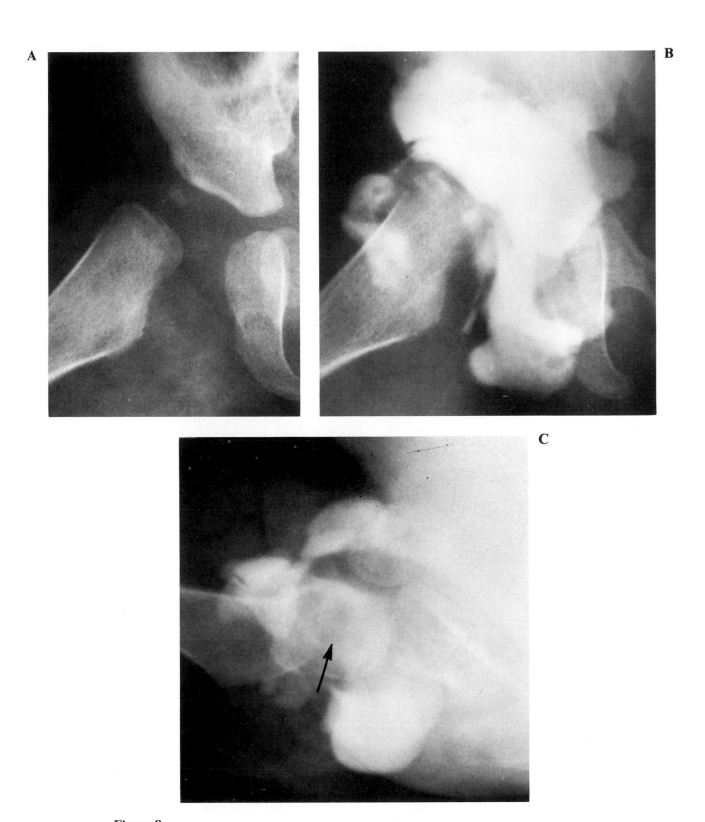

Figure 8
A. In a neonatal septic arthritis, a plain radiograph demonstrates dislocation of the femur and juxta-articular osteoporosis.
B, C. An arthrogram performed following the aspiration of purulent fluid shows multiple communicating extracapsular abcesses and sinus tracts and a partially destroyed femoral capital epiphysis (arrow).

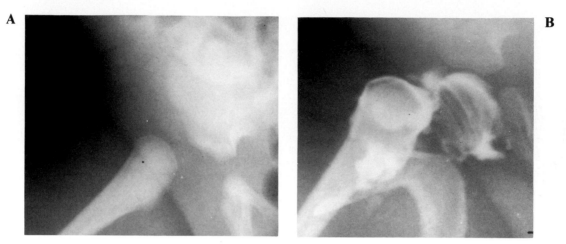

Figure 9
A. In a neonatal septic hip the plain roentgenogram was interpreted as showing a hip dislocation. Following aspiration of pus, contrast medium was injected.
B. The arthrogram demonstrated a pathologic epiphyseal fracture with the cartilaginous head located in the acetabulum. Cultures grew *Staphylococcus aureus.* Radiographs made two weeks later showed osteomyelitis of the femur.

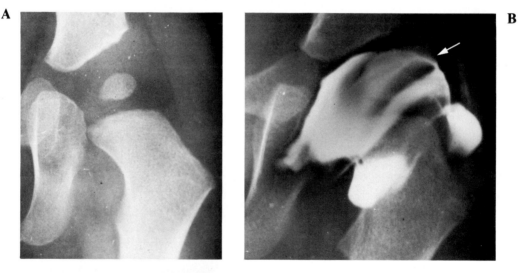

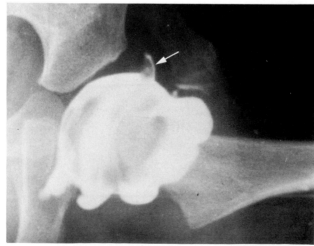

Figure 10
A. In an infant with a dysplastic subluxed hip, a conventional radiograph with the hip in neutral position demonstrates the ossific nucleus of the femoral head slightly displaced superolaterally.
B, C. The arthrogram confirmed the subluxation and showed elevation of the limbus thorn (arrows) and incomplete coverage of the cartilaginous head by the acetabulum.

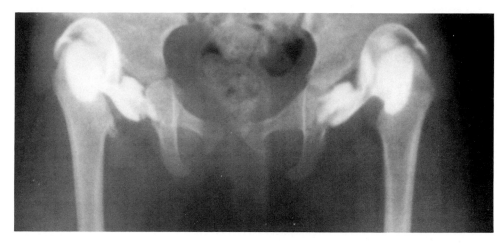

Figure 11
In a frank congenital hip dislocation, the arthrogram shows the femoral head displaced superolaterally and completely uncovered by the acetabulum. The capsule is stretched superiorly by the dislocated femoral head and indented by the infolded cartilaginous limbus producing the typical hourglass deformity. The ligamentum teres is visible and the femoral head is flattened on its medial aspect.

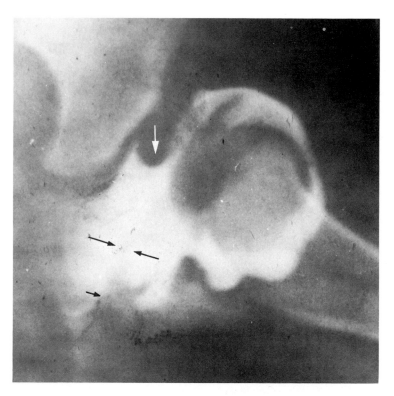

Figure 12
A frank hip dislocation shows an infolded limbus (white arrow) and thickened ligamentum teres (black arrows) which interfered with closed reduction.

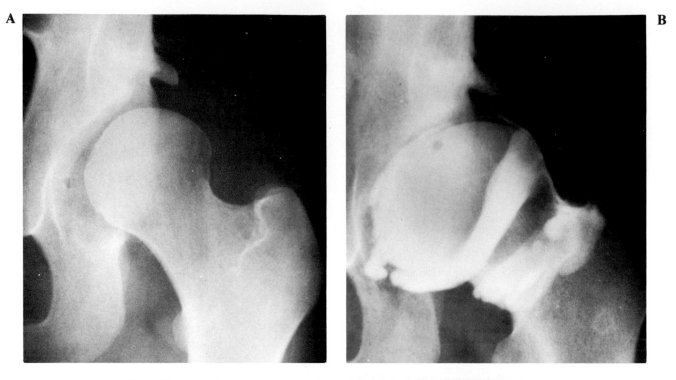

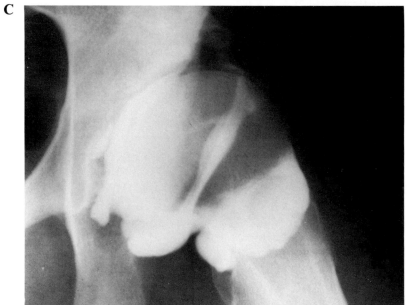

Figure 13
A. In hip dysplasia with joint incongruity, the femoral head is seen displaced superolaterally within a shallow acetabulum.
B, C. Abnormal pooling of contrast material at the inframedial aspect of the joint space indicates incongruity of joint surfaces. Some thinning of the articular cartilage near the superior aspect of the femoral head is also apparent.

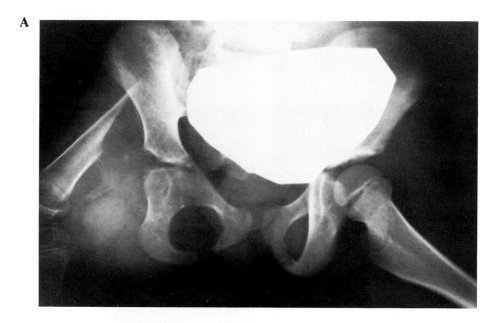

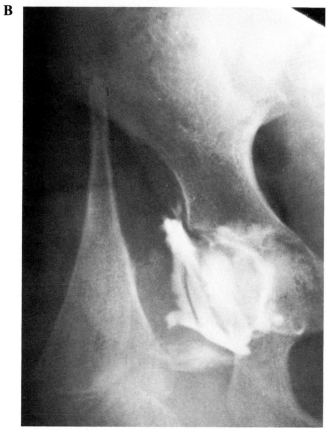

Figure 14
A. An infant with proximal focal femoral deficiency shows absence of an ossified proximal femoral shaft, femoral neck, and femoral head on conventional roentgenograms.
B. The arthrogram shows a cartilaginous femoral head within the acetabulum. These arthrographic findings help in determining prognosis and treatment.

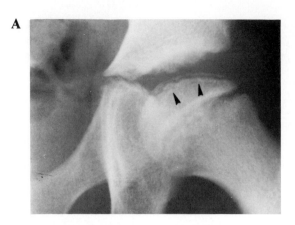

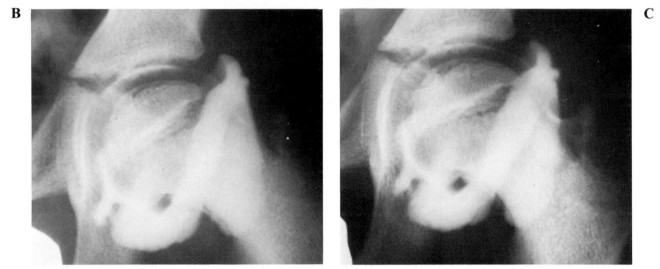

Figure 15
A. In Legg Calve Perthes disease, the plain radiograph demonstrates a subchondral crescent sign (arrowheads).
B, C. The arthrogram shows a mild deformity of the articular surface of the femoral head and minimal incongruence of the joint, demonstrated by slight pooling of contrast in the joint space above the area of subchondral collapse.

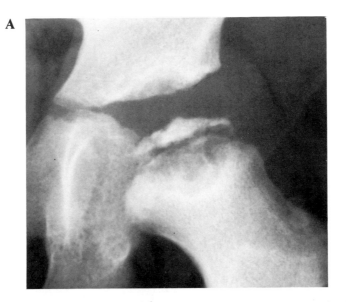

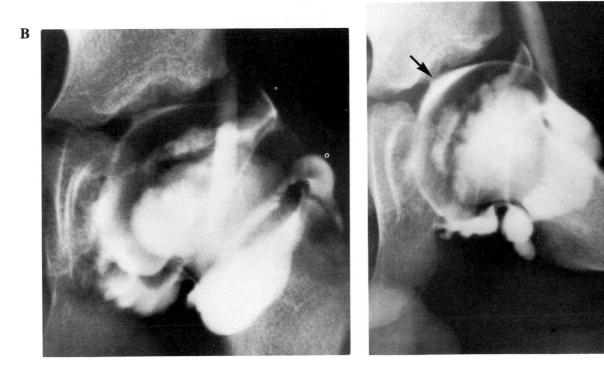

Figure 16
A. Standard radiographs of a child with Legg Calve Perthes disease show fragmentation and collapse of the femoral capital epiphysis and a large metaphyseal cyst.
B, C. The arthrogram demonstrates flattening and broadening of the cartilaginous portion of the femoral head with incongruity of joint surfaces as evidenced by accumulation of contrast agent at the superomedial aspect of the joint (arrow).

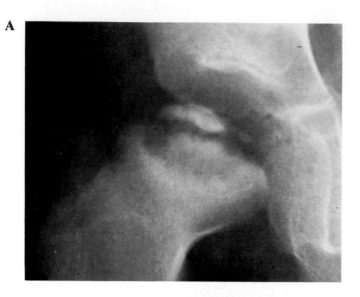

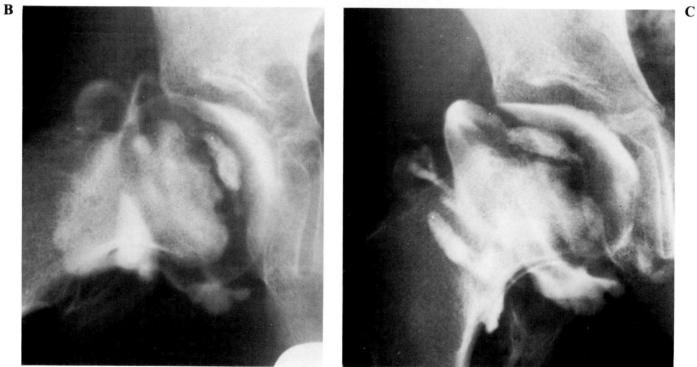

Figure 17
A. A conventional radiograph shows a late stage of Legg Calve Perthes disease.
B, C. The arthrogram shows considerable incongruity of joint surfaces with marked distortion of the cartilaginous femoral head.

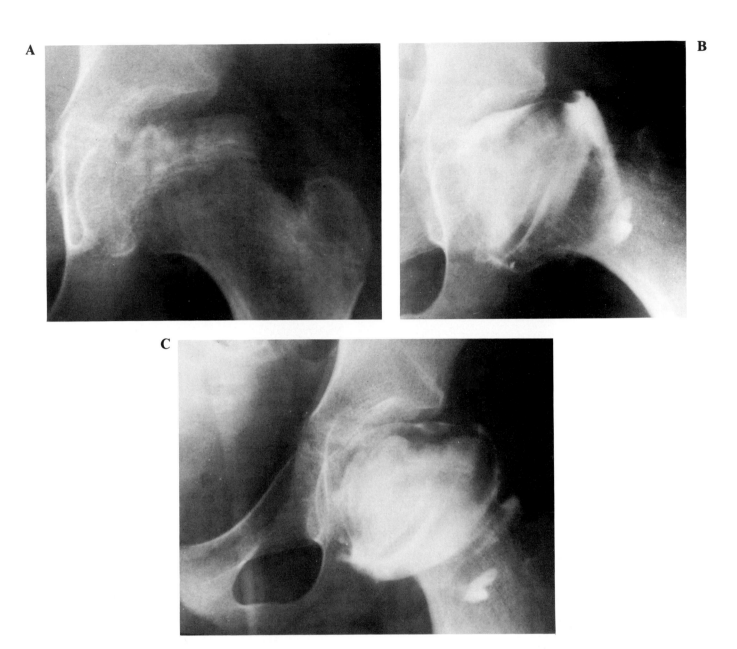

Figure 18
A. The plain radiograph shows the late stage of Legg Calve Perthes disease.
B, C. The arthrogram shows flattening of the cartilaginous femoral head and irregularity of the superior articular cartilage of the femoral head and of the articular cartilage of the acetabulum. The limbus is blunted. The femoral head is incompletely covered by the acetabulum, and there is pooling of contrast agent in the joint space indicating marked incongruity. These findings indicate a poor prognosis.

A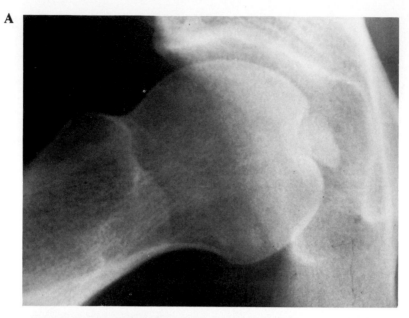

B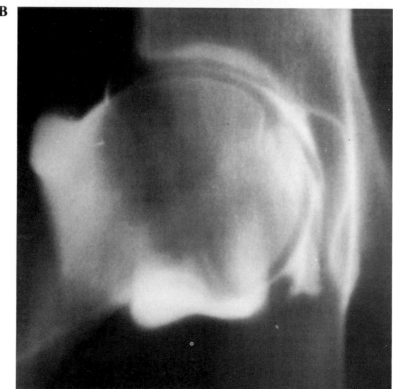

Figure 19
A. In a 16-year-old patient who had had Legg Calve Perthes disease, standard radiographs show an ununited osseous fragment of the femoral head.
B. An arthro-tomogram demonstrates that the cartilage overlying the osseous fragment is intact and that the fragment is not loose within the joint.

A

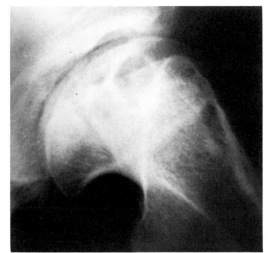

B

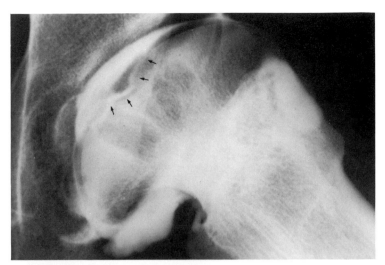

C

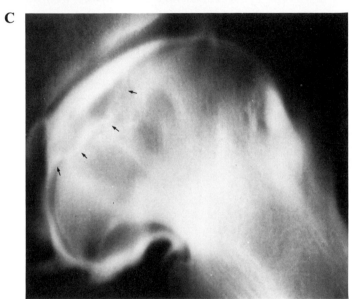

Figure 20
A. In a 22-year-old patient who had Legg Calve Perthes disease as a child, the routine radiographs demonstrate early degenerative joint disease.
B. An arthrogram shows a large osteochondral fragment which appears completely surrounded by contrast material (arrows) and is therefore loose within the joint.
C. The tomogram confirms that contrast medium (arrows) is between the osseous fragment and the femoral head.

11

The Ankle

Jeremy J. Kaye

Ankle sprains are common and may result in chronic instability and prolonged disability. In the acutely injured patient, stress films, particularly if done without anesthesia, may be unreliable in determining ligamentous instability because false-negative studies may be due to muscle spasm.

Ankle arthrography is a simple procedure that can assess the integrity of the ligamentous structures of the acutely injured ankle, evaluate the articular cartilages, and detect and localize loose bodies. The procedure is safe and reliable.

TECHNIQUE

Ankle arthrography is technically simple. When the examination is performed to assess the integrity of the ankle ligaments, single positive contrast arthrography is used. When the examination is designed to evaluate the articular cartilages, double contrast arthrography is better. When the presence or absence of loose bodies is in question, then air arthrography, double contrast arthrography, or single positive contrast arthrography can be utilized.

The patient is placed in the recumbent position on a fluoroscopic table with the ankle in the lateral position and the front of the ankle facing the examiner. The dorsalis pedis artery is palpated and its course is marked in order to avoid its puncture. A lead marker is placed on the front of the ankle with a small piece of tape, and under fluoroscopic observation it is moved to the selected needle entrance point, which is then marked with indelible ink (Fig. 1). The ideal needle path is near the midline and has a slightly cranial direction in order to avoid the overhanging anterior margin of the tibia. The standard arthrographic tray is used, to which is added a 22-gauge, 1- to 1½-in. needle.

The skin over the ankle is prepared with a solution of povidone-iodine and draped with a sterile towel with a small center hole. Using a 2 cc syringe and a 25-gauge ⅝-in. needle, a skin wheal of local anesthetic (1 percent lidocaine hydrochloride) is raised. Joint puncture with the 22-gauge needle is then performed using brief intermittent fluoroscopy (Fig. 2). When the tip of the needle is seen to project between the anterior margin of the tibia and the dome of the talus, it is in an intra-articular location (Fig. 3).

The use of the lateral projection and fluoroscopy facilitates this joint puncture since the joint space seen fluoroscopically in the anteroposterior projection represents the highest point of the tibiotalar articulation and not its anterior portion. Thus, the needle directed toward the projected joint space (Fig. 4A), strikes the overhanging anterior margin of the tibia (Fig. 4B).

Prior to the injection of contrast material, any fluid within the joint should be aspirated. If no fluid can be aspirated, a drop or two of contrast medium can be injected (Fig. 5). If the needle is intra-articular, the contrast medium flows away from the needle tip (Fig. 6). If the arthrogram is performed to assess the ligamentous structures, approximately 6 to 8 cc of meglumine diatrizoate is injected. If a double contrast examination is desired, approximately 0.5 to 1 cc of meglumine diatrizoate is injected, followed by 6 to 8 cc of room air. If air alone is used, approximately 6 to 8 cc is sufficient. If tomography is contemplated during a double contrast arthrogram, the addition of 0.1 to 0.2 cc of 1:1000 solution of epinephrine delays absorption of the positive contrast material. When either a double contrast or an air arthrogram is being done, it is advisable, prior to removing the needle, to check fluoroscopically for tendon sheath or subtalar joint filling, as supplemental air or positive contrast material may be needed if the tendon sheaths fill.

Following the injection, the needle is removed and the ankle is manipulated briefly. Standard overhead tube films are taken in the anteroposterior, the lateral, and both oblique projections. The patient then exercises the ankle and, after the initial set of films is reviewed, a second set is obtained. If the examination is performed to assess the articular cartilage or to detect loose bodies, stress roentgenograms made under fluoroscopic control and tomography may be useful.

ANATOMY FOR ANKLE ARTHROGRAPHY

The strongest of the lateral ligaments is the calcaneofibular ligament. This ligament takes its origin from the posteromedial aspect of the distal fibula and passes posteriorly, slightly medially, and downward to insert upon the calcaneus near its upper margin (Fig. 7). The calcaneofibular ligament lies immediately beneath and is contiguous to the tendon sheaths of the peroneus longus and brevis muscles.

The most commonly injured of the lateral supporting ligaments of the ankle is the anterior talofibular ligament. Roughly trapezoidal in shape, it originates from the anterolateral aspect of the most distal fibula and passes anteriorly and medially to insert onto the neck of the talus (Fig. 8). The anterior talofibular ligament forms a nearly straight line with the calcaneofibular ligament. Of the two, the calcaneofibular ligament is stronger.

A third lateral supporting ligament is the posterior talofibular ligament. It originates from the medial aspect of the distal fibula and inserts onto the talus above the posterior subtalar joint (Fig. 9). Another lateral ligament of importance for arthrography is the distal an-

terior tibiofibular ligament. It takes its origin from the anterior aspect of the distal tibia just above the tibiotalar joint and passes downward, posteriorly, and laterally to insert onto the anterior aspect of the distal fibula. The distal anterior tibiofibular ligament lies above the anterior talofibular ligament (Fig. 10).

On the medial side of the ankle, the only important ligamentous structure is the deltoid ligament. The deltoid ligament blends intimately with the tendon sheaths of the posterior tibial tendon and the flexor hallucis longus and flexor digitorum longus tendons. When this ligament is isolated, it is seen as a roughly fan-shaped structure extending downward from the medial malleolus and sending fibers to the talus and calcaneus (Fig. 11).

THE NORMAL ARTHROGRAM

In the normal ankle, the injected contrast material forms an umbrella over the articular surface of the talus (Fig. 12). An upward extension of contrast material is seen between the distal tibia and fibula, filling the syndesmotic recess. It can be best appreciated on the anteroposterior and oblique projections (Figs. 12A, B). On the lateral projection, the anterior and posterior recesses of the joint are well visualized (Fig. 12C).

In approximately 10 percent of patients examined, there is a communication between the tibiotalar joint and the posterior subtalar joint which fills with contrast material. It is not known to be of clinical significance. The arthrographic appearance is that of a double umbrella in the anteroposterior and oblique projections (Figs. 13A, B). In the lateral projection, the contrast material forming the lower umbrella is in the posterior subtalar joint (Fig. 13C).

In approximately 20 percent of patients, injected contrast material fills the tendon sheaths of the flexor hallucis longus and the flexor digitorum longus posteriomedially to the ankle (Fig. 14A). It is of no known clinical significance. The opacified flexor tendon sheaths are seen beneath the sustentaculum tali on the lateral view of the ankle (Fig. 14B).

There should be no tendon sheath filling on the lateral side of a normal ankle.

THE ABNORMAL ARTHROGRAM

Anterior Talofibular Ligament Tears

Anterior talofibular ligament tears are the most common of all ligament tears at the ankle. This injury is typically produced by forced inversion of the foot.

When an ankle arthrogram is performed within 48 hours of a tear, leakage of contrast material from the joint around the tip of the distal fibula and into the soft tissues is seen (Figs. 15–18, 22–25). The amount of leakage is not directly related to the severity of the tear. It depends in part on the time elapsed since the injury and on the degree of filling of extra-articular structures, most notably the posterior subtalar joint and the long flexor tendon sheaths, which reduce the intra-articular pressure of the injected contrast substance. With anterior talofibular ligament tears, a small leak of contrast agent may be seen best on an external oblique projection (Fig. 17B).

Tears of the anterior talofibular ligament can become watertight about 48 hours after the injury, even though the ligament is not structurally intact. It is therefore important to perform ankle arthrograms for diagnosis of ligamentous injuries shortly after the injury.

It is also advisable to obtain roentgenograms both before (Fig. 18A) and after (Fig. 18B) exercise. Occasionally only the films obtained after exercise demonstrate the leakage of contrast material indicating a tear of the anterior talofibular ligament (Fig. 18B).

Calcaneofibular Ligament Tears

Acute calcaneofibular ligament tears are almost invariably associated with tears of the anterior talofibular ligament. When the calcaneofibular ligament is torn, a communication is established between two synovial-lined structures, the ankle joint and the peroneal tendon sheaths, which fill with contrast agent. Opacification of the peroneal tendon sheaths on the lateral side of the ankle indicates that a calcaneofibular ligament tear has occurred (Figs. 19–24). If the ankle arthrogram is performed within 48 hours of the injury, and there is no associated tear of the anterior talofibular ligament, it can be presumed that the calcaneofibular ligament tear is due to an old injury with a persistent communication between the joint and the tendon sheaths.

Posterior Talofibular Ligament Tears

Although the posterior talofibular ligament is structurally the smallest of the lateral ligaments, isolated tears do not seem to occur. The posterior talofibular ligament lies between the posterior recess of the ankle joint and the posterior subtalar joint. Some instances of opacification of the posterior subtalar joint, a finding regarded as normal, may be due to an old tear of the posterior talofibular ligament.

Distal Anterior Tibiofibular Ligament Tears

Tears of the distal anterior tibiofibular ligament are not seen as isolated injuries. When the ligament is torn, the arthrogram shows leakage of contrast material upward, through and out of the syndesmotic recess (Fig. 25B). An abnormal separation between the distal tibia and fibula may be seen on plain roentgenograms.

Combined Lateral Ligament Tears

Combined lateral ligament tears are common. When there are tears of the anterior talofibular ligament and the calcaneofibular ligament, the arthrogram shows leakage of contrast material around the distal end of the fibula and filling of the peroneal tendon sheaths (Figs. 22–25). In tears of the anterior talofibular ligament and the distal anterior tibiofibular ligament, there is leakage of contrast material around the tip of the fibula (Fig. 25A) as well as contrast material between the distal tibia and fibula above the syndesmotic recess (Fig. 25B).

Deltoid Ligament Tears

Isolated deltoid ligament tears are uncommon. They are usually associated with a fracture of the distal fibula or with a disruption of the distal tibiofibular syndesmosis. When the deltoid ligament is torn, the arthrogram shows leakage of contrast material beneath the medial malleolus (Fig. 26). A medial leak of contrast may be difficult to identify since it may be partially obscured by the normal opacification of the tendon sheaths of the flexor hallucis longus and the flexor digitorum longus.

Articular Cartilage and Loose Bodies

When assessing the integrity of the articular cartilage, air arthrography (Fig. 27B) or double contrast arthrography (Fig. 28) may be utilized. Of the two, double contrast arthrography seems to give better delineation of the articular cartilage. Tomography, used to supplement either air arthrography or double contrast arthrography, allows more precise evaluation of the integrity of the articular cartilage. Large osseous intra-articular bodies may be apparent on positive contrast arthrography, preferably performed with tomography.

Anteriorly and posteriorly the capsule of the ankle is loose in order to allow for dorsiflexion and plantarflexion of the foot. Folds of a lax capsule should not be misinterpreted as an attached radiolucent body within the joint. Prone and supine cross-table lateral radiographs are useful during arthrography in identifying loose cartilaginous bodies and excluding artifacts caused by inadvertently injected air bubbles.

Adhesive Capsulitis

Occasionally, following ankle trauma and particularly following immobilization for an ankle sprain or fracture, an adhesive capsulitis develops, causing the patient persistent pain, limitation of ankle motion, and disability. This condition, similar to that occurring in the shoulder, is probably more common than generally appreciated, and can be detected by ankle arthrography. The arthrogram shows a marked diminution in the size of the capsular space (Figs. 29A, B). The margins of the capsular insertions are retracted and irregular. Adhesive capsulitis is usually associated with periarticular demineralization.

PITFALLS

Occasionally, when the ankle joint is overdistended, some contrast material may leak from the needle puncture hole. Leakage of contrast is usually best seen on the lateral radiograph and is easily distinguished from a tear of the anterior talofibular ligament. Care must be taken that air bubbles and the normal synovial irregularities are not mistakenly interpreted as loose bodies.

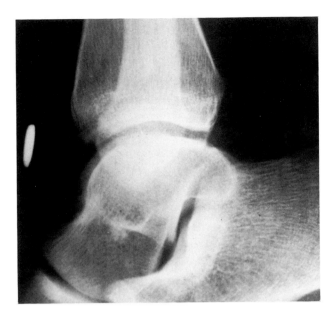

Figure 1
The patient is recumbent on a fluoroscopic table with the ankle in the lateral position. Using brief intermittent fluoroscopy, a lead marker is placed on the front of the ankle at a site where the needle can slide easily beneath the anterior lip, the tibia. This point is then marked on the skin with indelible ink.

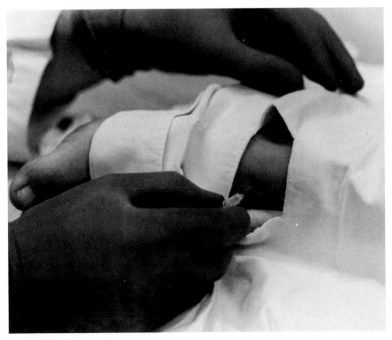

Figure 2
After the skin has been prepared with povidone-iodine solution, the ankle is draped. Using aseptic technique, a skin wheal of local anesthetic is raised at the point marked on the skin. The 1½-in., 22-gauge needle used for joint puncture is directed slightly cranially.

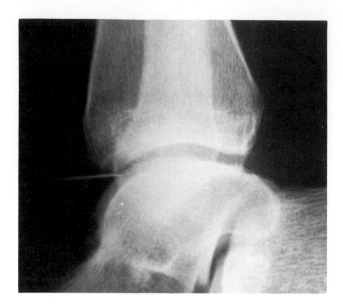

Figure 3
Using intermittent fluoroscopy, the needle is advanced until its tip is seen between the distal tibia and the talus. This position of the needle tip confirms its intra-articular location.

A 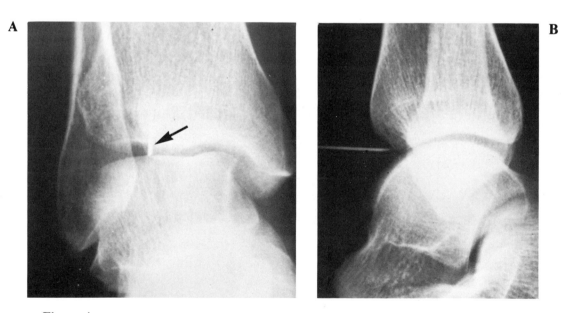 B

Figure 4
A. Incorrect needle tip placement occurs frequently when the needle (arrow) is directed toward the joint space as it is seen fluoroscopically in the anteroposterior projection.
B. The lateral projection reveals that the tip of the needle is impinging on the anterior margin of the tibia and is not intra-articular.

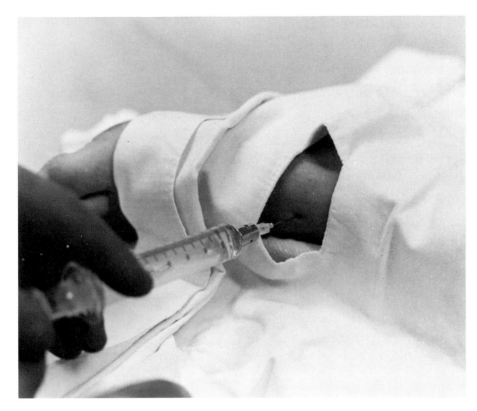

Figure 5
Contrast medium is injected into the ankle by connecting a syringe directly to the needle.

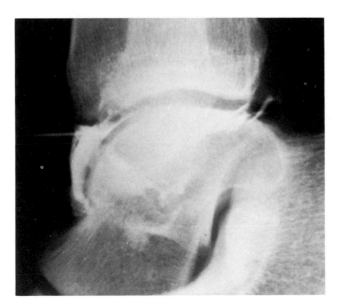

Figure 6
When no fluid can be aspirated from the joint, an injection of a very small amount of contrast material confirms the intra-articular location of the needle tip. The injected contrast material flows away from the needle tip, outlining portions of the tibiotalar articulation.

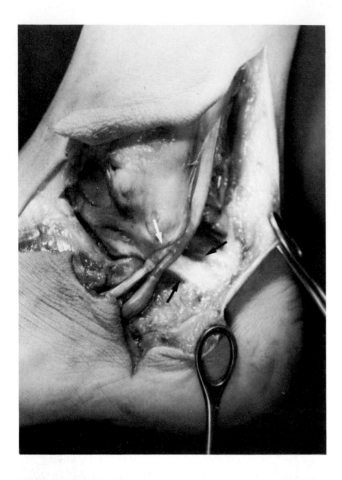

Figure 7
The calcaneofibular ligament (black arrows) originates from the medial aspect of the fibular tip and inserts onto the upper aspect of the calcaneus. The ligament is in close contact with the peroneal tendon sheaths (white arrow).

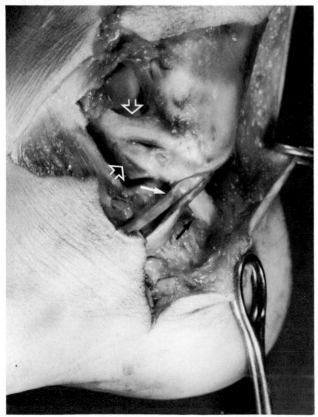

Figure 8
The anterior talofibular ligament (open white arrows) extends from the anterolateral aspect of the most distal fibula to the neck of the talus. It is the most frequently injured ankle ligament. The calcaneofibular ligament (black arrow) and the peroneal tendons (white arrow) are visible on the anatomic specimen.

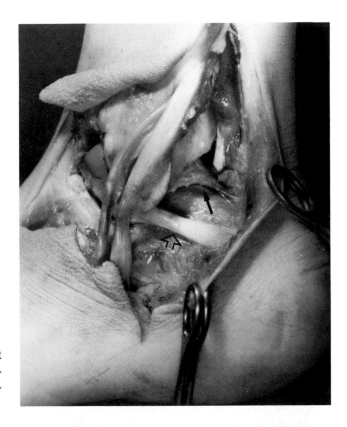

Figure 9
The roughly triangular posterior talofibular ligament (arrow) is seen when the peroneal tendons are reflected anteriorly. The anatomic specimen shows the course of the calcaneofibular ligament (open arrow).

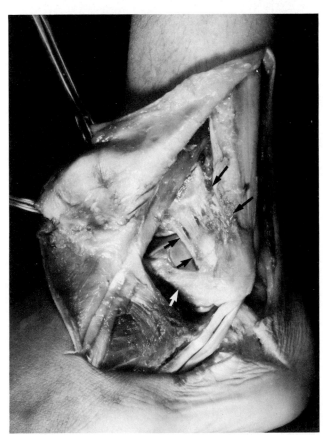

Figure 10
The distal anterior tibiofibular ligament (black arrows) often consists of several bands. They originate from the anterolateral aspect of the distal tibia and pass downward to insert on the anterolateral aspect of the distal fibula. This ligament lies above the anterior talofibular ligament (white arrow).

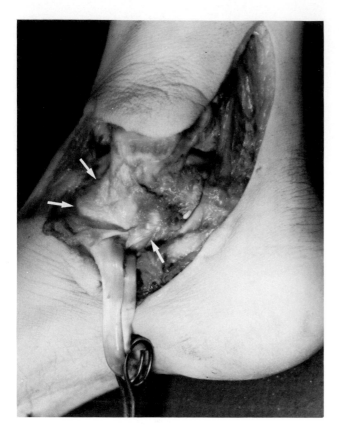

Figure 11
The deltoid ligament (arrows) can be seen after the posterior tibial and long flexor tendons and their surrounding synovial sheaths have been removed. It originates from the medial aspect of the medial malleolus and passes downward, sending fibers to the talus and calcaneus.

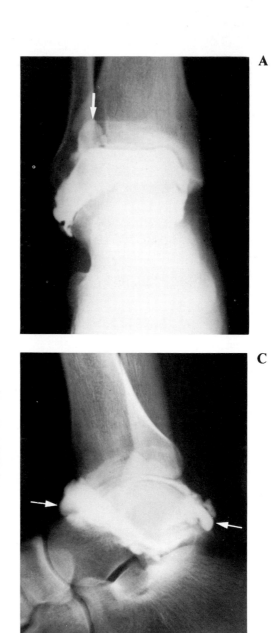

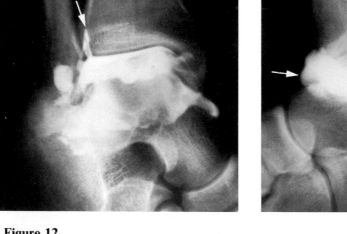

Figure 12
A normal ankle arthrogram is shown (**A**) in the anteroposterior projection, (**B**) in the oblique projection, and (**C**) in the lateral projection. The injected contrast material appears like an umbrella over the articular surface of the talus. In the anteroposterior and oblique projections, a streak of contrast material (arrows) is seen extending up between the distal tibia and fibula in the sydesmotic recess. In the lateral projection the anterior and posterior recesses of the ankle joint are seen (arrows).

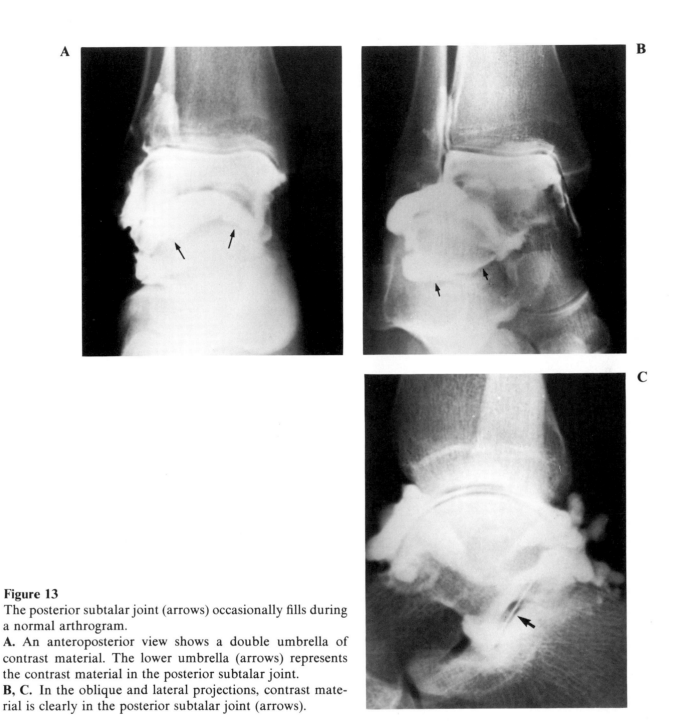

Figure 13
The posterior subtalar joint (arrows) occasionally fills during
a normal arthrogram.
A. An anteroposterior view shows a double umbrella of
contrast material. The lower umbrella (arrows) represents
the contrast material in the posterior subtalar joint.
B, C. In the oblique and lateral projections, contrast material is clearly in the posterior subtalar joint (arrows).

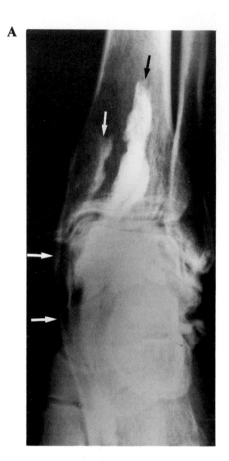

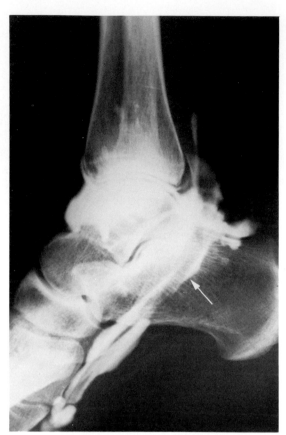

Figure 14
Contrast filling of the long flexor tendon sheaths (arrows) is a normal variant.
A. In the anteroposterior projection the opacified tendon sheaths are seen on the medial side of the ankle.
B. In the lateral projection the opacified tendon sheaths (arrow) are below the sustentaculum tali.

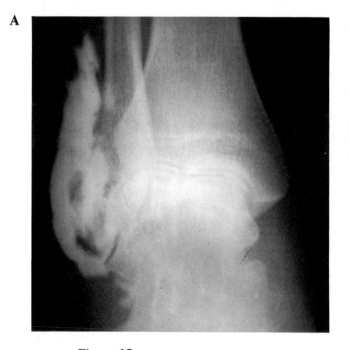

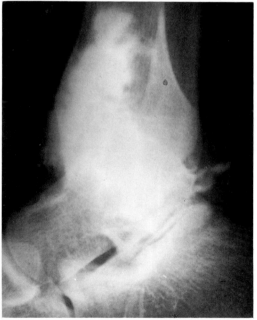

Figure 15
After an anterior talofibular ligament tear, the arthrogram shows that contrast material has leaked through the tear into the surrounding soft tissues.
A. In the anteroposterior projection the leaked contrast material is projected around the tip of the fibula and lateral to the fibula.
B. In the lateral projection the leaked contrast material is in front of the fibula.

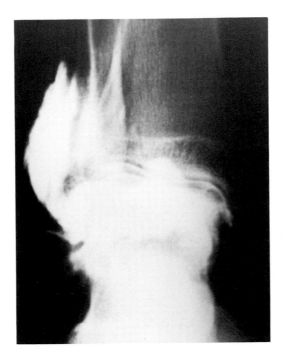

Figure 16
In this arthrogram of a patient with an anterior talofibular ligament tear, the contrast material has leaked from the joint through the tear and surrounds the distal fibula.

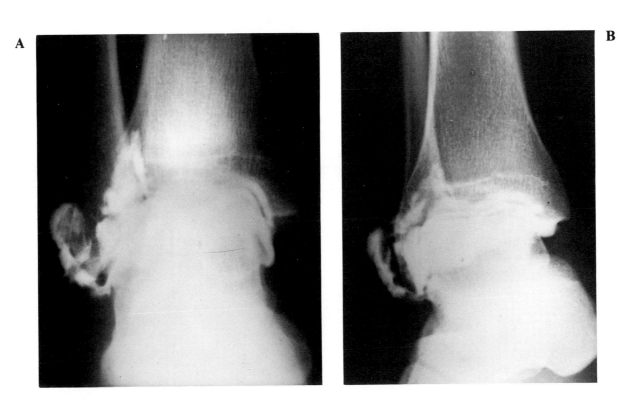

Figure 17
A. With an anterior talofibular ligament tear, the contrast material leaks through the tear and is identified on the anteroposterior projections.
B. A tear of the anterior talofibular ligament is sometimes seen better on radiographs made in the external oblique projection.

A

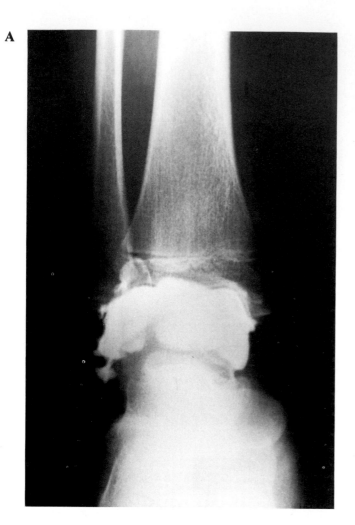

B

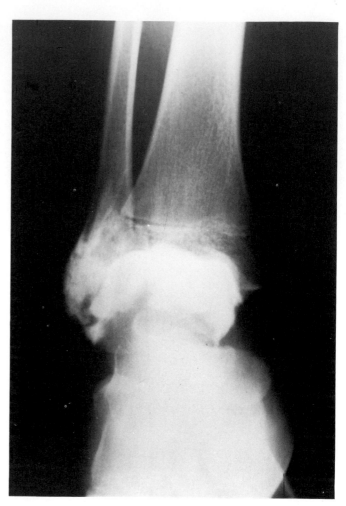

Figure 18
A. With an anterior talofibular ligament tear, initial radiographs may show no evidence of leakage of contrast material from the joint.
B. A second set of roentgenograms, after exercise, demonstrates that contrast material has leaked through a tear in the anterior talofibular ligament and collected around the tip of the distal fibula.

A
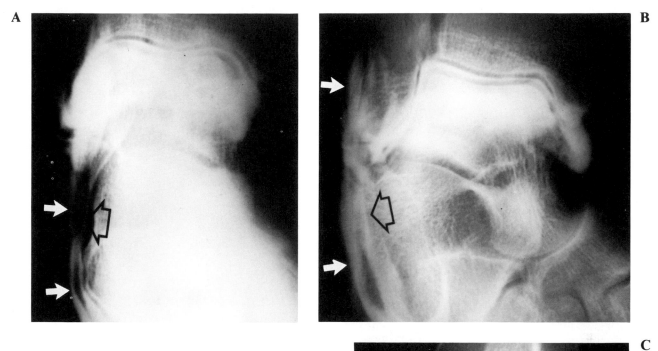
B

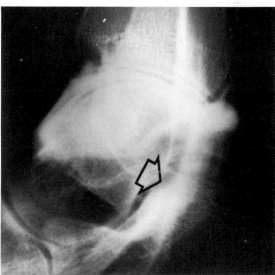
C

Figure 19
When the calcaneofibular ligament is torn, an arthrogram shows that injected contrast material fills the synovial sheaths around the peroneal tendons on the lateral side of the ankle (arrows) and can be identified in the (**A**) antero-posterior, (**B**) oblique, and (**C**) lateral projections. In the lateral projection, the contrast medium in the peroneal tendon sheaths is projected over the sustentaculum tali. Opacification of the peroneal tendon sheaths in the absence of a demonstrable associated anterior talofibular ligament tear implies that the injury to the calcaneofibular ligament is not acute.

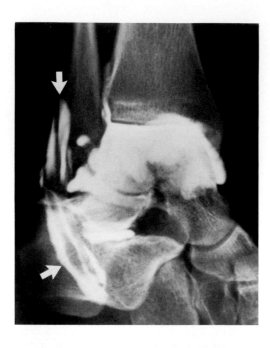

Figure 20
A calcaneofibular ligament tear is best demonstrated on the oblique projection by filling of the peroneal tendon sheaths (arrows).

A

B

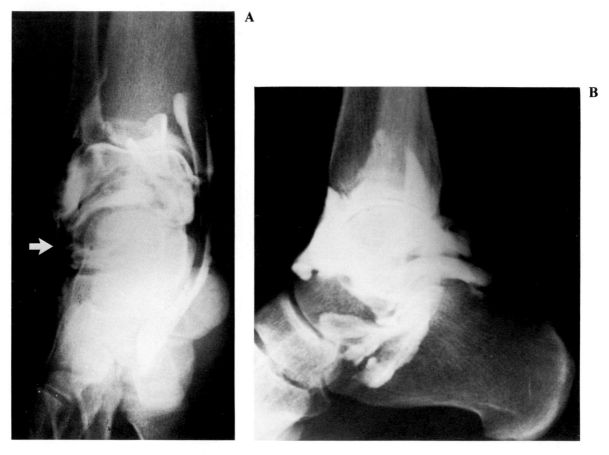

Figure 21
A. Careful inspection of the anteroposterior radiograph is necessary to see the minute amount of contrast material in the peroneal tendon sheaths (arrow), indicating a calcaneofibular ligament tear.
B. In the lateral projection, the contrast material in the long flexor tendon sheaths obscures the opacified peroneal tendon sheaths.

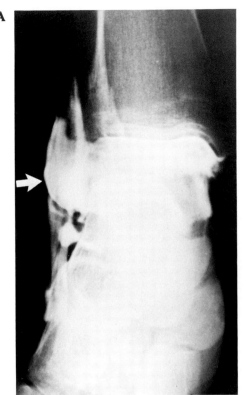
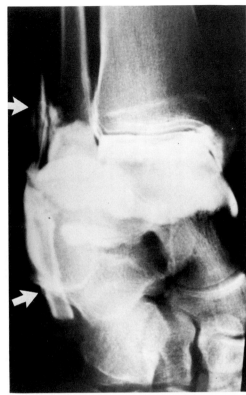

Figure 22
A. In the anteroposterior projection of an arthrogram, contrast material has leaked from the joint through a tear in the anterior talofibular ligament (arrow). Contrast material also fills the peroneal tendon sheaths, indicating a calcaneofibular ligament tear.
B. In the oblique projection, the peroneal tendon sheath filling is more clearly visible (arrows).

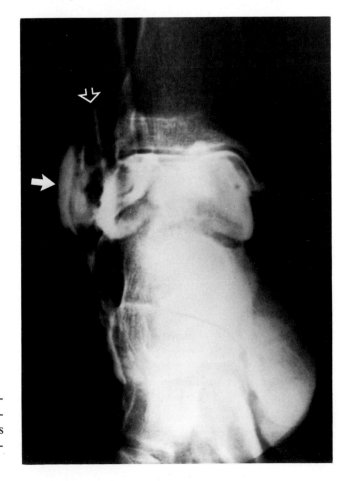

Figure 23
Injected contast material has leaked through a tear in the anterior talofibular ligament and is seen in the soft tissues adjacent to the lateral margin of the fibula (arrow). There is also filling of the peroneal tendon sheath (open arrow), indicative of a torn calcaneofibular ligament.

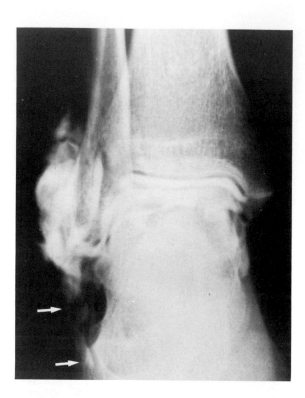

Figure 24
An arthrogram shows leakage of contrast material around the tip of the fibula, indicating an anterior talofibular ligament tear. Peroneal tendon sheath filling (arrows) indicates a calcaneofibular tear.

A

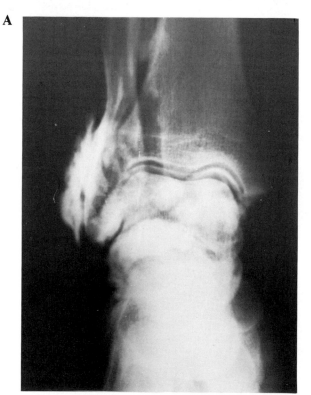

B

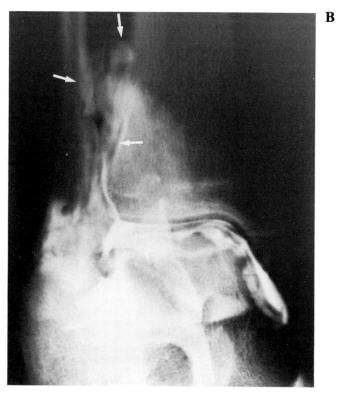

Figure 25
A. An abnormal distance between the distal tibia and fibula is evident in the anteroposterior projection of an arthrogram. The arthrogram shows leakage of contrast material around the tip of the fibula, indicating an anterior talofibular ligament tear.
B. In an oblique projection, leaked contrast material from the syndesmotic recess (arrows) is seen, indicating a distal anterior tibiofibular ligament tear.

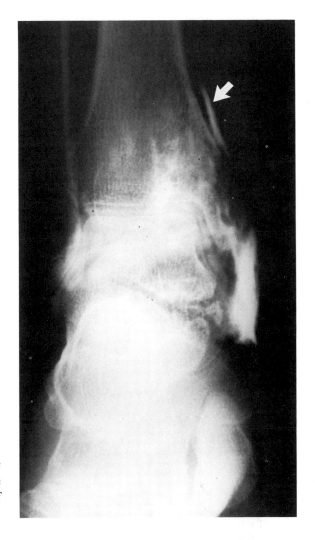

Figure 26
A deltoid ligament tear is demonstrated arthrographically by a small leak of contrast material on the medial side of the ankle. There is also a fracture of the distal fibula. Filling of the long flexor tendon sheaths (arrow) is a normal variant.

A

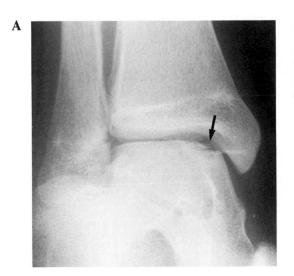

B

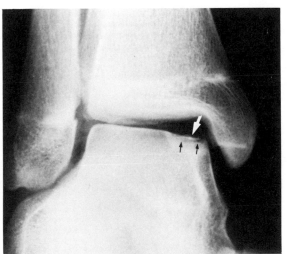

Figure 27
A. Osteochondritis dissecans or subchondral fracture of the talus (arrow) is shown on a plain radiograph.
B. The air-only arthrogram shows air (black arrows) beneath the small separate ossicle (white arrow), indicating that it is at least partially loose.

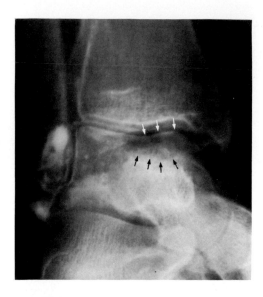

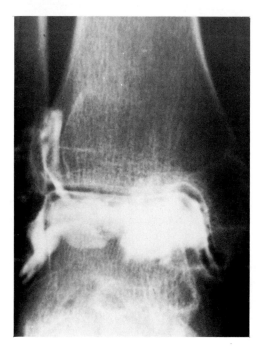

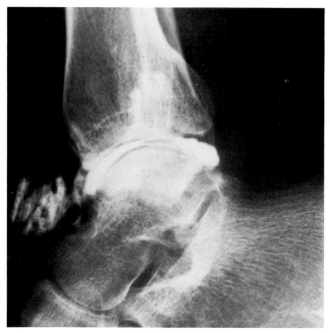

Figure 28
A double contrast arthrogram shows that the articular cartilage (white arrows) overlying a subchondral osseous fragment of the talus (black arrows) is intact.

Figure 29
A, B. With adhesive capsulitis, there is marked retraction and irregularity of the capsule with reduced joint capacity seen in both frontal and lateral projections. The lateral projection shows that some of the injected contrast agent has leaked out through the puncture site anteriorly.

12
Talo-calcaneonavicular Arthrography

Helene Pavlov

Tarsal coalitions can produce a painful, rigid flat foot, often requiring operative procedures for relief of pain. Coalitions between the calcaneus and the navicular or between the calcaneus and talus at the sustentacular–talar joint are the most common. Coalitions can be osseous or fibrous. Calcaneonavicular coalitions are easily seen on routine plain roentgenograms. Sustentacular–talar coalitions are usually not adequately seen, even with tangential or Harris views of the calcaneus. The presence or absence of sustentacular–talar coalition can be confirmed by performing an arthrogram.

TECHNIQUE

After antiseptic and anesthetic preparation and draping, a 22-gauge, 1½-in. needle is inserted into the talonavicular joint under fluoroscopic guidance by a dorsal and medial approach with the foot in the lateral position. Following the injection of 2 to 3 cc of positive contrast agent, routine anteroposterior, lateral, and oblique views of the hindfoot and ankle, in addition to Harris views with 35°, 45°, and 55° tube angulation are obtained. Lateral tomograms may be performed when indicated.

ANATOMY

The head of the talus articulates with the navicular and the anterior portion of the calcaneus including the sustentaculum tali. The articulation extends from the navicular across the plantar calcaneonavicular ligament to the sustentaculum tali, forming a ball and socket joint. Thus, the talonavicular and anterior talocalcaneal joints are continuous, and contrast agent injected into the talonavicular joint fills a normal sustentacular–talar joint.

ARTHROGRAPHIC FINDINGS

The normal sustentacular–talar joint is best seen on the Harris view (Fig. 1A) and can also be seen on the lateral view superior to the subtalar joint (Fig. 1B). The presence of positive contrast within the sustentacular–talar joint excludes a tarsal coalition. The absence of an opacified sustentacular–talar joint confirms the diagnosis of a coalition (Figs. 2A, B). Tomography in the lateral projection can be useful in identifying contrast agent within the sustentacular–talar articulation (Figs. 3A, B).

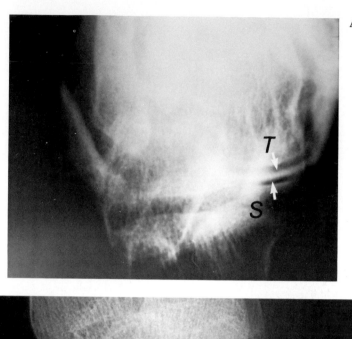

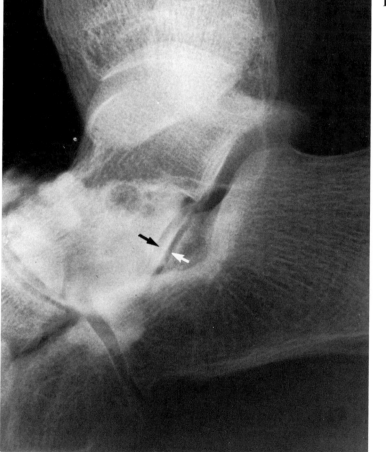

Figure 1
A. Normal sustentacular–talar articulation is seen on the Harris view, where a thin contrast line (arrows) is visible between the talus (T) and the sustentaculum (S).
B. On a lateral view, the contrast (arrows) is again seen between the talus and the sustentaculum.

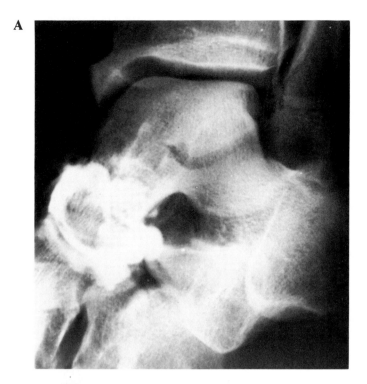

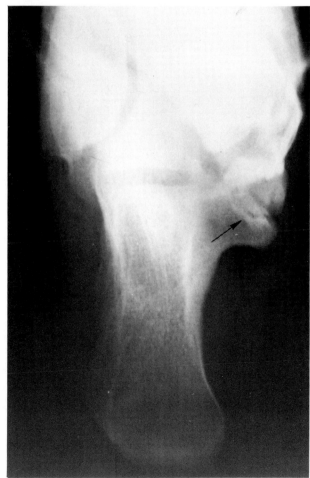

Figure 2
A. An oblique view of the hindfoot demonstrates the lack of opacification in the sustentacular–talar joint. There is no osseous bridge, as the coalition is completely fibrous.
B. A fibrous sustentacular–talar tarsal coalition is seen on the Harris view which demonstrates an irregular, deformed sustentacular–talar joint unopacified by contrast (arrow).

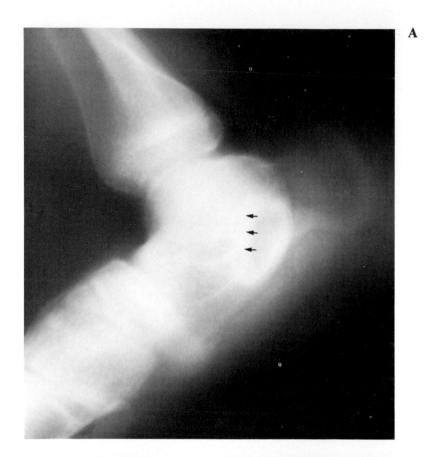

A

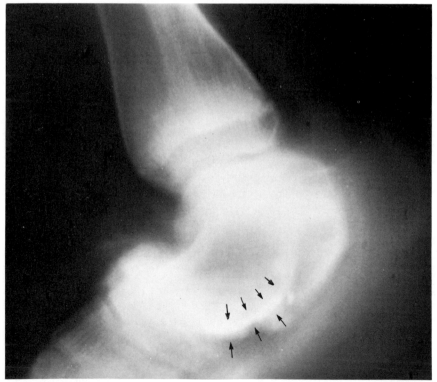

B

Figure 3
A. On a lateral tomogram, the sustentacular-talar joint (arrows) is abnormal.
B. Following the injection of contrast agent into the talonavicular joint, a lateral tomogram shows contrast agent in the anterior subtalar joint (arrows), but not in the sustentacular-talar joint. This confirms a sustentacular-talar coalition.

13

The Elbow

Terry Hudson

Arthrography can be useful in evaluating patients with painful or functionally impaired elbows. Injection of contrast medium into the elbow is not difficult, but arthrograms must be carefully positioned and of high quality. Also, tomography is often required for a complete evaluation.

Most commonly, elbow arthrography is performed to detect or confirm the presence of intra-articular loose bodies or to evaluate the surfaces of the articular cartilages. Elbow arthrography can also opacify synovial cysts, verify correct needle position during diagnostic joint aspiration, or demonstrate the hypertrophied, irregular synovial tissue of rheumatoid arthritis or pigmented villonodular synovitis. A rare application is to search for intra-articular tumor extension from adjacent bone or soft tissue. The contracted capsule associated with capsular fibrosis can be demonstrated, as can acute traumatic capsular tears and capsular distortions associated with recurrent elbow dislocations.

Known or suspected infection of the elbow joint is not a contraindication to arthrography, which is usually performed in conjunction with diagnostic arthrocentesis. As with other joints, when pyarthrosis is not suspected, a periarticular infection is a contraindication to arthrography because of the risk of infecting the joint during needle insertion.

EQUIPMENT

The standard arthrographic tray is used with the addition of a 22-gauge, 1½-in. needle. A larger diameter needle should not be used because it may result in leakage of contrast agent from the puncture site into the soft tissues after the injection. A smaller diameter needle is not used because it would not allow aspiration of viscous joint fluid.

The ideal radiographic unit for this examination has image-amplified fluoroscopy with a fractional millimeter focal spot for spot filming. It should also be equipped for tomography, which is frequently required for a complete examination. A unit with an overhead X-ray tube and under-table image amplifier is preferred because there is adequate space between the tube and the patient to work under sterile conditions. When a conventional fluoroscope with an image amplifier on the tower is used, the spot film unit and image intensifier are locked in the highest position above the elbow to permit injection without moving the fluoroscopic tower. Such positioning allows control of the injection by intermittent fluoroscopy. If a fluoroscopic unit with a fractional millimeter focal spot is not available, the patient can be injected under fluoroscopic guidance and arthrographic films can be made with an overhead tube at a 40-in. distance with the smallest focal spot available.

TECHNIQUE

Preliminary plain roentgenograms of the elbow are examined and, if necessary, additional films are made. If an exposure technique has not been established, proper exposure factors should be determined by making preliminary fluoroscopic spot films and tomograms of the elbow prior to injection. In general, positive contrast arthrograms require more exposure than plain roentgenograms, whereas air or double contrast arthrograms require the same or slightly less exposure. For an adult of average size the factors will be approximately 50 kVp and 6 mAs using a three-phase generator and High Plus (Dupont) screens.

The patient is positioned sitting next to the table or lying prone with the arm parallel to the X-ray table, lateral side up, and the elbow flexed to 90° (Figs. 1A, B). Radiolucent sponges can be placed to facilitate a comfortable and correct position. A lead marker is placed on the skin and then fluoroscopically positioned directly over the radiocapitellar joint (Fig. 2A), and that point is marked with indelible ink that will not wipe off when the skin is antiseptically prepared. Alternatively, the puncture site may be located with a sterile marker after skin preparation. The skin is prepared with three applications of povidone-iodine solution; the elbow is then covered with a sterile drape sheet with a 2 × 2 in. hole. The injection procedure is carried out under aseptic conditions, with the examiner wearing sterile gloves. Using a 25-gauge needle, the skin and subcutaneous tissues at the marked point are anesthetized with a 1 percent lidocaine hydrochloride solution. A 22-gauge, 1½-in. needle is then inserted perpendicular to the elbow at the marked point (Fig. 2B). The needle is advanced deeply enough so that it will stand upright. Fluoroscopy should show the needle perpendicular at the radiocapitellar joint space (Fig. 2C). The needle is advanced using intermittent fluoroscopy to ensure that it remains in its vertical position above the joint space. If the needle deviates from its intended path, it should be withdrawn to the subcutaneous tissues and redirected. Resistance is felt as the needle enters the fibrous joint capsule and sometimes a "give" is felt when the needle perforates the capsule completely and its tip enters the joint. The needle should then be advanced 1 or 2 mm further. In most patients the needle tip is within the joint cavity when the tip is 1 cm from the skin surface.

If fluid is present within the elbow it should be aspirated as completely as possible. If infection is suspected but no fluid can be aspirated, a specimen for culture can be obtained by injecting sterile saline without a bacteriostatic agent, followed by reaspiration of that fluid for culture and smear. When no fluid is present, intra-articular position can be confirmed by injecting a drop or two of contrast solution. A 1- or 2-cc syringe, preferably glass to reduce friction, is filled with methylglucamine diatrizoate contrast agent and is attached to the needle. A drop is injected with fingertip pressure. Alternatively, the syringe may be attached to the needle by a length of sterile plastic tubing filled with contrast agent. If the needle tip is in the joint, contrast medium will flow quickly away from the needle tip (Fig. 2D). This is followed by injection of the complete amount of positive contrast agent, and if a double contrast study is desired, it is followed by air (Fig. 2E). If the contrast agent puddles at the needle tip, it is outside the joint and the needle should be repositioned.

Although the flow of contrast agent can be observed fluoroscopically during the injection when plastic tubing is used (Fig. 2E), the direct attachment of a small syringe to the needle appears preferable because it is easier to judge injection pressure. With proper intra-articular needle placement there should be practically no resistance to the injection. The injection of local anesthetic solution to test for free flow indicating intra-articular needle placement is not recommended when a double contrast or air study of the elbow joint is planned, since excess fluid in this small joint reduces the clarity of the subsequent arthrogram. Similarly, since residual fluid will almost surely remain in the joint after injection of saline, a subsequent air or double contrast arthrogram may not be entirely satisfactory. Therefore, when diagnostic joint lavage has been performed, single positive contrast studies are preferable to the others.

After the injection of contrast agents the needle is removed (Fig. 2F) and the elbow is gently moved to distribute the contrast media throughout the joint. Vigorous exercise should be avoided because it may cause rupture of the distended capsule or, in a double contrast study, may produce confusing air bubbles.

Selection of the method of elbow arthrography depends on the clinical setting. The single positive contrast method is best used following diagnostic aspiration. It shows abnormalities of the synovial lining and may be useful in demonstrating the size and extent of synovial cysts. Since positive contrast medium may obscure small radiolucent or calcified bodies, the double contrast technique using 0.5 to 1.5 cc of a meglumine positive contrast agent and 8 to 12 cc of air is preferred for such cases. Articular surfaces are also well shown by this technique. When the patient has had a severe reaction to previous injections of radiographic contrast media, contraindicating such injections, 8 to 12 cc of air alone may be used, although the intra-articular surfaces are not seen as well by this method. In inflammatory joint disease, absorption of positive contrast agent occurs more rapidly than in a normal joint, leading to a rapid loss of sharp detail in the arthrographic films. The resorption of contrast media can be delayed by the addition of 0.1 to 0.2 cc of a 1:1000 solution of epinephrine. The addition of epinephrine is also advisable in examinations that are lengthened by tomography. Epinephrine is of no value when air alone is injected.

Once contrast media have been injected, radiographs must be obtained quickly before the sharp details of the contrast-coated intra-articular surface begins to disappear. The number and types of exposures that constitute a complete study depend on the suspected pathology. Those arthrograms to confirm needle position for diagnostic aspiration and those performed with single positive contrast medium alone may require only a few films to demonstrate synovial cysts or proliferative synovial disease. Similarly, the tight joint space of capsular fibrosis (frozen elbow) or the lax capsule associated with recurrent dislocation of the elbow can be documented with a few arthrographic exposures. Usually lateral, internal, and external oblique views and an anteroposterior view of the elbow suffice. If a synovial cyst is suspected and initial films are normal, or if these films show partial filling of a cyst, a second set of films should be taken after the elbow has been vigorously exercised for a few minutes to possibly force contrast agent into the cyst.

Arthrography performed to demonstrate loose bodies or to evaluate articular cartilages requires many projections and is best performed by the double contrast method. Immediately after joint injection, fluoroscopic spot films are taken in anteroposterior, lateral, and oblique projections with varying degrees of flexion and extension of the elbow. If these films allow a definite diagnosis, the study is complete. Most of the time, however, the spot films will not be definitive and tomography will be necessary. The elbow is then placed in the optimal position, as determined from the previous spot films, and tomograms are made. Exposure settings are based on previous experience or on the preliminary tomograms made before injection. The lateral projection has been found to be the most informative. Tomograms should be made with the thinnest possible sections on available equipment and at 2- to 4-mm intervals. A pluridirectional tube movement is optimal.

ANATOMY AND THE NORMAL ARTHROGRAM

The articular cartilage surfaces are convex over the capitellum and trochlea of the distal humerus and concave in the central portion of the radial head and at the radial notch of the ulna (Figs. 3, 4). These cartilages normally have smooth, intact surfaces and are thicker in a child (Fig. 5) than in an adult. The distensible joint capsule may be divided into three compartments: anterior, posterior, and annular recesses (Figs. 3–6). The anterior recess extends over the anterior surface of the trochlea and capitellum of the humerus. Distended by contrast medium, this recess is clearly visible. It is

shallow over the anterior surfaces of the trochlea and capitellum and more capacious over the radial and coronoid fossae, where prominent radial and coronoid recesses are evident. The posterior recess of the joint extends over the posterior surface of the distal humerus and is shallow as it overlies the condyles and the posterior surface of the smoothly curved capitellum. Two areas of the posterior recess are quite deep. One is the olecranon recess lying within the olecranon fossa and partially surrounding the olecranon process of the ulna. The other is posterior to the radial head. Both recesses balloon out when the elbow is extended (Fig. 6). The posterior recess, particularly the olecranon recess, is difficult to evaluate on routine arthrography and adequate visualization usually requires a combination of arthrography and tomography. The annular recess (Fig. 7) is the most distal extension of the synovial cavity of the elbow; it encircles the radial neck, passing under and bulging beyond the annular ligament (Figs. 3–5). The annular ligament attaches at the margins of the radial notch of the ulna, encircling and stabilizing the radial head articulation. The sacciform or radioulnar recess extends distally from the annular recess, lying between the radius and ulna proximal to the bicipital tubercle of the radius (Fig. 4).

On the lateral view, the anterior synovial surface may form folds, especially with flexion of the elbow and incomplete distension of the capsule (Fig. 3A). This surface is flatter and smoother with the elbow extended or more fully distended by injected contrast media (Fig. 3B).

The normal defect in the articular cartilage and subchondral cortex at the midportion of the ulnar notch is seen particularly well on tomography. It should not be mistaken for osteochondritis dissecans (Figs. 3A, 8C).

Lateral tomograms show the radiocapitellar and ulnar–trochlear articulations more clearly than plain films. The capitellum is a direct extension of the lateral column of the humerus, extending anteriorly in a smooth curve (Fig. 3B). The trochlea, on lateral tomography, appears as a knob attached to the medial humeral column where the humerus is markedly thinned or occasionally completely fenestrated between the olecranon and coronoid fossae (Figs. 3A, 8C). The radial head and radioulnar articulations are best seen on plain or tomographic roentgenograms in the slight external oblique projection (Figs. 4A, B).

THE ABNORMAL ARTHROGRAM

Loose Bodies

The exact location of a calcification or a noncalcified loose body in the vicinity of the elbow joint can usually be determined accurately on double contrast or air arthrograms. Some chondromatous or osteochondromatous bodies may indeed be loose; others may be attached to the adjacent synovial membrane making it difficult to distinguish them from hypertrophied synovial tissue or synovial chrondromatosis.

The diagnostic criterion for an intra-articular loose body is that it be entirely surrounded by contrast media, preferably a thin coating of positive contrast medium enveloped by air on a double contrast study (Figs. 8, 9). When a chrondromatous or osteochondromatous body lies deep in the olecranon or coronoid fossa, its adequate evaluation usually requires tomography because these regions are hidden by overlying bone (Figs. 8A, B). Since the fossae lie between the medial and lateral humeral condyles, they cannot be projected entirely free of overlying bone. Even with thin tomographic sections, blurred condyles may produce confusing superimposed shadows. Tomography may also demonstrate multiple loose bodies where only one was suspected. They may be remote from the area of primary interest (Fig. 8D).

Osteochondritis Dissecans

When plain roentgenograms indicate osteochondritis dissecans or osteochondral fracture, arthrography can show whether or not the articular cartilage overlying the subchondral bony defect is intact. In early stages of osteochondritis dissecans, the overlying cartilage is usually intact (Figs. 10A–C). Later, the cartilage may fracture with the osteocartilaginous fragment remaining in place. It is shown by contrast agent seeping into the chondral fracture, completely or partially surrounding the osteochondral fragment. Still later, the cartilaginous or osteocartilaginous fragment may separate completely from its bed and lie free within the joint cavity. Then the arthrogram shows the defect in the articular cartilage as well as the loose body within the joint (Fig. 11). Thin section tomography is usually necessary for precise evaluation.

Synovial Cysts

Synovial cysts can arise from arthritic joints, especially in patients with rheumatoid arthritis. Such cysts often present with swelling and signs of inflammation in the antecubital fossa and proximal forearm. They are readily demonstrated by positive contrast arthrography of the elbow (Figs. 12A, B). A large quantity of contrast agent is necessary for adequate filling of the cyst. Active or passive motion of the elbow facilitates filling of the cyst. The study is not complete until films are made after vigorous exercise of the elbow, because some cysts may not fill initially. Direct injection of the cyst may fail to demonstrate its communication with the joint. Leakage of contrast agent from the elbow into the soft tissues of the forearm with or without synovial cysts can occur in patients with rheumatoid arthritis.

Synovial Abnormalities

Abnormally irregular synovial membranes can be demonstrated by positive contrast arthrography. Tomography is usually not necessary. Although the synovial lining of the anterior recess may be normally irregular in flexion, marked irregularity persisting in extension is abnormal. Hypertrophied synovial membranes are seen in rheumatoid arthritis, septic arthritis, pigmented villonodular synovitis (Figs. 13A, B), lipoma arborescens, uncalcified synovial chondromatosis, and hemangioma of the synovial tissues. The arthrographic appearance is similar in all of these entities and a specific diagnosis is not made by the arthrogram alone.

Capsular Abnormalities

Abnormal laxity of recesses and detachment of the joint capsule from its normal bony attachments is demonstrated arthrographically in patients with recurrent dislocation of the elbow. The tight capsule associated with posttraumatic limitation of elbow motion, analogous to adhesive capsulitis of the shoulder, can also be demonstrated. The diagnosis of rupture of the elbow capsule can be made arthrographically (Fig. 14), but surgical repair of such capsular tears is rarely undertaken.

PITFALLS

Inadvertent extra-articular injection or leakage of contrast medium along the needle track may be misinterpreted as a torn capsule. Care should be taken not to mistake normal synovial folds or air bubbles for intra-articular bodies. The normal defect in the trochlear notch of the ulna should not be misinterpreted as an abnormality.

The wrong contrast method may be selected if preliminary X-ray examinations are not carefully inspected. Failure to perform tomography can in some cases lead to an incomplete examination.

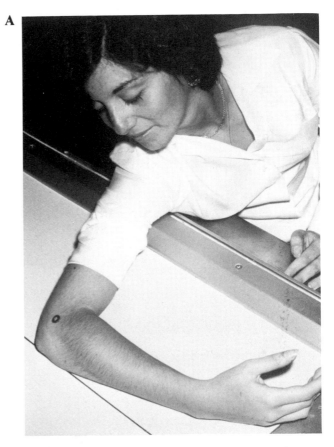

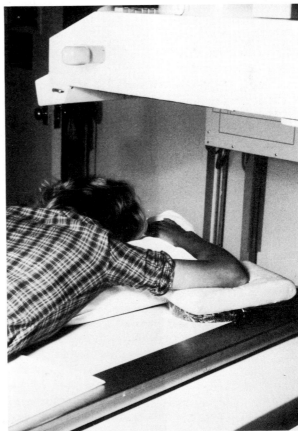

Figure 1
A. The patient is seated with the arm abducted and placed on the radiographic table. An overhead X-ray tube and under-table image intensifier provide ample space to maintain sterile technique during injection. A lead marker has been placed over the radiohumeral joint.
B. Alternately, the patient can be placed prone, with the elbow flexed and the arm placed parallel to the table top. Using a conventional fluoroscope, the tower should be locked in its highest position to allow ample working space. The protective lead curtains have been removed to illustrate the technique.

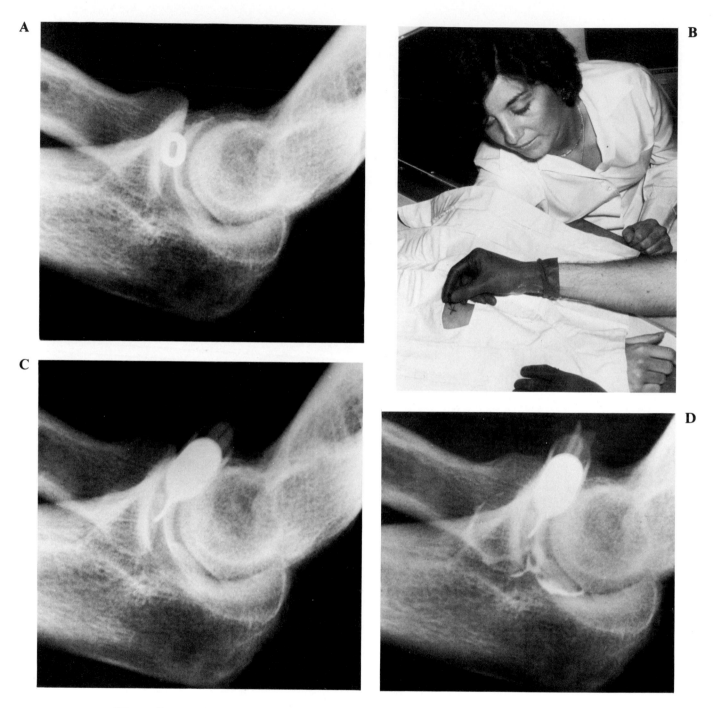

Figure 2
A. A lead marker is placed over the radiocapitellar joint with fluoroscopic guidance and its location is marked on the skin with indelible ink.
B. After the elbow is prepared with povidone-iodine solution, draped, and anesthetized, a 22-gauge, 1½-in. disposable needle is placed vertically into the radial capitellar joint under fluoroscopic guidance.
C. The point of the needle is seen in the correct position at the radiocapitellar articulation.
D. After the needle has been advanced into the radiocapitellar joint, a 2-cc syringe filled with meglumine diatrizoate is attached to the needle. A few drops of contrast agent have been injected and are seen within the elbow joint, verifying correct needle position.

E

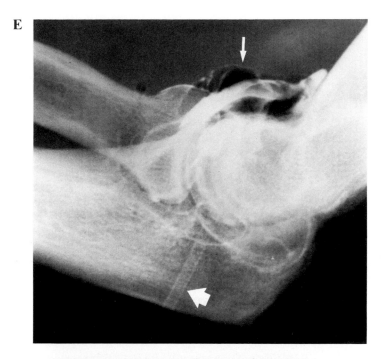

F

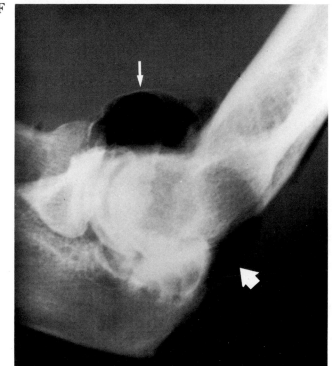

Figure 2
E. After the injection of positive contrast agent has been completed, sterile plastic connecting tubing (large arrow) is attached to the needle and air is injected under fluoroscopic observation. The anterior recess of the joint is distended by air (small arrow).
F. After the injection is completed, the needle is removed. The well-distended anterior (small arrow) and posterior (large arrow) recesses are shown with the elbow flexed.

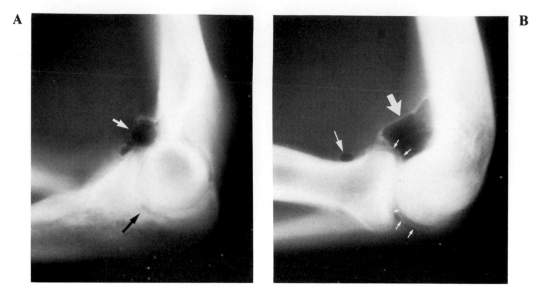

Figure 3
A. A lateral tomogram through the ulnar–trochlear joint shows the coronoid recess anteriorly (white arrow) and the minimally distended olecranon recess posteriorly. The small defect in the ulnar notch (black arrow) is normal.
B. A lateral tomogram through the radiocapitellar joint shows a distended anterior recess (large arrow), a part of the annular recess (medium arrow), and the articular cartilage (small arrows).

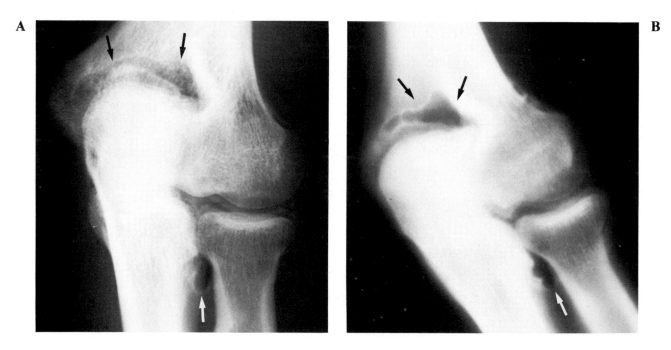

Figure 4
An arthrogram (**A**) and arthrotomogram (**B**) in slight external oblique projection show the olecranon recess (black arrows), the radioulnar or sacciform recess (white arrow) and the articular cartilage surfaces of the radiocapitellar joint.

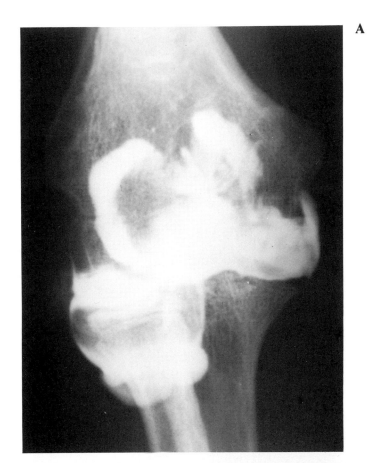

A

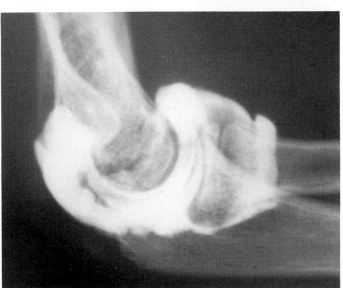

B

Figure 5
The anteroposterior (**A**) and lateral (**B**) projections of a normal positive contrast arthrogram of a child show the joint recesses filled by positive contrast medium. The articular cartilage, particularly that of the radial head, is much thicker and the annular recess is more prominent than they are in an adult. The anterior and posterior recesses are partially superimposed on the anteroposterior projection.

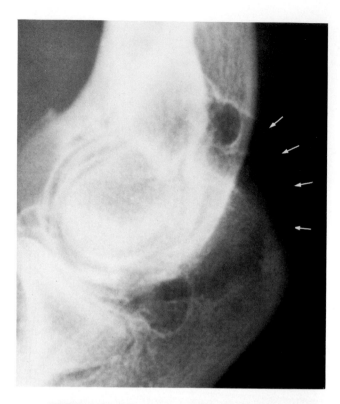

Figure 6
With the elbow in an extended position, the stretched anterior tissues compress the anterior synovial recess and cause distention of the posterior recess (arrows).

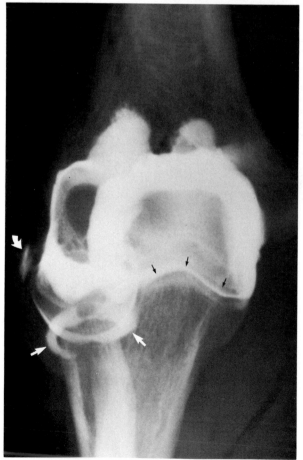

Figure 7
The anteroposterior view shows the superimposed anterior and posterior recesses, the annular recess (white arrows), and the ulnar–trochlear articular cartilage surfaces (black arrows). The radiocapitellar joint is not well seen because the elbow is slightly flexed. There is a slight leak of contrast medium at the site of needle puncture (curved arrow).

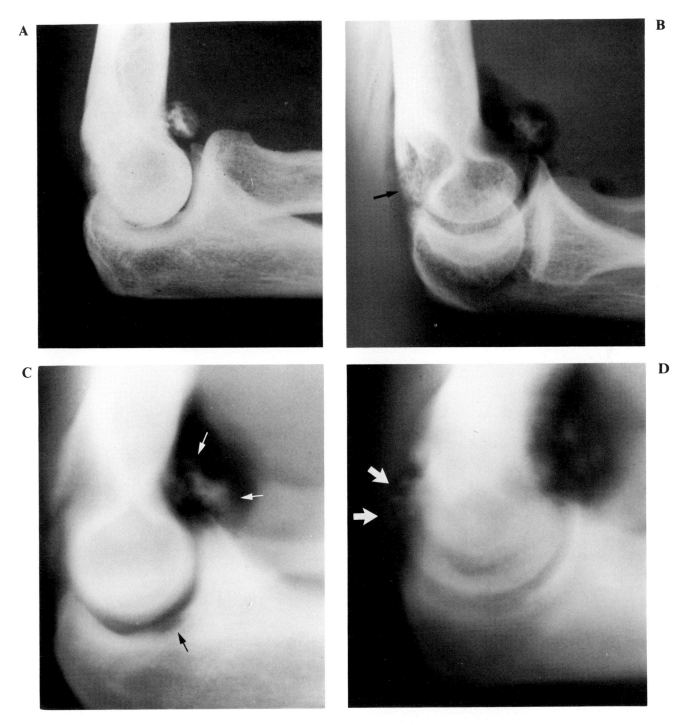

Figure 8
A. A single calcific density is seen anterior to the elbow on the plain roentgenogram.
B. A lateral projection of an air arthrogram shows the calcified body surrounded by air, verifying its intra-articular position. There is also a poorly seen density in the posterior recess (arrow).
C. A lateral tomogram through the trochlea shows several calcified loose bodies in the anterior recess (white arrows). The ulnar notch defect is normal (black arrow).
D. A slightly more lateral tomographic section shows several more calcified loose bodies in the posterior recess (arrows).

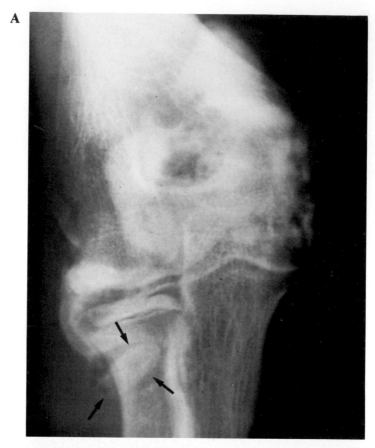

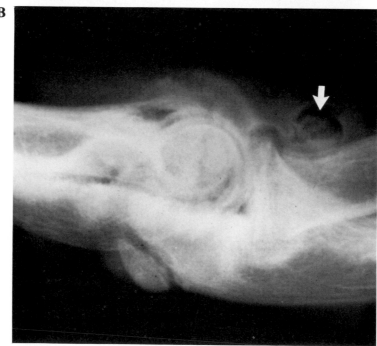

Figure 9
A. A double contrast arthrogram shows a large, loose body (arrows) in the annular recess.
B. A cross-table lateral projection of the arthrogram also provides excellent visualization of the loose body in the annular recess (arrow).

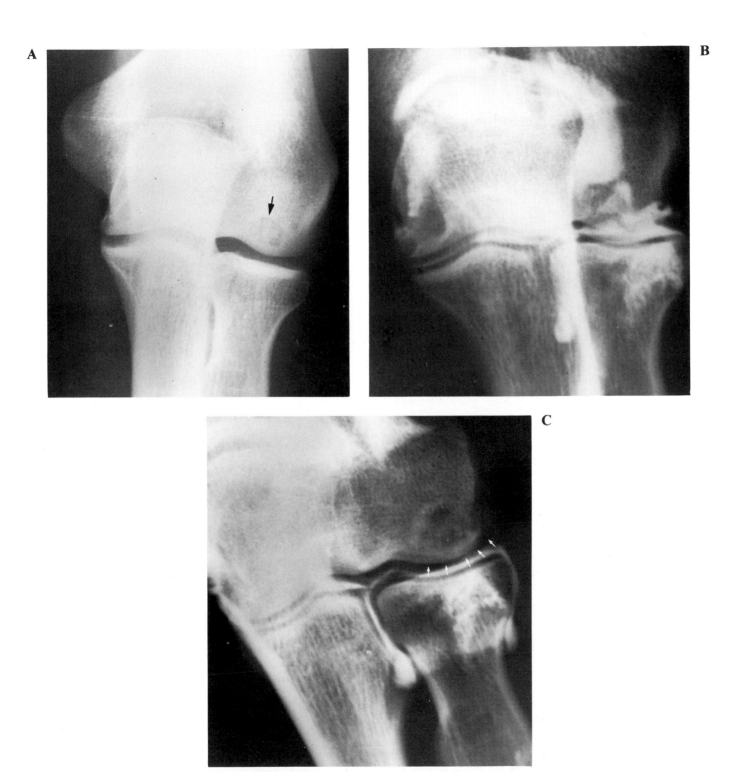

Figure 10
A. Osteochondritis dissecans of the capitellum (arrow) is shown on a plain anteroposterior roentgenogram of the elbow.
B. The anteroposterior arthrogram shows an overlying recess obscuring the area of interest.
C. The external oblique view projects the capitellum free of opacified recesses and demonstrates its intact articular cartilage (arrows).

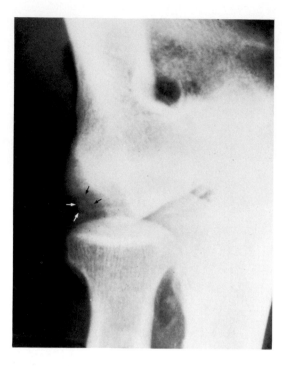

Figure 11
Osteochondritis dissecans of the capitellum with a loose fragment is seen on the oblique view of a double contrast arthrogram. Air completely surrounds the fragment (arrows), indicating that it is loose.

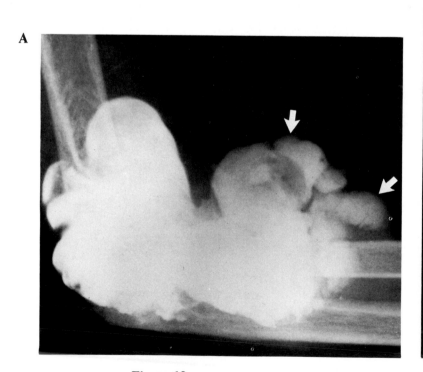

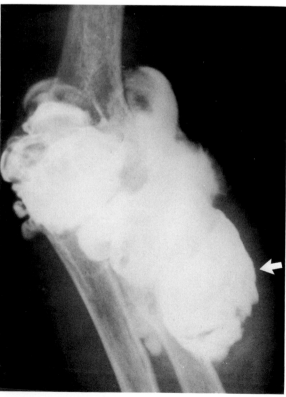

Figure 12
A, B. A synovial cyst (arrows), extending into the forearm was caused by rheumatoid arthritis. (Courtesy of Dr. J. Leland Sosman and Dr. Barbara Weissman.)

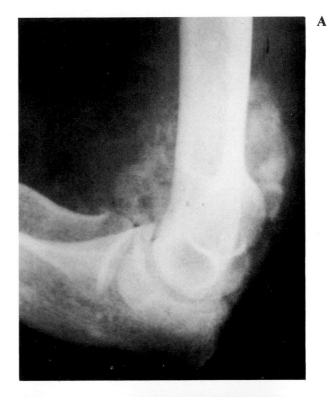

A

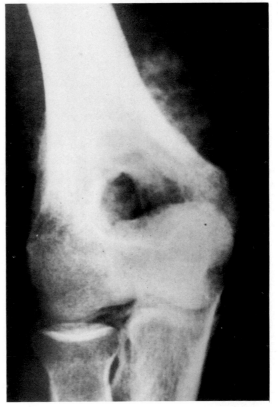

B

Figure 13
A, B. Pigmented villonodular synovitis causes distention of the joint capsule. Synovial proliferation produces multiple filling defects in the positive contrast substance within the joint. (Courtesy of Dr. J. Leland Sosman and Dr. Barbara Weissman.)

A

B

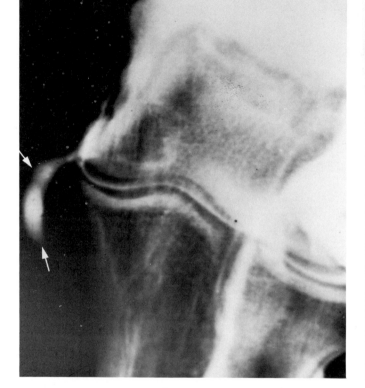

Figure 14
A, B. A fluoroscopic spot film (**A**) and a post-exercise roentgenogram show contrast agent leaking (arrows) through a posttraumatic capsular tear on the ulnar aspect of the elbow. (Courtesy of Dr. J. H. Milsap, Jr.)

14

The Wrist

Amy Beth Goldman

Wrist arthrography is used to evaluate structures that cannot be seen on plain radiography. These structures include the synovium, the intra-articular ligaments, and the articular cartilages including the triangular fibrocartilage.

The most common indication is persistent pain or limitation of motion after trauma. In patients with an injured wrist and normal plain radiographs and in those with clearly united fractures, the arthrogram can reveal tears of the triangular fibrocartilage, disruptions of the intercarpal ligaments, or posttraumatic synovitis. Rarely, when plain roentgenograms demonstrate a persistent lucent line at a scaphoid fracture, the arthrogram may differentiate a fibrous union from a complete nonunion.

The documentation and evaluation of inflammatory arthritis is another indication for contrast arthrography. Since the inflammatory arthritides, particularly rheumatoid arthritis, are primarily synovial abnormalities, the arthrogram provides a means of documenting early soft tissue changes. The cartilaginous and osseous findings demonstrable on plain radiographs occur later in the course of the disease. Moreover, the aspiration performed prior to arthrography may establish the etiology of the synovitis. The contrast arthrogram may also document the degree of cartilage damage and assist the surgeon in the selection of candidates for synovectomy.

TECHNIQUE

The patient is seated next to the fluoroscopic table with the arm resting on it. The hand is placed palm down with the wrist flexed over a triangular radiolucent sponge (Fig. 1A). The forearm is positioned to make the normal ventral tilt of the distal radial articular surface parallel to the vertical fluoroscopic X-ray beam. Under fluoroscopic control, a lead "O" is moved into position over the radiocarpal joint, to select the projected puncture point, preferably just lateral to the scapholunar joint. The point is marked on the skin with indelible ink (Fig. 1B). If the joint puncture is too close to the scapholunar articulation, the needle could inadvertently enter the midcarpal compartment instead of the radiocarpal space.

The skin is prepared with a povidone-iodine solution and the wrist is draped. Following the administration of a small amount (0.5 to 1 cc) of local anesthetic at the skin mark, a 22-gauge, 1½-in. needle is passed vertically into the radiocarpal joint (Fig. 1C). If the wrist is quite thin, and arthrocentesis is not contemplated, the 25-gauge, ½-in. needle used to inject the anesthetic is used for joint puncture. As in other joints, aspiration is attempted prior to any test injection since iodinated contrast material is slightly bacteriostatic. Unaspirated fluid tends to dilute the contrast material. If infection is suspected, and no joint fluid can be aspirated, 1 or 2 cc of sterile saline can be injected into and aspirated from the joint for smear and culture.

When the needle tip is intra-articular, a test injection is made with a drop or two of positive contrast material. If the needle is intra-articular, the contrast flows freely away from the needle tip and outlines a portion of the radiocarpal joint (Fig. 1D). Then about 2 to 4 cc of meglumine diatrizoate is injected and the needle and the pillow are removed. The wrist is briefly and gently manipulated to distribute the contrast material, and the filming is quickly begun.

The routine arthrogram includes anteroposterior, lateral, and both oblique projections. If initial roentgenograms fail to demonstrate extension of contrast material into the distal radioulnar or midcarpal compartments, the patient is asked to exercise the wrist again and the radiographs are repeated. If the indication for arthrography is to document an ununited fracture of the scaphoid, tomographic studies are added.

The patient should have little or no discomfort during or following the examination.

ANATOMY

The wrist joint has four main compartments: the radiocarpal articulation (where the contrast material is injected), the distal radioulnar joint, the midcarpal space, and the common carpometacarpal joints (Fig. 2). In addition to these major divisions, the first carpometacarpal joint has its own separate capsule and there is a separate pisotriquetral joint space.

The radiocarpal articulation lies between the distal articular surface of the radius and the proximal row of the carpal bones. It is separated from the distal radioulnar joint by a triangular fibrocartilage, which is also known as the meniscus or articular disk or triangular cartilage. This fibrocartilage is shaped like two triangles that are fused at their apices toward the radial third of the disk. The base of the larger triangle is fixed to the ulnar styloid and that of the smaller one is attached to the distal radial margin at the ulnar notch. The narrow isthmus where the apices of the triangles are fused is less than 1 mm wide.

The radiocarpal and midcarpal compartments are separated by the synovial-lined intercarpal ligaments.

The capsule of the wrist joint is surrounded and reinforced by strong extra-articular ligaments which include the volar and dorsal components of the radiocarpal ligament and the two collateral ligaments. The extensor and flexor tendons at the wrist pass over the capsule where they are covered by synovial sheaths.

THE NORMAL ARTHROGRAM

The normal wrist arthrogram shows the radioulnar articulation as a smooth, cup-shaped, contrast-filled sac

that is bordered proximally by the articular cartilage of the distal radius and the triangular fibrocartilage (Figs. 3, 4). Distally, it is bounded by the articular cartilages of the proximal carpal row and the interosseous ligaments (Fig. 3A). The radiocarpal joint has two small outpouchings. The first is the volar recess which is on the anterior aspect of the wrist (Figs. 3B, 4B). On the anteroposterior radiograph, the volar recess is projected through the distal radius and the radiocarpal joint (Figs. 3A, 4A). The second outpouching is the prestyloid recess. It is located laterally, distal to the tip of the ulnar styloid (Figs. 3A, 4A). In some individuals the pisiform-triquetrial compartment fills through a normal communication (Fig. 4).

The distal radioulnar joint, the midcarpal joints, the tendon sheaths, and the lymphatics do not fill when a normal radiocarpal joint is injected.

THE ABNORMAL ARTHROGRAM

Tears of the Triangular Fibrocartilage

When there is a tear of the triangular fibrocartilage, the wrist arthrogram shows extension of the injected contrast material from the radiocarpal joint into the distal radioulnar compartment (Fig. 5). Tears of the triangular fibrocartilage may occur as isolated injuries or may accompany a fracture of the distal radius when there is no fracture of the ulnar styloid.

Partial tears of the triangular fibrocartilage are very unusual and are seen as tiny pools of contrast material extending into the disk (Fig. 6).

Although an arthrogram may document a tear in the triangular fibrocartilage, it does not indicate whether the lesion is old or new.

There is some disagreement about perforations of the triangular fibrocartilage and whether they are a normal variant. Communications have been reported in 16 to 40 percent of the cases. Of these, the highest incidences occurred in autopsy series, suggesting that the incidence of incompetent disks may be related to the age of the patient and previous trauma.

Traumatic Intercarpal Communications

When the interosseous intercarpal ligaments are ruptured, the wrist arthrogram shows the contrast material injected into the radiocarpal space extending into the midcarpal space (Fig. 7). The midcarpal joint may communicate with the common carpometacarpal joint, and this, too, may fill (Fig. 7). The first carpometacarpal joint does not fill.

Interruptions of the intercarpal ligaments are reported to occur in 13 to 26 percent of cases. A communication between the radiocarpal and pisotriquetral joint is reported to occur in 34 percent of wrists. The incidence of both of these communications also increases with age and is probably related to trauma or degenerative change. It is possible that these findings are not clinically significant.

If an abnormal communication is demonstrated between the radiocarpal and midcarpal joints, anteroposterior films, with the hand in radial and ulnar deviation, are indicated to exclude abnormal alignment of the proximal carpal row (Fig. 8A). In cases of rotatory subluxation of the carpal scaphoid, stress radiographs demonstrate the abnormal communication, with contrast material filling the gap between the scaphoid and lunate (Fig. 8B).

Scaphoid Fractures

Fractures of the carpal scaphoid are frequently complicated by delayed union. The arthrogram is rarely used to distinguish between a true nonunion and a fibrous union (Fig. 9A). In this unusual clinical situation, only small amounts of contrast should be injected since excessive positive contrast agent can obscure a thin line of contrast extending through the bone (Fig. 9B). Tomography is also helpful.

Posttraumatic Synovitis and Degenerative Joint Disease

When chronic synovitis follows wrist trauma, the arthrogram shows irregularity of the margins of the joint capsule (Fig. 10). Intercompartmental communications, abnormal opacification of tendon sheaths, and filling of communicating cysts (Fig. 11) may also be seen. Lymphatic filling and laxity of the capsule usually are not observed.

In degenerative joint disease or neuropathic arthropathy, the arthrogram shows irregularity and thinning of the articular cartilages and may show the multiple filling defects of loose bodies. Synovial irregularity and tendon sheath communications can be demonstrated.

Inflammatory Arthritides

The arthrographic appearance of rheumatoid arthritis is better known than that of other inflammatory synovial diseases, but the arthrographic findings of rheumatoid arthritis are nonspecific and are shared by other arthritides.

Rheumatoid arthritic wrist arthrograms usually demonstrate several coexisting abnormalities. A common and early arthrographic abnormality is a diffuse corrugated appearance of the synovial-lined joint capsule (Figs. 12, 13). It has been observed in wrists with entirely normal plain roentgenograms. The corrugation is demonstrated best on the lateral view (Fig. 13B) and is usually seen in the region of the prestyloid recess.

The next most frequent finding is abnormal intercompartmental communication (Figs. 14–16). Communication with the distal radioulnar compartment is caused by destruction of the triangular fibrocartilage. The arthrogram shows contrast medium extending between the distal radius and ulna, or contrast material nearly surrounding the distal end of the ulna (Figs. 14–16). The latter finding has been described only after six months of clinical complaints, suggesting that it takes time to destroy the disk. A communication between the midcarpal and radiocarpal joints is also a sequel of rheumatoid arthritis and is due to the destruction of the fine interosseous, intercarpal ligaments (Figs. 15, 16). Plain radiographs obtained in radial and ulnar deviation may demonstrate a rotatory subluxation of the carpal scaphoid. The contrast study directly demonstrates an abnormal extension of contrast material into the spaces between the distal carpal row (Figs. 15, 16).

Lymphatic opacification is noted in one-third of rheumatoid wrists (Fig. 13). It reflects the hyperemia and activity of the synovium or the excessive production of synovial fluid.

Less common findings are abnormal communications between the radiocarpal joint and the flexor or extensor tendon sheaths (Figs. 15, 16) or communications with extracapsular synovial cysts (Fig. 16). Synovial pouches become enlarged.

Infectious arthritis is also inflammatory, and the arthrographic findings are essentially the same as those seen in rheumatoid arthritis. In infectious arthritis the progress of the destructive inflammatory changes is rapid in pyogenic arthritis and slower in granulomatous arthritis. The differential diagnosis is made by aspiration and culture.

PITFALLS

An extra-articular or partially extra-articular injection may accidentally fill an extensor tendon sheath. Selection of a needle puncture site too near the scapholunar articulation may allow inadvertent injection of the midcarpal joint, mimicking a tear of the intercarpal ligament.

A

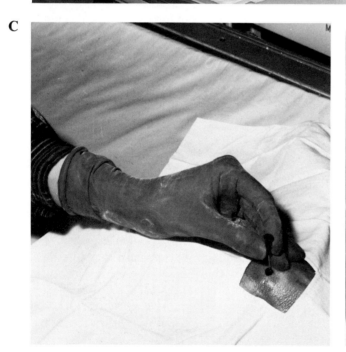

B

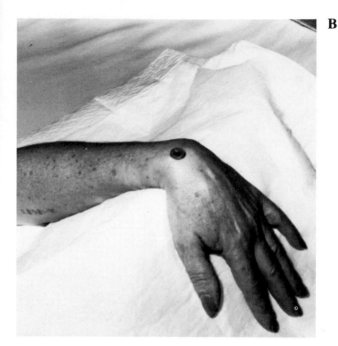

C

D

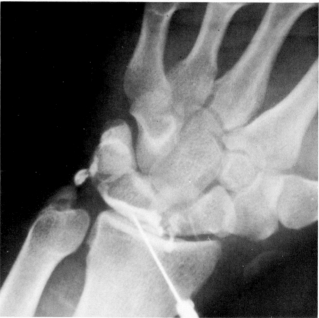

Figure 1
A. For the injection the hand is placed palm down with the wrist flexed over a triangular sponge.
B. Under fluoroscopic control, a lead marker is placed over the radiocarpal joint between the scaphoid and the radial styloid. This point is marked on the skin with indelible ink.
C. Following antiseptic skin preparation and injection of local anesthesia, a 22-gauge, 1½-in. needle is directed from the skin mark into the joint space.
D. The intra-articular location of the needle tip is verified by seeing a small quantity of injected contrast agent within the joint.

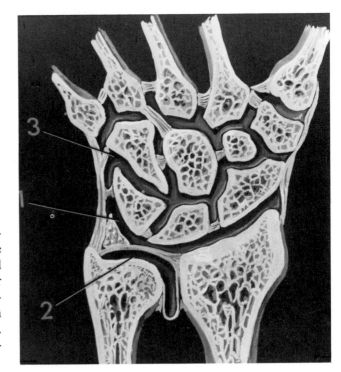

Figure 2
There are three major compartments in the wrist. The radio-carpal joint (1) is bordered proximally by the radius and the triangular cartilage, and the distal ulna, and it is bordered distally by the proximal carpal row. The distal radioulnar joint (2) is separated from the radiocarpal joint by the trian-gular cartilage. The midcarpal joints (3) are separated from the radiocarpal joint by inter-carpal interosseous ligaments. The midcarpal joints usually communicate with the com-mon carpo-metacarpal joint.

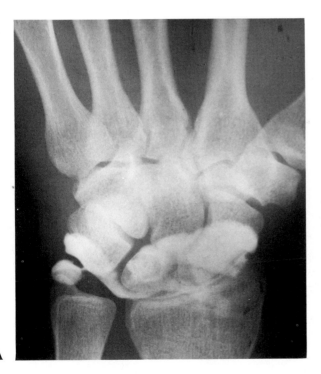

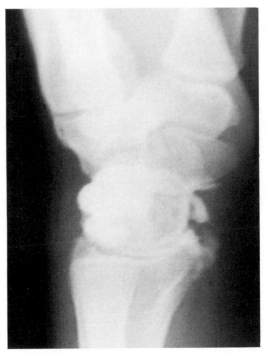

A

B

Figure 3
A. In a normal wrist arthrogram the anteroposterior view shows the opacified radio-carpal joint with its prestyloid recess and also its volar pouch which is superimposed on the radius.
B. The lateral view shows the contrast-filled capsule and volar pouch.

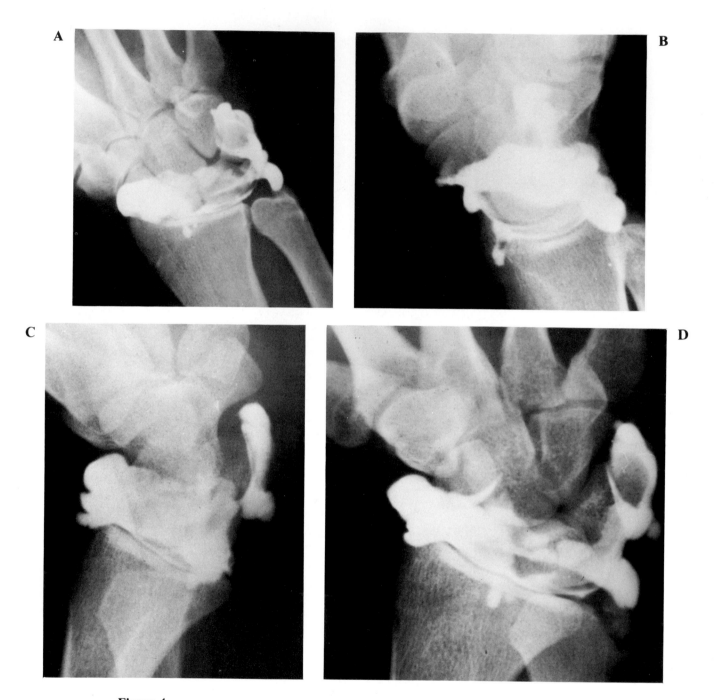

Figure 4
A normal wrist arthrogram shows a communicating pisiform bursa on (**A**) the postero-anterior view, (**B, C**) the oblique views, and (**D**) the lateral view.

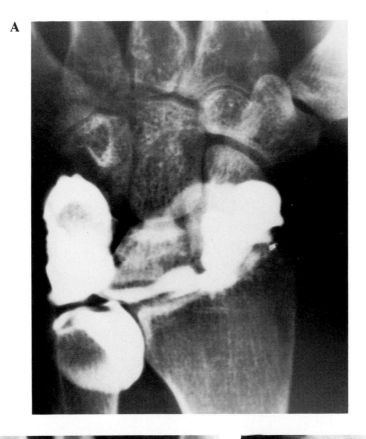

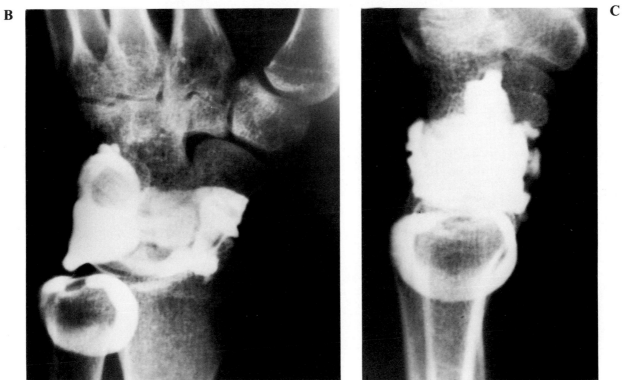

Figure 5
A tear of the triangular cartilage allows contrast to extend into the distal radioulnar joint. The opacified distal radioulnar joint can be identified on (**A**) the postero-anterior view, (**B**) the oblique view, and (**C**) the lateral view.

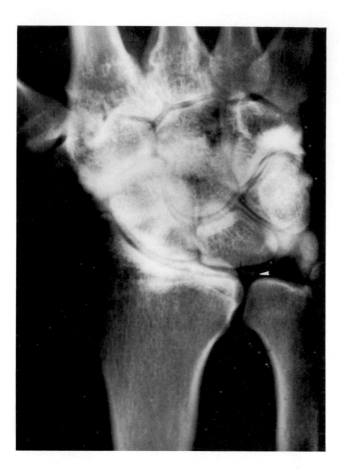

Figure 6
Contrast agent extending into but not through the triangular cartilage indicates a partial tear (arrowhead). Opacification of the midcarpal joint indicates that there is also a complete tear of at least one of the interosseous ligaments of the proximal carpal row.

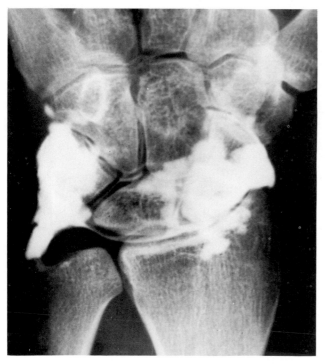

Figure 7
An abnormal communication between the radiocarpal and midcarpal joints is demonstrated.

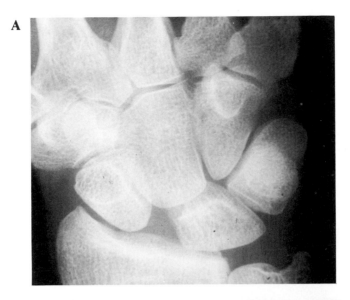

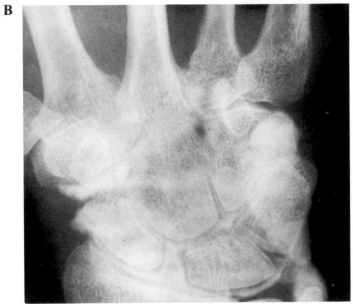

Figure 8
A. A postero-anterior roentgenogram of the wrist shows a rotatory subluxation of the scaphoid.
B. A postero-anterior view of the arthrogram shows opacification of the abnormally wide scapholunate joint caused by rupture of the scapholunate ligament.

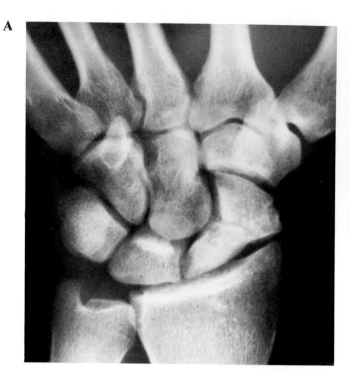

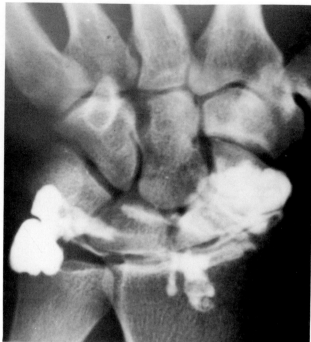

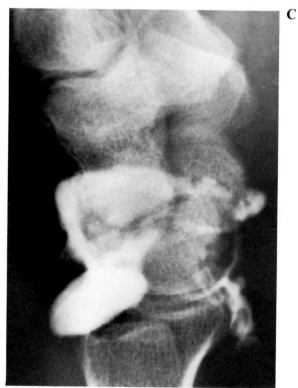

Figure 9
A. A plain radiograph of the wrist shows an ununited scaphoid fracture.
B. On the arthrogram, contrast agent opacifying the fracture line indicates that there is not even a fibrous union.
C. The corrugated appearance of the synovial-lined capsule is consistent with post-traumatic synovitis.

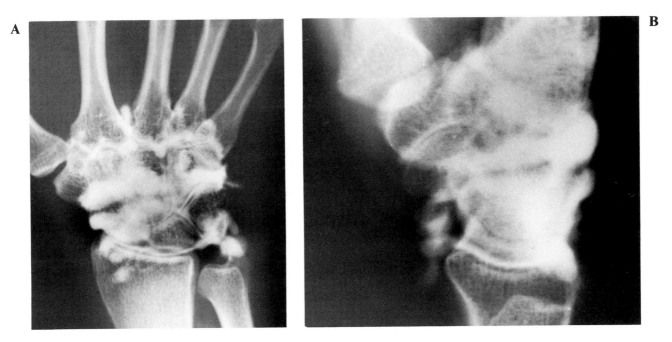

Figure 10
A, B. Irregularity of the synovium and intercarpal ligament tears allowing midcarpal joint opacification were caused by trauma.

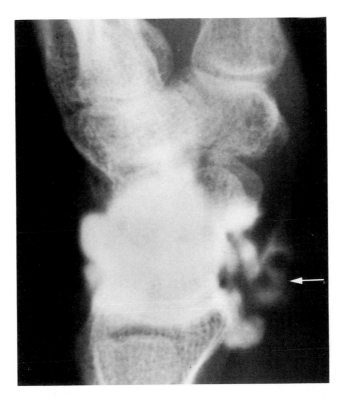

Figure 11
A communicating posttraumatic cyst (arrow) on the volar aspect of the wrist is seen partially opacified on the lateral view of a wrist arthrogram.

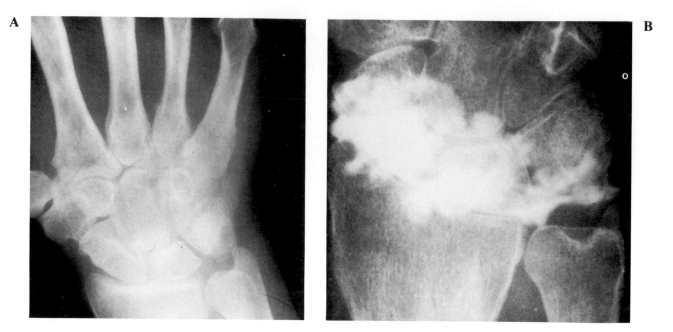

Figure 12
A. In an early stage of rheumatoid arthritis, a plain radiograph of the wrist shows no bony abnormalities.
B. The arthrogram demonstrates a corrugated outline of the synovium, indicating an inflammatory arthritis.

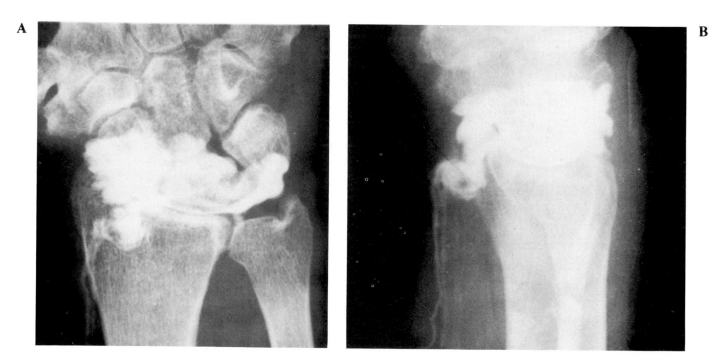

Figure 13
In an early stage of rheumatoid arthritis (**A**) the postero-anterior view and (**B**) the lateral view show a corrugated outline of the joint capsule. The volar pouch is enlarged and irregular in outline. Opacified lymphatics extend into the soft tissues of the forearm.

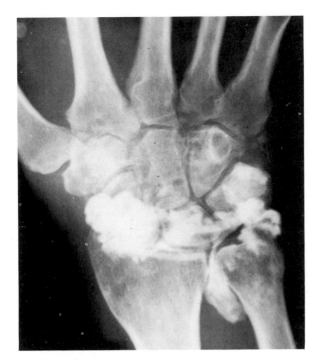

Figure 14
In moderately advanced rheumatoid arthritis, the arthrogram reveals erosion and perforation of the triangular cartilage causing opacification of the distal radioulnar joint. The synovium has a corrugated outline.

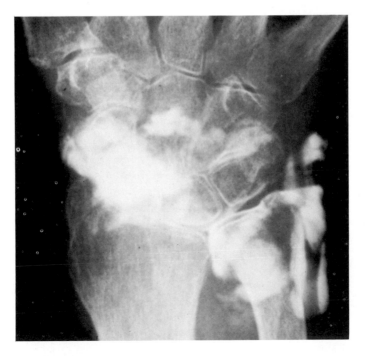

Figure 15
In an advanced stage of rheumatoid arthritis, communication of the radiocarpal joint with the distal radioulnar joint and the midcarpal joints is shown. There is also an abnormal communication between the wrist joint and a tendon sheath.

A

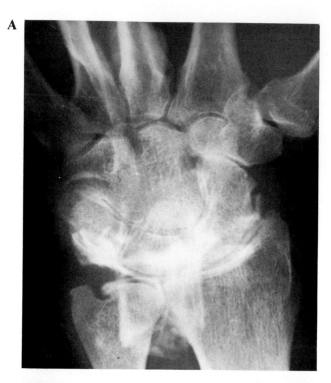

B

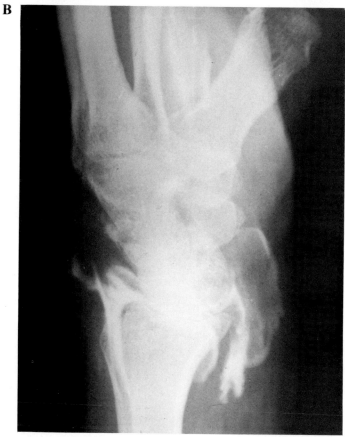

Figure 16
(**A**) A postero-anterior view and (**B**) a lateral view of an arthrogram reveal the abnormal communications of the radiocarpal with the distal radioulnar and intercarpal joints, as well as with the flexor tendon sheath. The patient had rheumatoid arthritis.

SUGGESTED READING

Chapters 1–4

Andrén L, Wehlin L: Double contrast arthrography of the knee with horizontal roentgen ray beam. Acta Orthop Scand 29:307–314, 1960

Angell FL: Fluoroscopic technique of double contrast arthrography of the knee. Radiol Clin N Am 9:85–98, 1971

Burgon, DW: Arthrographic findings in meniscal cysts. Radiology 101:579–581, 1971

Butt WP, McIntyre JL: Double contrast arthrography of the knee. Radiology 92:487–499, 1969

Dalinka MK, Coren GS, Wershba M: Knee arthrography. CRC Crit Rev Clin Radiol Nucl Med 4:1059, 1973

Flynn M, Kelly JP: Local excision of cyst of lateral meniscus of knee without recurrence. J Bone Joint Surg 58B:88–89, 1976

Freiberger RH, Killoran PJ, Cardona G: Arthrography of the knee by double contrast method. Am J Roentgenol Radium Ther Nucl Med 97:736–747, 1966

Furuya M, Harrison-Stubbs MO, Freiberger RH: Arthrography of the knee: analysis of 2101 arthrograms and 623 surgical findings. Rev Hosp Spec Surg 2. 11–21, 1972

Gallo GA, Bryan RS: Cysts of the semilunar cartilages of the knee. J Bone Joint Surg, 116:65–68, 1968

Hall FM: Epinepherine enhanced knee arthrography. Radiology 11:215–217, 1974

Hall FM: Pitfalls in knee arthrography. Radiology 118:55–62, 1976

Hall FM: Further pitfalls in knee arthrography. J Can Assoc Radiol 29:179–184, 1978

Harley JD: An anatomic-arthrographic study of the relationship of the lateral meniscus and the popliteus tendon. Am J Roentgenol Radium Ther Nucl Med 128:181–187, 1977

Jelasco DV: The fascicles of the lateral meniscus. An anatomic-arthrographic correlation. Radiology 114:335–339, 1975

Kaplan EB: Discoid lateral meniscus of the knee joint—nature, mechanism and operative treatment. J Bone Joint Surg 39:77–87, 1957

Kaye JJ, Freiberger RH: Arthrography of the knee. Clin Orthop 107:73–80, 1975

Kaye, JJ, Ghelman B, Freiberger RH: Arthrography of the knee. MEDCOM, New York, New York, 1975.

Lewin JR, Mulhern LM: Lymphatic visualization during contrast arthrography of the knee. Radiology 103:577–579, 1972

Lindblom K: Arthrography of the knee, roentgenographic and anatomic study. Acta Radiol [Suppl] 74:1–112,1974

McIntyre, JL: Arthrography of the lateral meniscus. Radiology 105:531–536, 1972

Montgomery CE: Synovial recesses in knee arthrography. Am J Roentgenol Radium Ther Nucl Med 121:86–88, 1974

Murdock G: Congenital discoid semilunar cartilage. J Bone Joint Surg 38:564–566, 1956

Nathan PA, Cole SC: Discoid meniscus. A clinical and pathologic study. Clin Orthop 64:107–113, 1969

Nicholas JA, Freiberger RH, Killoran PJ: Double contrast arthrography of the knee: its value in the management of two hundred and twenty-five knee derangements. J Bone Joint Surg 52A:203–220, 1970

Resnick D, Goergen TG, Kaye JJ, Ghelman B, Woody PR: Discoid medial meniscus. Radiology 121:575–576, 1976

Ricklin R, Ruttimann A, DelBuono MS: Meniscus Lesions: Practical Problems of Clinical Diagnosis, Arthrography and Therapy. New York, Grune and Stratton, 1971

Russell E, Hamm R, LePage JR, Schoenbaum SW, Satin R: Some normal variations of knee arthrograms and their anatomical significance. J Bone Joint Surg 60A: 66–74, 1978

Smillie IS: The congenital discoid meniscus. J Bone Joint Surg 30:671–682, 1948

Symeonides PP, Eoannides G: Ossicles in the knee menisci. J Bone Joint Surg, 54A:1288–1292, 1972

Wickstrom KT, Spitzer RM, Olsson HE: Roentgen anatomy of the posterior horn of the lateral meniscus. Radiology 116:617–619, 1975

Chapter 5

Dalinka MK, Garofola J: The infrapatellar synovial fold—a helpful aid in the evaluation of the anterior cruciate ligament. Am J Roentgenol Radium Ther Nucl Med 127:589–591, 1976

Dalinka MK, Gohel VK, Rancier L: Tomography in the evaluation of the cruciate ligament. Radiology 108:31–33, 1973

Liljedahl SO, Lindvall N, Wetterford J: Roentgen diagnosis of rupture of anterior cruciate ligament. Acta Radiol 4:225–239, 1966

Mittler S, Freiberger RH, Harrison-Stubbs M: A method of improving cruciate ligament visualization in double contrast arthrography. Radiology 102:441–442, 1972

Pavlov H, Freiberger RH: An easy method to demonstrate the cruciate ligaments by double contrast anthrography. Radiology 126:817–818, 1978

Pavlov H, Torg, JS: Double contrast arthrographic evaluation of the anterior cruciate ligament. Radiology 126:661–665, 1978

Wang JB, Marshall JL: Acute ligamentous injuries of the knee. Single contrast arthrography—a diagnostic aid. J Trauma 15:431–440, 1975

Chapter 6

Aichroth P: Osteochondritis dissecans of the knee. J Bone Joint Surg 53:440–446, 1971

Anderson PW, Maslin P: Tomography applied to knee arthrography. Radiology, 110:271–275, 1974

Burgon DW: Lipoma arborescens of the knee—another cause of filling defects on a knee arthrogram. Radiology, 101:583–584, 1971

Doppman JL: Baker's cyst and the normal gastrocnemius-semimembranosus bursa. Am J Roentgenol Radium Ther Nucl Med 94:646–652

Lapayowker MS, Cliff MM, Tourtellotte CD: Arthrography in the diagnosis of calf pain. Radiology, 95:319–323, 1970

Lewin JR, Mulhern LM: Lymphatic visualization during contrast arthrography of the knee. Radiology, 103:577–579, 1972

Lindgren PG: Gastrocnemius-semimembranosus bursa and its relation to the knee joint. Acta Radiol [Diagn] (Stockh) 18 (5):497–512, 1977

Horns JW: The diagnosis of chondromalacia by double contrast arthrography of the knee. J Bone Joint Surg 59:119–120, 1977

Horns JW: Single contrast knee arthrography in abnormalities of the articular cartilage. Radiology, 105:537–540, 1972

Insall J, Falvo KA, Wise DW: Chondromalacia patellae. J Bone Joint Surg 58A:1–8, 1976

Perri PG, Rodnan GP, Mankin HJ: Giant synovial cysts of the calf in patients with rheumatoid arthritis. J Bone Joint Surg 50A:709–719, 1968

Staple TW: Extrameniscal lesions demonstrated by double contrast arthrography of the knee. Radiology, 102: 311–319, 1972

Taylor AR: Arthrography of the knee in rheumatoid arthritis. Br J Radiol 42:493–497, 1969

Wang JB, Marshall JL: Acute ligamentous injuries of the knee. Single contrast arthrography—a diagnostic aid. Trauma 15:431–440, 1975

Wolfe RD, Colloff B: Popliteal cysts. J Bone Joint Surg 54A:1057–1063, 1972

Chapter 7

Ellis VH: The diagnosis of shoulder lesions due to injuries of the rotator cuff. J Bone Joint Surg 35B:72–74, 1953

Kernwein GA, Roseberg B, Sneed WR, Jr: Arthrographic studies of the shoulder joint. J Bone Joint Surg 39:1267–1279, 1957

Killoran PJ, Marcove RC, Freiberger RH: Shoulder arthrography. Am J Roentgenol Radium Ther Nucl Med 103:658–668, 1968

Lindblom K: Arthrography and roentgenography in ruptures of the tendons of the shoulder joint. Acta Radiol [Suppl] (Stockh) 20:548, 1939

Lundberg BJ: Arthrography and manipulation in rigidity of the shoulder joint. Acta Orthop Scand 36:35–44, 1965

Mosely HF: Shoulder Lesions. 3rd Ed., E. S. Livingstone, Edinburgh, 1969

Neviaser S: Arthrography of the Shoulder. The Diagnosis and Management of the Lesions Visualized. Charles C. Thomas, Springfield, 1975

Neviaser JS: Arthrography of the shoulder joint. J Bone Joint Surg 44A:1321–1330, 1962

Neviaser JS: Ruptures of the rotator cuff. Clin Orthop 3:92–98, 1953

Neviaser JS: Adhesive capsulitis of the shoulder. J Bone Joint Surg 27:211–222, 1945

Reeves B: Arthrography of the shoulder. J Bone Joint Surg 48B, 424–435, 1966

Samilson RL, Raphael RL, Post L: Shoulder arthrography. JAMA 175:773–778, 1961

Schneider R, Ghelman B, Kaye JJ: A simplified injection technique for shoulder arthrography. Radiology 114:738–739, 1975

Weston WJ: The enlarged subdeltoid bursa in rheumatoid arthritis. Br J Radiol 42:481–486, 1969

Chapter 8

Andrén L, Lundberg BJ: Treatment of rigid shoulders by joint distension during arthrography. Acta Orthop Scand 36:45–53, 1965

Bankart ASB: The pathology and treatment of recurrent dislocation of the shoulder joint. Br J Surg 26:29, 1938

Bost FC, Inman VT: The pathological changes in recurrent dislocation of the shoulder. A report of Bankart's operative procedure. J Bone Joint Surg [Am] 24:595–613, 1942

Debeyre J, Patie D, Elemelik E: Repair of ruptures of the rotator cuff of the shoulder with a note on advancement of the supraspinatus muscle. J Bone Joint Surg [Br] 47:36–42, 1965

Ghelman B, Goldman AB: The double contrast shoulder arthrogram: evaluation of rotator cuff tears. Radiology 124:251–254, 1977

Hitchcock HH, Bechtol CO: Painful shoulder, observations on the role of the tendon of the long head of the biceps brachii in its causation. J Bone Joint Surg [Am] 30: 263–273, 1948

Lindblom K, Palmer J: Ruptures of the tendon aponeurosis of the shoulder joint—the so-called supraspinatus ruptures. Acta Chir Scand 82:133–142, 1939

McLaughlin HL: Rupture of the rotator cuff. J Bone Joint Surg [Am] 41:979–983, 1963

Schneider R, Ghelman B, Kaye JJ: A simplified injection technique for shoulder arthrography. Radiology 114: 738–739, 1975

Wolfgang GL: Surgical repair of tears of the rotator cuff of the shoulder. Factors influencing the result. J Bone Joint Surg [Am] 57:14–26, 1974

Chapter 9

Anderson LS, Staple TC: Arthrography of total hip replacements using subtraction technique. Radiology 109:470, 1973

Brown CS, Knickerbocker WJ: Radiologic studies of the investigation of causes of total hip replacement failures. J Can Assoc Radiol 24:245–253, 1973

Dolinskas C, Campbell RE, Rothman RH: The painful Charnley total hip replacement. Am J Roentgenol Radium Ther Nucl Med 121:61, 1974

Dussault RG, Goldman AB, Ghelman B: Roentgenographic diagnosis of loosening and/or infection in hip prostheses. Correlation between roentgen and surgical findings. J Can Assoc Radiol 28:119, 1977

Guerra J, Jr, Armbuster TG, Resnick D, et al: The adult hip: an anatomic study. Radiology 128:11, 1978

Mullins MF, Sutton RN, Lodwick GS: Complications of total hip replacement. Am J Roentgenol Radium Ther Nucl Med 121:55, 1974

Murray WR, Rodrigo JJ: Arthrography for the assessment of pain after total hip replacement. J Bone Joint Surg [Am] 57:1060, 1975

Razzano, CD, Nelson CL, Wilde AH: Arthrography of the adult hip. Clin Orthop 99:86, 1974

Salvati EA, Freiberger RH, Wilson PD, Jr: Arthrography for complications of total hip replacement. J Bone Joint Surg [Am] 53:701, 1971

Salvati EA, Ghelman B, McLaren T, Wilson PD, Jr: Subtraction technique in arthrography for loosening of total hip replacement fixed with radiopaque cement. Clin Orthop 101:105–109, 1974

Warren R, Kaye JJ, Salvati EA: Arthrographic demonstration of an enlarged iliopsoas bursa complicating osteoarthritis of the hip. Case Report, J Bone Joint Surg [Am] 57:413, 1975

Chapter 10

Artz TD, Levine DB, Lim WN, Salvati EA, Wilson PD, Jr: Neonatal diagnosis, treatment and related factors of congenital dislocation of the hip. Clin Orthop 110:112, 1975

Barnett JC, Arcomano JP: Hip arthrography in children, with renografin. Radiology, 73:245, 1958

Canale ST, D'Anea AF, Catler JM, Snedder HE: Innominate osteotomy in Legg-Calve Perthes disease. J Bone Joint Surg [Am] 54:25, 1972

Freiberger RH, Ghelman B, Kaye JJ, Spragge JW: Hip disease of infancy and childhood. Curr Probl Radiol 5:1, 1973

Glassburg GB, Ozonoff MB: Arthrographic findings in septic arthritis of the hip in infants. Radiology, 128:151, 1978

Goldman AB, Schneider R, Martel W: Acute chondrolysis complicating slipped capital femoral epiphysis: roentgen diagnosis and differential diagnosis. Am J Roentgenol Radium Ther Nucl Med 130:945, 1978

Goldman AB, Schneider R, Wilson PD, Jr: Proximal focal femoral deficiency: roentgen diagnosis and differential diagnosis. J Can Assoc Radiol 29:101, 1978

Goldman AB, Hallel T, Salvati EM, Freiberger RH: Osteochondritis dissecans complicating Legg Perthes Disease. Radiology 121:561, 1976

Grech P: Hip Arthrography. Chapman and Hall Ltd., London, 1977.

Heublein GW, Greene GS, Conforti VP: Hip joint arthrography. Am J Roentgenol Radium Ther Nucl Med 68:736, 1952

Jonsäter S: Coxa plana. A histo-pathologic and arthrographic study. Acta Orthop Scand [Suppl] 12, 1953

Katz JF: Arthrography in Legg-Calve Perthes disease. J Bone Joint Surg [Am] 50:467, 1968

Kaye JJ, Winchester PH, Freiberger RH: Neonatal septic "dislocation" of the hip: true dislocation or pathological epiphyseal separation? Radiology 114:671–674, 1975

Kenin A, Levine J: A technique for arthrography of the hip. Am J Roentgenol Radium Ther Nucl Med 68:197, 1952

Ozonoff MB: Controlled arthrography of the hip: a technique of fluoroscopic monitoring and recovery. Clin Orthop 93:260, 1973

Severin E: Arthrography in congenital dislocation of the hip. J Bone Joint Surg 21:304, 1939

Severin E: Arthrograms of hip joints of children. Surg, Gynecol Obstet 72:601, 1941

Severin E: Arthrography in sequelae to acute infections. Acta Orthop Scand 93:389, 1946

Chapter 11

Ala-ketola L, Puranen J, Koivisto E, Puuperä M: Arthrography in the diagnosis of ligament injuries and classification of ankle injuries. Radiology 125:63–68, 1977

Arner O, Ekengren K, Hulting B, Lindholm A: Arthrography of the talo-crural joint. Anatomic, roentgenographic, and clinical aspects. Acta Chir Scand 113:253–259, 1957

Berridge FR, Bonnin JG: The radiographic examination of the ankle joint including arthrography. Surg Gynecol Obstet 79:383–389, 1944

Broström L: Sprained ankles. I. Anatomic lesions in recent sprains. Acta Chir Scand 128:483–495, 1964

Broström L, Liljedahl SO, Lindvall N: Sprained ankles. II. Arthrographic diagnosis of recent ligament ruptures. Acta Chir Scand 129:485–499, 1965

Broström L: Sprained ankles. III. Clinical observations in recent ligament ruptures. Acta Chir Scand 130:560–569, 1965

Broström L, Sundelin P: Sprained ankles. IV. Histologic changes in recent and "chronic" ligament ruptures. Acta Chir Scand 132:248–253, 1966

Broström L: Sprained ankles. V. Treatment and prognosis in recent ligament ruptures. Acta Chir Scand 132:537–550, 1966

Broström L: Sprained ankles. VI. Surgical treatment of "chronic" ligament ruptures. Acta Chir Scand 132:551–565, 1966

Fordyce AJW, Horn CV: Arthrography in recent injuries of the ligaments of the ankle. J Bone Joint Surg 54B:116–121, 1972

Fussell ME, Godley DR: Ankle arthrography in acute sprains. Clin Orthop 93:278–290, 1973

Goldman AB: Katz M, Freiberger RH: Post-traumatic adhesive capsulitis of the ankle. Am J Roentgenol Radium Ther Nucl Med 127:585–588, 1976

Gordon RB: Arthrography of the ankle joint. J Bone Joint Surg 52A:1623–1631, 1970

Hansson CJ: Arthrographic studies on the ankle joint. Acta Radiol 22:281–287, 1941

Kaye JJ, Bohne WH: A radiologic study of the ligamentous anatomy of the ankle. Radiology 125:659–667, 1977

Mehrez M, El Geneidy S: Arthrography of the ankle. J Bone Joint Surg 52B:308–312, 1970

Olson RW: Arthrography of the ankle: its use in the evaluation of ankle sprains. Radiology 92:1439–1446, 1969

Percy, EC, Hill RO, Callaghan JE: The "sprained ankle." J Trauma 9:972–985, 1969

Spiegel PK, Staples OS: Arthrography of the ankle joint: problems in diagnosis of acute lateral ligament injuries. Radiology 114:587–590, 1975

Staples OS: Result study of ruptures of lateral ligaments of the ankle. Clin Orthop 85:50–58, 1972

Staples OS: Ruptures of the fibular collateral ligaments of the ankle. J Bone Joint Surg 57A:95–100, 1975

Chapter 12

Harris R, Beath T: Etiology of peroneal spastic flat foot. J Bone Joint Surg [Br] 30:624–634, 1948

Kaye J, Ghelman B, Schneider R: Talocalcaneonavicular joint arthrography for sustentacular-talar tarsal coalitions. Radiology 115:730–731, 1975

Chapter 13

Arviddson H, Johansson O: Arthrography of the elbow-joint. Acta Radiol 43:445–452, 1955

Eppwright RH, Wilkins KE: Fractures and dislocations of the elbow. In Charles A Rockwood, Jr., and David P. Green, Fractures, J.B. Lippincott, Philadelphia, 1975, pp. 529–531.

Ehrlich GE: Antecubital cysts in rheumatoid arthritis—a corollary to popliteal (Baker's) cysts. J Bone Joint Surg 54A:165–169, 1972

Eto RT, Anderson PW, Harley JD: Elbow arthrography with the application of tomography. Radiology 115:283–288, 1975

Goode JD: Synovial rupture of the elbow joint. Ann Rheum Dis 27:604–609, 1968

Trias A, Comeau Y: Recurrent dislocation of the elbow in children. Clin Orthop 100:74–77, 1974

Chapter 14

Harrison MO, Freiberger RH: Arthrography of the rheumatoid wrist joint. Am J Roentgenol Radium Ther Nucl Med 112:480–487, 1971

Kessler L, Silberman Z: An experimental study of the radiocarpal joint by arthrography. Surg Gynecol Obstet 112:33–40, 1961

Liebolt FL: Surgical fusion of the wrist joint. Surg Gynecol Obstet 66:1008–1023, 1938

Ranawat CS, Freiberger RH, Jordan LR, Straub LR: Arthrography in the rheumatoid wrist joint. J Bone Joint Surg 51A:1269–1281, 1969

Resnick D: Rheumatoid arthritis of the wrist: why the ulnar styloid? Radiology 112:29–35, 1974

Resnick D: Arthrography in the evaluation of the arthritic disorders of the wrist. Radiology 113:331–340, 1974

INDEX

X-Ray Department
Royal United Hospital
Bath